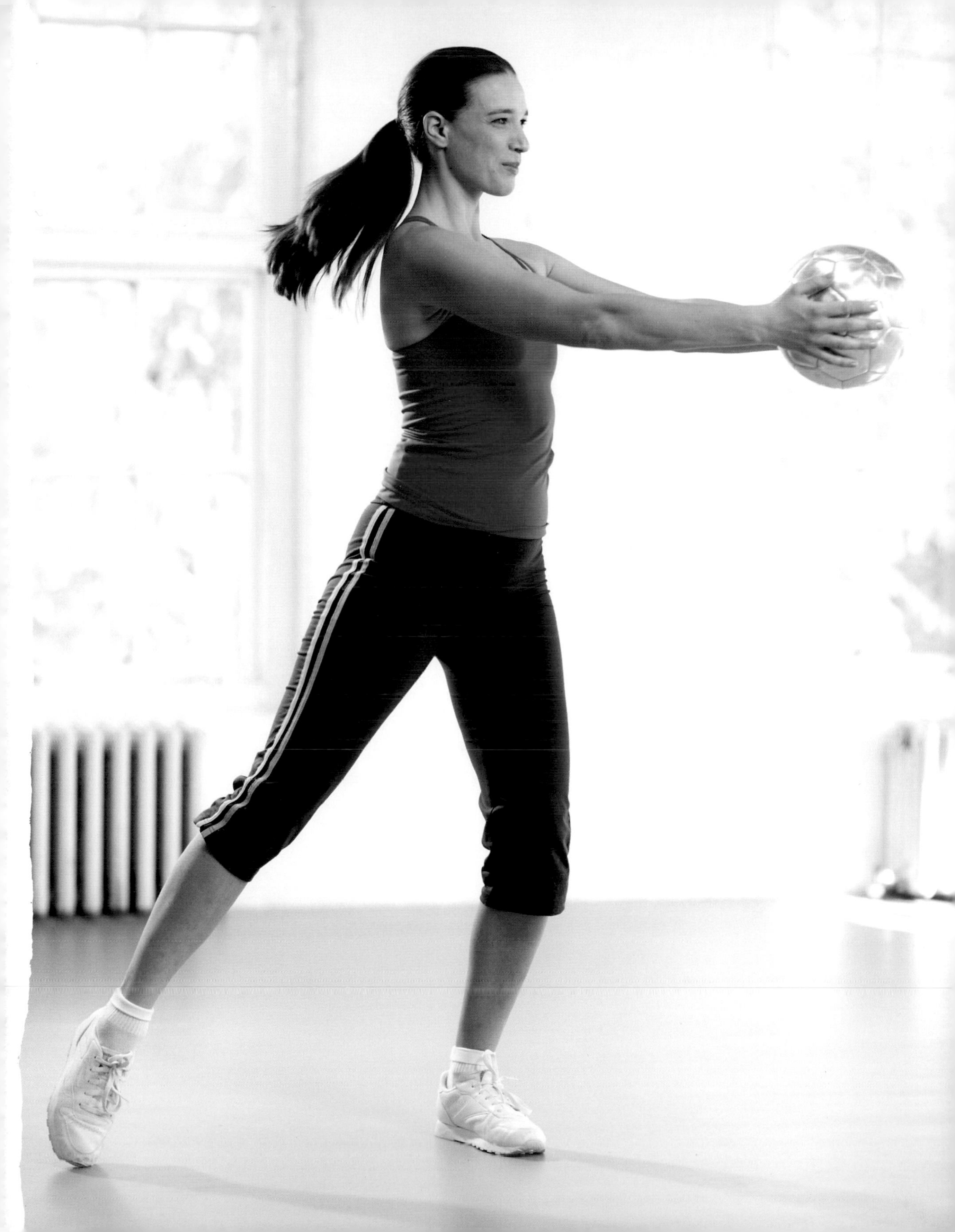

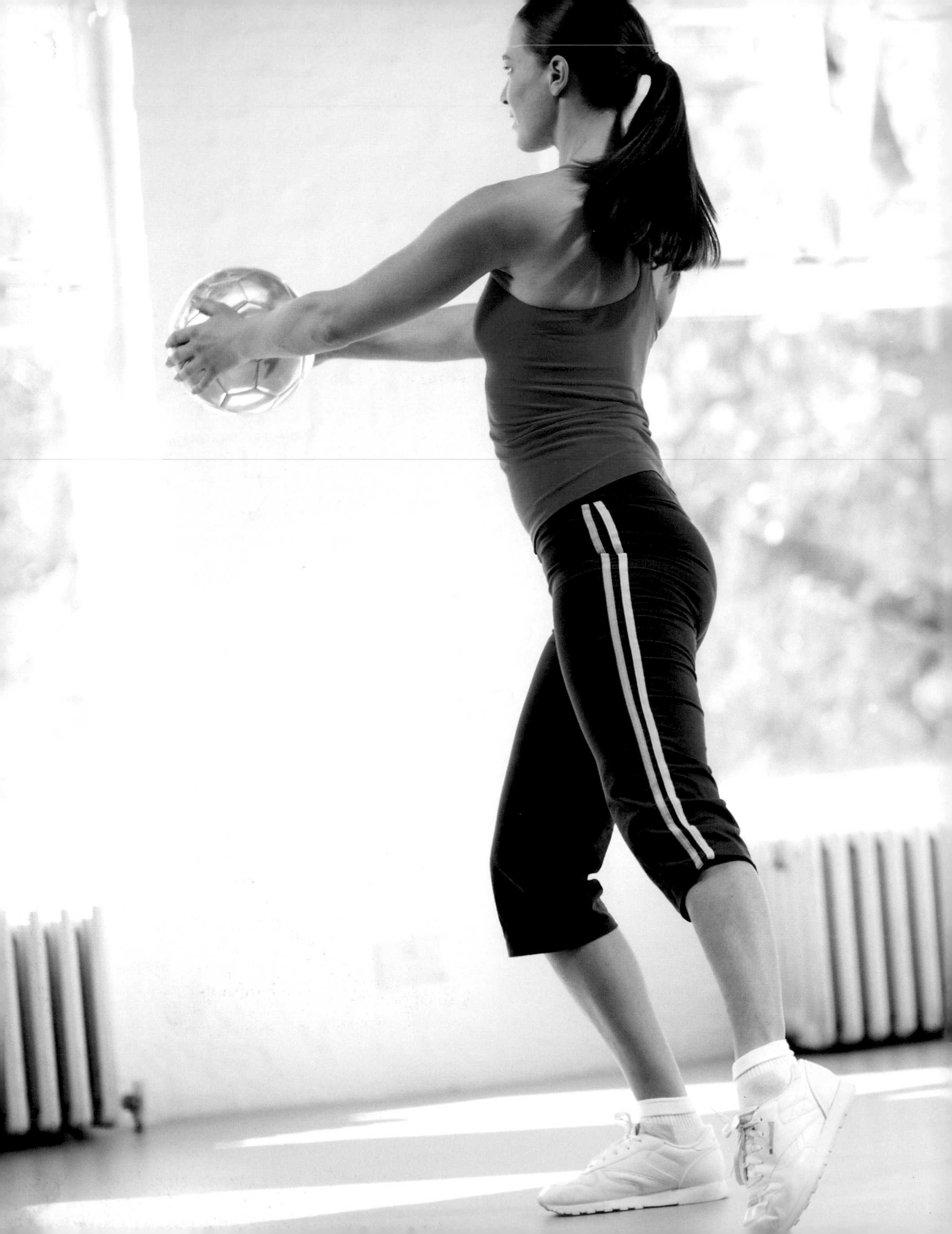

>> 15 minute total body workout

Joan Pagano

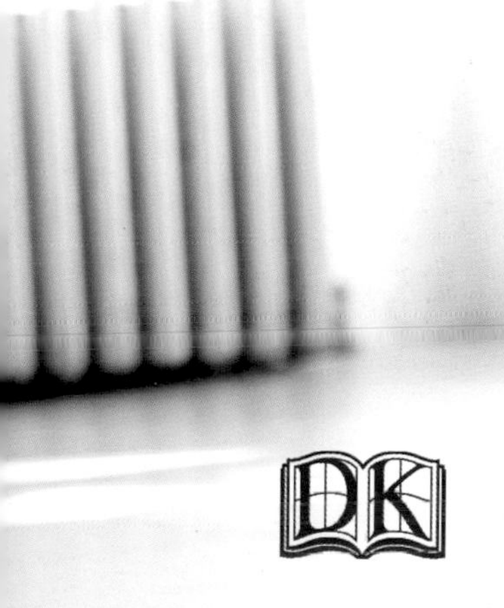

DK

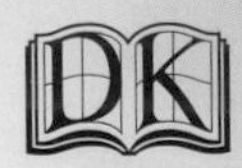

London, New York, Melbourne, Munich, Delhi

For my clients and all those who put their trust in me

Project Editor Helen Murray
Project Art Editor Anne Fisher
Senior Editors Jennifer Latham, Jo Godfrey Wood
Senior Art Editor Peggy Sadler
Managing Editor Penny Warren
Managing Art Editor Marianne Markham
Art Director Peter Luff
Publishing Director Mary-Clare Jerram
Stills Photography Ruth Jenkinson
DTP Designer Sonia Charbonnier
Production Controller Rebecca Short
Production Editor Luca Frassinetti
Jacket Designer Neal Cobourne

DVD produced for Dorling Kindersley by
Chrome Productions www.chromeproductions.com

Director Gez Medinger
DOP Marcus Domleo, Matthew Cooke
Camera Marcus Domleo, Jonathan Iles
Production Manager Hannah Chandler
Production Assistant Azra Gul, Tom Robinson
Grip Pete Nash
Gaffer Paul Wilcox, Johann Cruickshank
Music Chad Hobson
Hair and Makeup Victoria Barnes, Roisin Donaghy
Voice-over Suzanne Pirret
Voice-over Recording Ben Jones

First American Edition, 2008

Published in the United States by
DK Publishing
375 Hudson Street
New York, New York 10014

08 09 10 9 8 7 6 5 4 3 2 1

BD567-Jan 08

Health warning
Always consult your doctor before starting a fitness program if you have any health concerns, and especially if you are pregnant, have given birth in the last six weeks, or have a medical condition such as high blood pressure, arthritis, or asthma. This book is not intended for people suffering from back problems; it provides programs to strengthen the back and prevent back problems from occurring. If you have any pain while exercising, stop immediately.

Every effort has been made to ensure that the information contained in this book is complete and accurate. However, neither the publisher nor the author is engaged in rendering professional advice or services to the individual reader. The ideas, information, and suggestions contained in this book are not intended as a substitute for consulting with your physician. All matters regarding your health require medical supervision. Neither the author nor the publisher shall be liable or responsible for any loss or damage allegedly rising from any information or suggestion in this book.

Published in Great Britain by Dorling Kindersley Limited.

A catalog record for this book is available from the Library of Congress

ISBN 978-0-7566-3356-1

Printed and bound by Sheck Wah Tong, China

Discover more at
www.dk.com

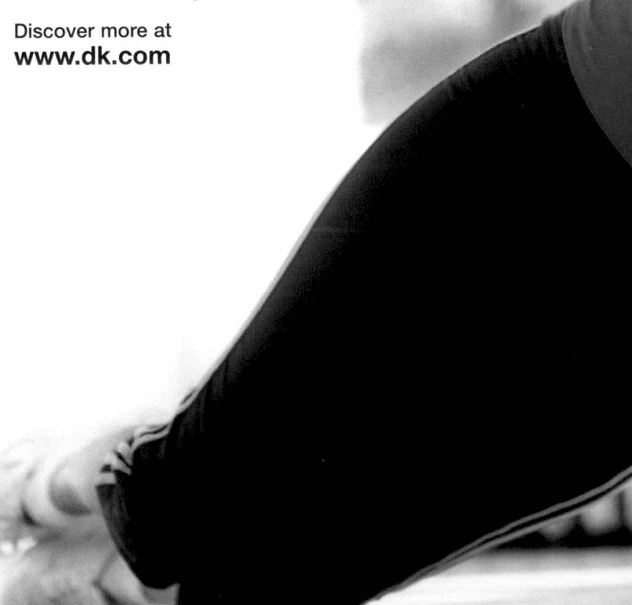

contents

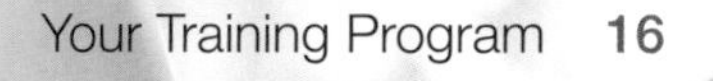

author foreword

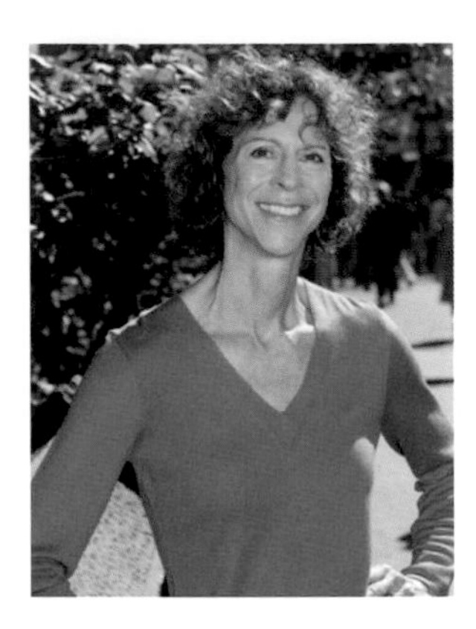

In 20 years' experience as a personal fitness trainer, I have often been asked the same key question: What is the best exercise? And the answer is easy: The best exercise is the one that you will do! What works for you is as unique as your own personality, your personal likes and dislikes, your goals in an exercise program, and your individual resources—such as your available time, money, and space.

The best exercise is the one that suits a lifestyle. Convenience and efficiency have always been important factors for me personally. With a busy work schedule of training clients in their homes or private gyms, I enjoy working out in the comfort of my own home, avoiding additional travel time. I like the freedom of doing my exercise whenever time permits, and I prefer using minimal equipment to challenge my capabilities.

Like our own fingerprints, goals in an exercise program are very individual. To be successful, we must develop realistic, attainable goals. It is far better to start small, achieve the initial goals we set for ourselves, and build a foundation of success and confidence, which can be utilized in setting further goals.

If we are too ambitious in setting our targets at the outset, it is possible to become discouraged and give up.

One common goal we all share is to be able to maintain a comfortable level of activity throughout a lifetime, creating a "habit" of exercise. Exercising regularly for even just 15 minutes is an investment that will serve our bodies for life. Brief doses of exercise done consistently over time yield dramatic benefits in terms of reducing the risk of developing diseases such as diabetes and hypertension. Doing "a little bit a lot" has a dramatic effect on the appearance, too, allowing us to shed excess weight and keep muscle tone and flexibility.

Of course, the more you do, the more you benefit. The four 15-minute *Total Body Workout* routines offer you the option of doing from one to four routines in the course of a day; you have the choice of picking the ones that suit your mood and your starting level of fitness, as well as the variety to challenge yourself and keep your workouts fresh. So have fun developing and creating your own exercise habit!

Joan Pagano

>> **how to use** this book

This book combines cardio and strength training to give you a full-body workout with maximum benefits. Take time to study the exercises in detail and familiarize yourself with what you will need to do. Use the gatefold summary as a quick reminder.

The accompanying DVD is designed to be used with the book to reinforce the exercises shown there. As you watch the DVD, page references to the book flash up on the screen. Refer to these for more detailed instruction. In the book, some of the exercises have a starting position, shown in the inset, and the large photographs show the exercise. Annotations give you tips on proper positioning and white dotted-line "feel-it-here" patches hone in on specific body areas in the resistance training exercises.

Each program begins with a three-minute warm up sequence, which gradually builds in intensity. The main body of the workout is comprised of 10 minutes of resistance training exercises alternating with cardio intervals. The sequence ends with a two-minute cool down, providing full-body stretches. All the exercises are designed with the beginner in mind, although the fourth workout, Lunge Around the Clock, requires a little more skill, so if you are completely new to exercise, gradually build up to this workout. See the introductory spreads, the Frequently Asked Questions, and the Total Body Roundup for further advice for beginners. Each sequence takes 15 minutes, but refer to the Introduction for advice on combining them for a longer workout. Follow these workouts three times a week, alternating with a day of rest, if you can (as muscles need one full day of rest in between strength-training workouts). You can do cardio exercise, such as swimming, walking, or cycling on your "off" days.

The gatefolds

The gatefold summaries at the end of each workout help you to see each Total Body Workout program in full view. Once you've watched the DVD and examined each exercise, use the handy gatefolds as a quick reference to trim your exercise time down to a succinct 15 minutes.

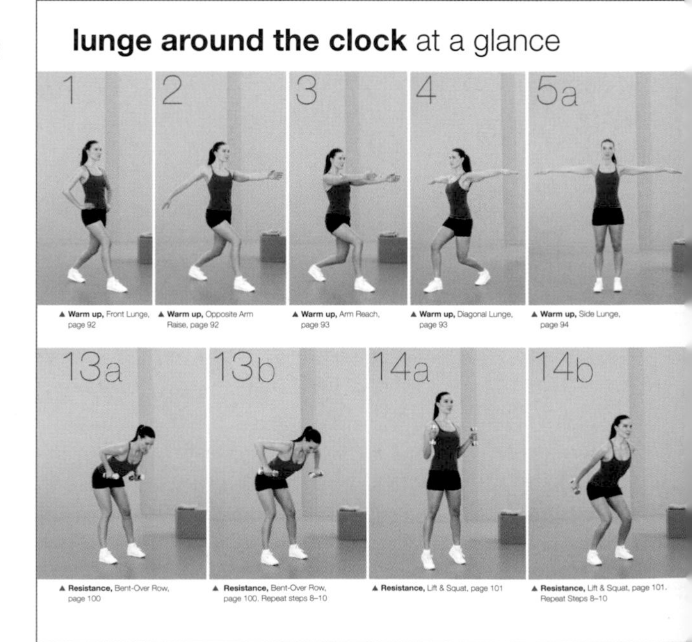

Gatefold The gatefold gives you a comprehensive demonstration of the entire program—an easy reference to make your workout quick and simple.

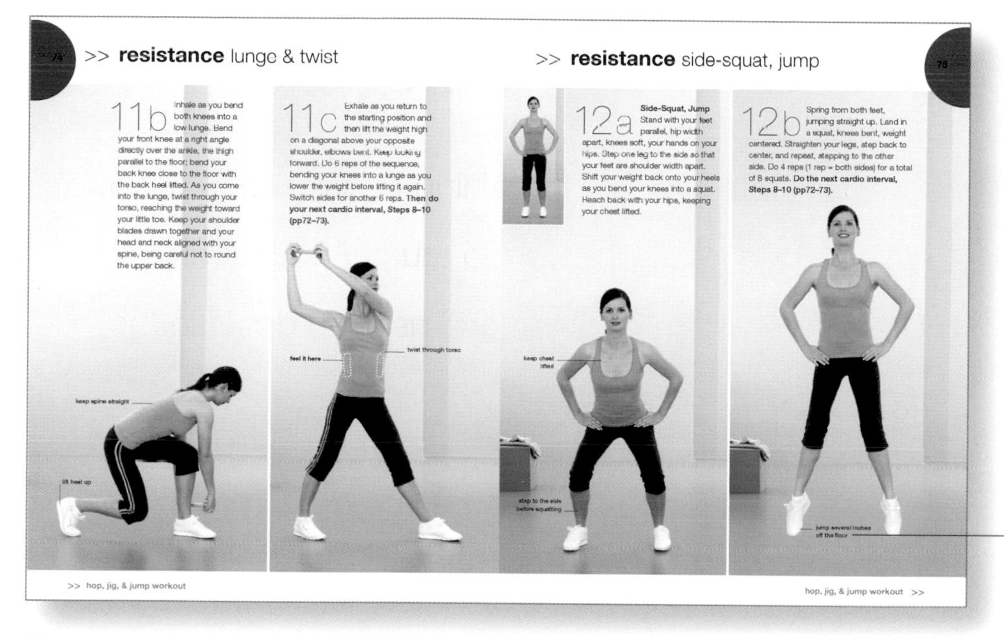

74

>> **resistance** lunge & twist

11b Inhale as you bend both knees into a low lunge. Bend your front knee at a right angle directly over the ankle, the thigh parallel to the floor; bend your back knee close to the floor with the back heel lifted. As you come into the lunge, twist through your torso, reaching the weight toward your little toe. Keep your shoulder blades drawn together and your head and neck aligned with your spine, being careful not to round the upper back.

11c Exhale as you return to the starting position and then lift the weight high on a diagonal above your opposite shoulder, elbows bent. Keep looking forward. Do 6 reps of the sequence, bending your knees into a lunge as you lower the weight before lifting it again. Switch sides for another 6 reps. **Then do your next cardio interval, Steps 8–10 (pp72–73).**

keep spine straight
lift heel up
feel it here
twist through torso

>> hop, jig, & jump workout

>> **resistance** side-squat, jump

75

12a **Side-Squat, Jump** Stand with your feet parallel, hip width apart, knees soft, your hands on your hips. Step one leg to the side so that your feet are shoulder width apart. Shift your weight back onto your heels as you bend your knees into a squat. Reach back with your hips, keeping your chest lifted.

12b Spring from both feet, jumping straight up. Land in a squat, knees bent, weight centered. Straighten your legs, step back to center, and repeat, stepping to the other side. Do 4 reps (1 rep = both sides) for a total of 8 squats. **Do the next cardio interval, Steps 8–10 (pp72–73).**

keep chest lifted
step to the side before squatting
jump several inches off the floor

hop, jig, & jump workout >>

annotations provide extra cues, tips, and insights

Step-by-step pages The inset photograph at the upper left gives you the starting position for the exercise, where necessary. The large photographs give you the steps required to complete it.

the gatefold shows all the main steps of the program

b
6
7
8a
8b
9a
9b
10a
10b
11
12
▲ Warm up, Reverse Lunge, page 95. Repeat Steps 5–1
▲ Resistance, Wood Chop Squat, page 95
▲ Cardio, Curtsy Lunge, page 96
▲ Cardio, Curtsy Lunge, page 96
▲ Cardio, Charleston Lunge, page 97
▲ Cardio, Charleston Lunge, page 97
▲ Cardio, Push-Off Lunge, page 98
▲ Cardio, Push-Off Lunge, page 98
▲ Resistance, Plié & Row, page 99. Repeat Steps 8–10
▲ Resistance, Balance Squat. Repeat Steps 8–10
16
17a
17b
18
19
20a
20b
▲ Cool down, Down Dog, page 102
▲ Cool down, Half Push-up & Side Plank, page 103
▲ Cool down, Child's Pose, page 104
▲ Cool down, Cross-Legged Stretch, page
▲ Cool down, Half Push-up & Side Plank, page 103
▲ Cool down, Kneeling Lunge, page 104
▲ Cool down, Cross-Legged Stretch, page 105

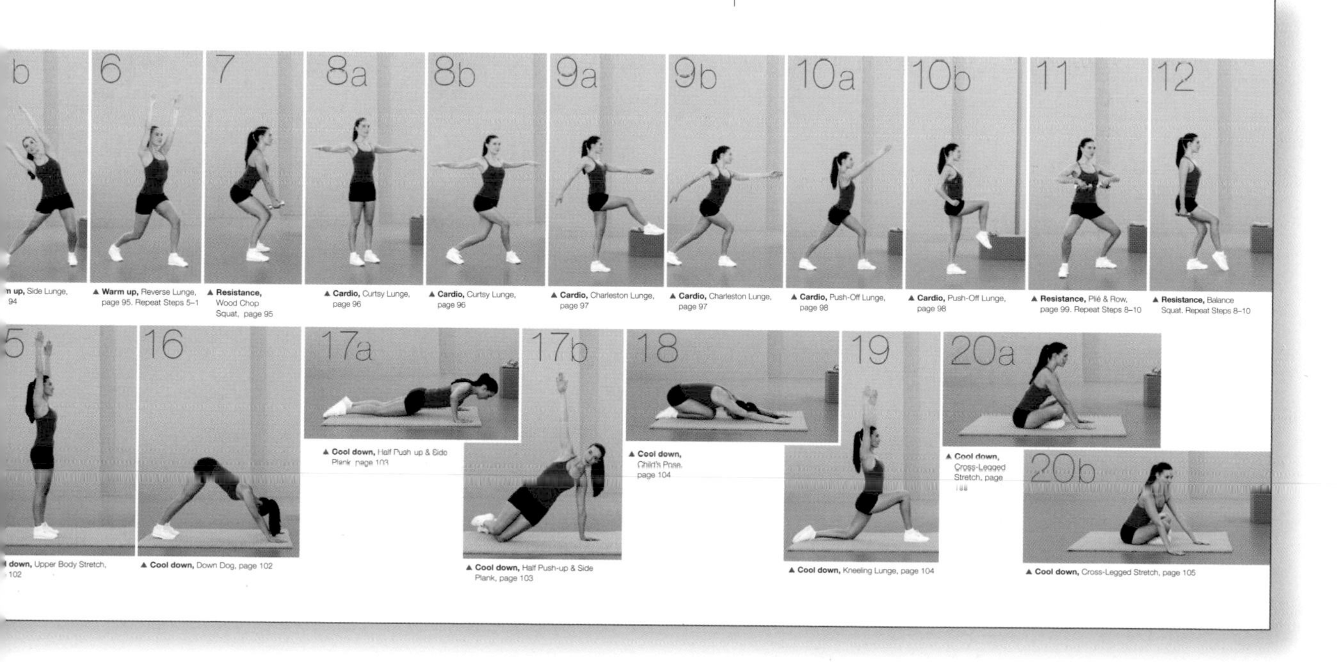

>> introduction

No more excuses! It's time to get moving. Do you think you're too busy, can't afford it, or don't have enough room or equipment to work out at home? Maybe you feel it's too boring, not fun, and you can't stick with it? Or that you're too lazy, old, fat, or out of shape to even begin?

The list of excuses not to get fit is endless, but the solution is simple: *Total Body Workout* provides the tools you need for an exercise program with minimal investment of time and resources, and from which you will definitely benefit.

15-minute workouts

The *Total Body Workout* exercise routines are designed to give you maximum benefit in the most efficient format, combining cardio and strength training. All it takes to complete a full-body routine is 15 minutes. Therefore, if 15 minutes is all you have, pick just one of them. Or, if you have more time, combine the routines for a 30-, 45-, or 60-minute workout. Choose your workout according to your level of fitness, energy, and available time.

Each of the four 15-minute workouts has a unique theme to make it more enjoyable and offer variety to your routines. They all challenge your body in different ways: Step-Touch (see p18) eases you into the habit of exercising. Beach Ball (see p42) uses a ball in a variety of sporty moves. Hop, Jig, and Jump (see p66) evokes the childlike joy of jumping. Lunge Around the Clock (see p90) requires the most skill and tests your limits a little bit more.

The formula for each workout is consistent: A three-minute warm up, 10 minutes of strength (or resistance) training exercises alternating with cardio intervals, and a two-minute cool down. These workouts have been selected to maximize your results by impacting all aspects of fitness.

>> **SMART tips** for success

Goal setting is one of the best ways to stay motivated to exercise. The SMART system states that goals should be:

- **Specific** What exactly do you want to achieve? Reduce fat, improve muscle tone, increase bone density? With clear goals, you can choose appropriate exercises.
- **Measurable** Unless your goal is measurable, you won't know if you've accomplished it. Specific goals are measurable: muscle tone can be measured by endurance exercises (see p14).
- **Action-oriented** An action plan breaking your long-term goal into weekly targets will give you the satisfaction of meeting short-term goals, and the opportunity to reassess whether your goals are reasonable.
- **Realistic** People often become disillusioned and stop exercising when they don't get their imagined results. Are your goals in sync with your body type? Do they match your personal preferences?
- **Timed** Setting a target date gives you the motivation to stick with an exercise program, but you must allow a realistic amount of time to achieve your goal.

Composition of a workout

The warm ups are a series of movements that gradually build in intensity, giving you the flavor of the workout and preparing your body for the exercises to come. The strength-training programs comply with fitness industry guidelines that target the major muscles of the hips, thighs, legs, back, chest, shoulders, arms, and abdomen. The one-minute cardio intervals carry out the theme of the workout, at a higher level of intensity to pump up your heart in between the resistance exercises.

The body of the workout is composed of standing exercises for the purpose of burning more calories and preserving bone density. Many of them are combination moves involving multiple muscle groups, such as Lunge and Row (see p51), and Squat with Knee Lift (see p50). Again, the purpose is to produce the best results for your efforts: to target the most muscle groups, burn the most calories, and improve coordination at the same time; training your muscles to work in patterns.

No workout is complete without a full-body stretch, and this is provided in the cool down. As opposed to more traditional stretches that isolate individual muscles, these positions target multiple muscle groups, often stretching the upper and lower body together. They provide a fluid sequence as you progress through the movements.

Integrating all of these aspects of training prepares your whole body to meet the demands of your day-to-day activities more effectively (i.e. functional training). You'll really appreciate it the next time you are walking home on a wet, windy day, an open umbrella in one hand, a tote bag over the opposite shoulder, with several shopping bags in the other hand, when you want to buy a newspaper without falling over. This is the payoff of functional training.

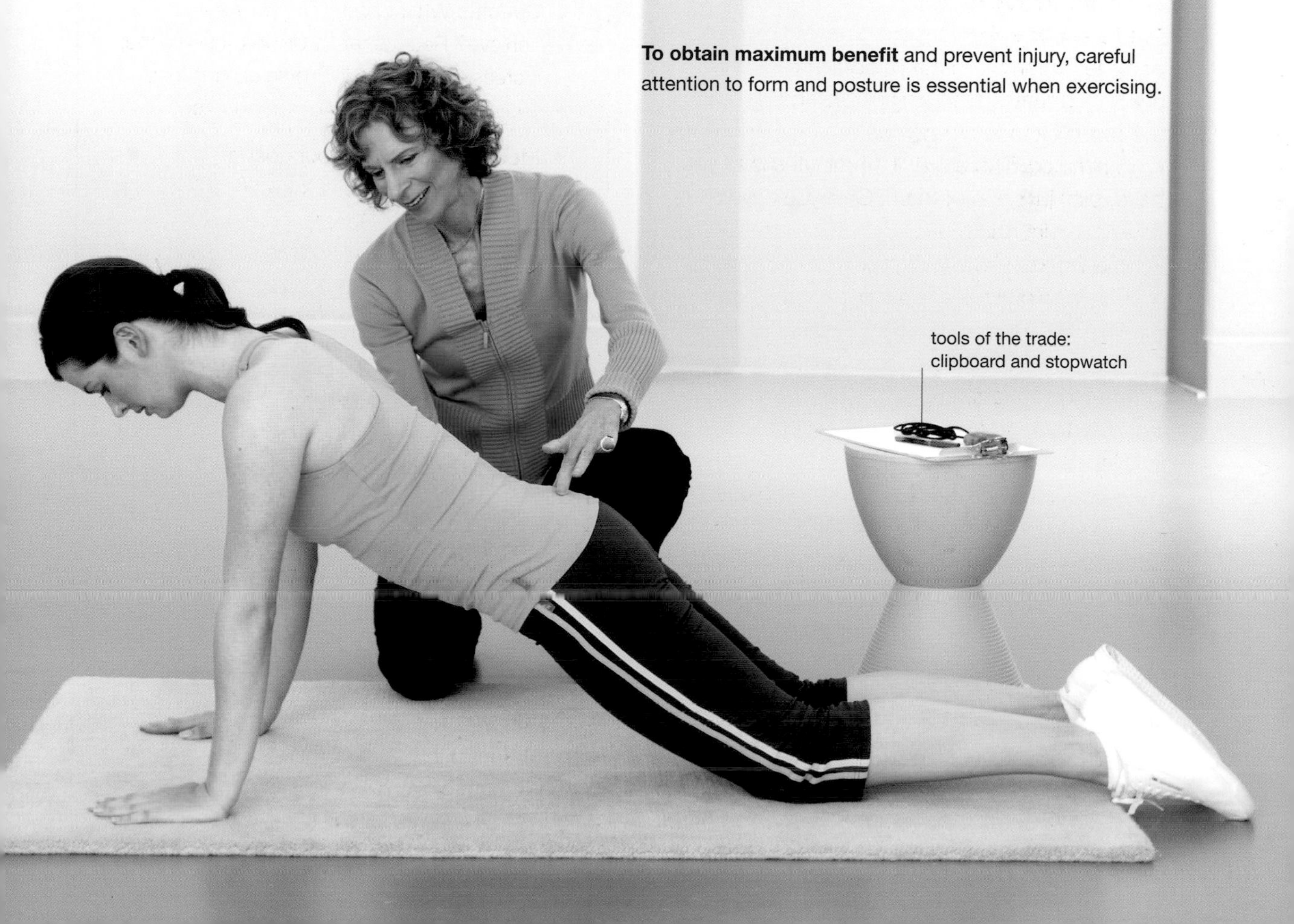

To obtain maximum benefit and prevent injury, careful attention to form and posture is essential when exercising.

tools of the trade: clipboard and stopwatch

>> **how healthy** are you?

A lean, well-toned figure is something that most of us aspire to, but body composition and shape are about more than just appearance: they are also closely related to fitness and health. Three simple measures are used to assess whether your body fat distribution is in a healthy range.

Studies show that a large waist circumference signals a greater risk of heart disease, high blood pressure, and diabetes than ample hips and thighs. This relationship between body shape and disease is sometimes summed up by the concept of "apples and pears." Unlike those who carry excess weight around the hips and thighs, people with apple-shaped figures are at increased risk of the diseases associated with abdominal obesity. Although your body type is inherited, you can minimize the associated health risks by controlling your weight and keeping fit.

Another simple way to determine body-fat distribution is the waist-to-hip ratio (see right). In women aged 20–39, a ratio of more than .79 is considered high; for women aged 40–59, the figure is .82; and for those aged 60–69, it is .84.

Body Mass Index (BMI), based on a ratio of weight to height, is used to assess the increased risk of weight-related health conditions. It may be inaccurate in some cases—for example, for someone with a lot of muscle mass, as muscle weighs more than fat—but the chart opposite is a simple way to check whether your weight is within healthy limits. If the result indicates that your weight poses a health risk, seek advice from your doctor.

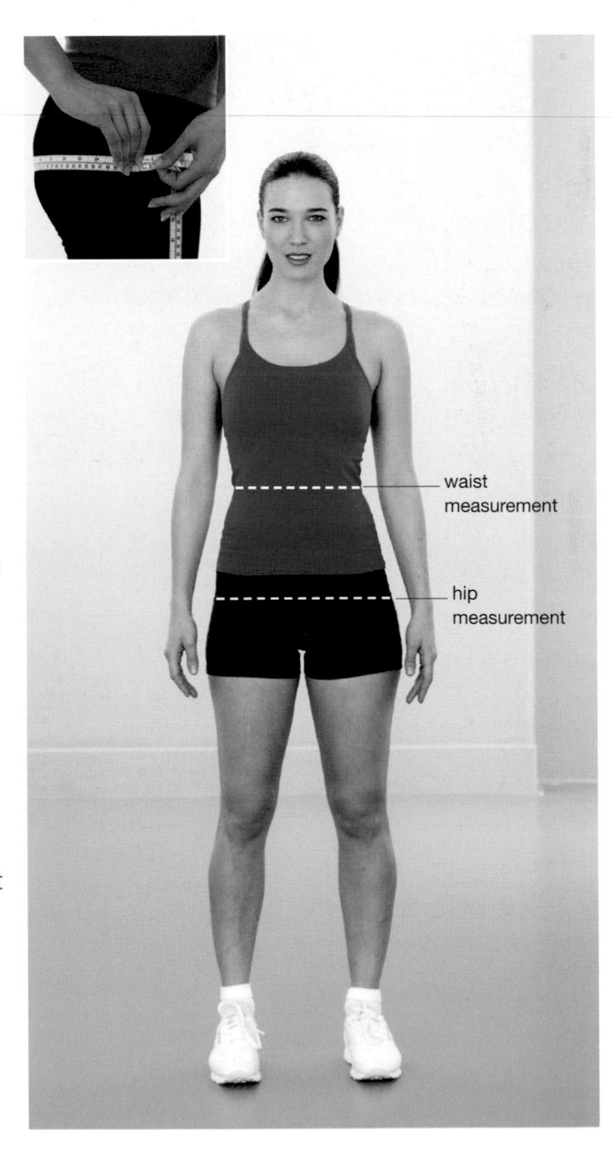

Waist-to-hip ratio is a very simple way to determine whether your body-fat distribution poses a health risk to you. Divide your waist measurement by your hip measurement to calculate the ratio.

Check your Body Mass Index (BMI)

Look down the column on the left-hand side of the table to find your weight (or the nearest to it); then look across that row until you see the column for your height. The number that appears where the two meet is your BMI score. To find out whether your score indicates that your weight is healthy for your height, go to the assessment underneath the table.

Weight	Height 58 in (1.47 m)	60 in (1.52 m)	62 in (1.57 m)	64 in (1.62 m)	66 in (1.68 m)	68 in (1.73 m)	70 in (1.78 m)	72 in (1.83 m)	74 in (1.88 m)	76 in (1.93 m)
120 lb (54 kg)	25	24	22	21	19	18	17	16	15	15
125 lb (57 kg)	26	24	23	22	20	19	18	17	16	15
130 lb (59 kg)	27	25	24	22	21	20	19	18	17	16
135 lb (61 kg)	28	26	25	23	22	21	19	18	17	16
140 lb (63 kg)	29	27	26	24	23	21	20	19	18	17
145 lb (66 kg)	30	28	27	25	23	22	21	20	19	18
150 lb (68 kg)	31	29	28	26	24	23	22	20	19	18
155 lb (70 kg)	32	30	28	27	25	24	22	21	20	19
160 lb (73 kg)	34	31	29	28	26	24	23	22	21	20
165 lb (75 kg)	35	32	30	28	27	25	24	22	21	20
170 lb (77 kg)	36	33	31	29	28	26	24	23	22	21
175 lb (79 kg)	37	34	32	30	28	27	25	24	23	21
180 lb (82 kg)	38	35	33	31	29	27	26	24	23	22
185 lb (84 kg)	39	36	34	32	30	28	27	25	24	23
190 lb (86 kg)	40	37	35	33	31	29	27	26	24	23
195 lb (88 kg)	41	38	36	34	32	30	28	27	25	24
200 lb (91 kg)	42	39	37	34	32	30	29	27	26	24
205 lb (93 kg)	43	40	38	35	33	31	29	28	26	25
210 lb (95 kg)	44	41	39	36	34	32	30	29	27	26
215 lb (98 kg)	45	42	39	37	35	33	31	29	28	26
220 lb (100 kg)	46	43	40	38	36	34	32	30	28	27
225 lb (102 kg)	47	44	41	39	36	34	32	31	29	27
230 lb (104 kg)	48	45	42	40	37	35	33	31	30	28
235 lb (107 kg)	49	46	43	40	38	36	34	32	30	29
240 lb (109 kg)	50	47	44	41	39	37	35	33	31	29
245 lb (111 kg)	51	48	45	42	40	37	35	33	32	30

What does your score mean?

Below 18.5	You are underweight, which may signal malnutrition
18.5–24.9	You are within a healthy weight range for your height
25–29.9	You are overweight, with an increased risk for health problems
30 and above	You are obese, with significantly increased risk for health problems

>> **test** your fitness

Before you start your training program, you must check that it is safe for you to begin. Take the PAR-Q questionnaire on the opposite page, and if you are in any doubt about the state of your health, please see your doctor before becoming more physically active. The three tests below will help you to assess your fitness.

Track your progress

One way to measure muscular fitness is to count how many repetitions you can perform, or how many seconds you can hold a contraction. To see how you measure up, do the three exercises shown, which will assess your muscular endurance in the lower, middle, and upper body. Record your results, noting the date, and after three months of training, repeat the tests. When you reassess yourself, perform the same version of the exercise.

If you are just beginning to exercise, or coming back to it after a long break, you may prefer to perform your first assessment after two or three months of exercising on a regular basis. Before attempting the exercises, warm up first by moving your arms and legs briskly for five minutes.

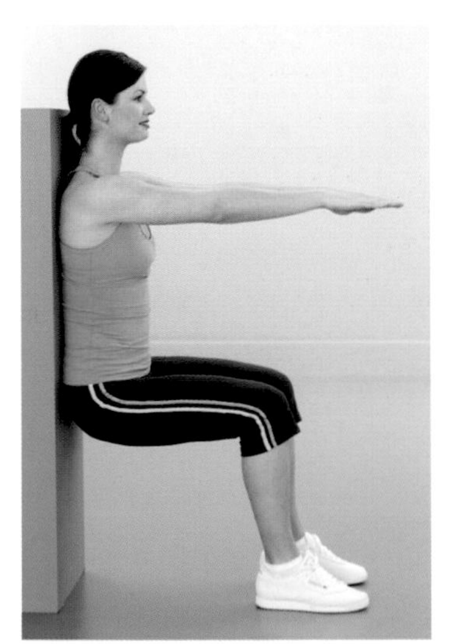

Lower body

Wall Squat

Slide down until your thighs are parallel to the floor and hold the position for as long as you can. (If you cannot slide all the way down, go as far as you can.)

Your score
Excellent 90 seconds or more
Good 60 seconds
Fair 30 seconds
Poor less than 30 seconds

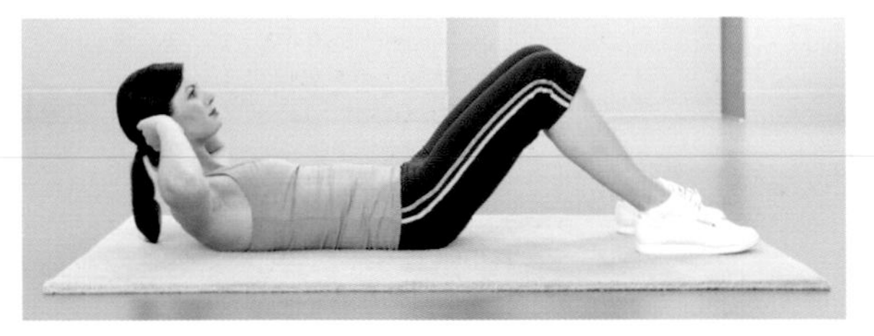

Middle body *Crunch with Scoop*

Count how many crunches you can do consecutively without resting. This is not a full sit-up. Lift your head and shoulders no higher than 30 degrees off the mat.

Your score	
Excellent	50 reps or more
Good	35–49 reps
Fair	20–34 reps
Poor	20 reps or less

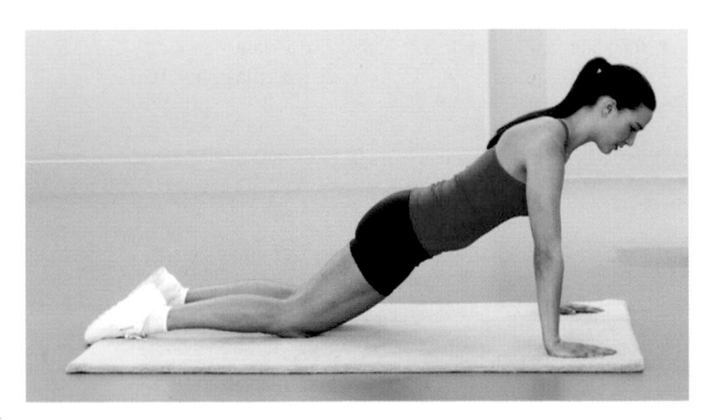

Upper body *Half Push-up*

Inhale as you bend your elbows, lowering your chest to the floor. Exhale as you push up to the starting position. Count how many you can do consecutively without a rest.

Your score	
Excellent	20 reps or more
Good	15–19 reps
Fair	10–14 reps
Poor	10 reps or less

PAR-Q AND YOU A questionnaire for people aged 15 to 69 Physical Activity Readiness Questionnaire – PAR-Q (revised 2002)

Regular physical activity is fun and healthy, and increasingly more people are starting to become more active every day. Being more active is perfectly safe for most people. However, some people should check with their doctor before they start becoming much more physically active than they are already.

If you are planning to become much more physically active than you are now, start by answering the seven questions in the box below. If you are between the ages of 15 and 69, the PAR-Q will tell you if you should check with your doctor before you start. If you are over 69 years of age, and you are not used to being very active, check with your doctor.

Common sense is your best guide when you answer these questions. Please read the questions carefully and answer each one honestly: check YES or NO.

YES	NO	
☐	☐	1 Has your doctor ever said that you have a heart condition and that you should only do physical activity recommended by a doctor?
☐	☐	2 Do you feel pain in your chest when you do physical activity?
☐	☐	3 In the past month, have you had chest pain when you were not doing physical activity?
☐	☐	4 Do you lose your balance because of dizziness or do you ever lose consciousness?
☐	☐	5 Do you have a bone or joint problem (for example, back, knee, or hip) that could possibly be made worse by a marked change in your physical activity?
☐	☐	6 Is your doctor currently prescribing drugs (for example, water pills) for your blood pressure or heart condition?
☐	☐	7 Do you know of any other reason why you should not do physical activity?

If you answered YES to one or more questions

Talk with your doctor by phone or in person BEFORE you start becoming much more physically active or BEFORE you have a fitness appraisal.
Tell your doctor about the PAR-Q and which questions you answered YES.
- You may be able to do any activity you want—as long as you start slowly and build up gradually. Or, you may need to restrict your activities to those which are safe for you. Talk with your doctor about the kinds of activities you wish to participate in and follow his/her advice.
- Find out which community programs are going to prove safe and helpful for you.

If you answered NO to all questions

If you answered NO honestly to all PAR-Q questions, you can be reasonably sure that you can:
- start becoming much more physically active—begin slowly and build up gradually. This is the safest and easiest way to go.
- take part in a fitness appraisal—this is an excellent way to determine your basic fitness so that you can plan the best way for you to live actively. It is also highly recommended that you have your blood pressure evaluated. If your reading is over 144/94, talk with your doctor before you start becoming much more physically active.

DELAY BECOMING MUCH MORE ACTIVE:
- if you are not feeling well because of a temporary illness such as a cold or a fever—wait until you feel better
- if you are or may be pregnant—talk to your doctor before you start becoming more active.

PLEASE NOTE:
If your health changes so that you then answer YES to any of the above questions, tell your fitness or health professional. Ask whether you should change your physical activity plan.

Informed use of the PAR-Q: The Canadian Society for Exercise Physiology, Health Canada, and their agents assume no liability for persons who undertake physical activity, and if in doubt after completing the questionnaire, consult your doctor prior to physical activity.

>> **your training** program

Now that you've assessed your current condition, you are ready to start making improvements to your personal level of fitness, as well as your health, appearance, energy levels, and overall mood. Each 15-minute workout combines cardio with resistance training and stretching.

Cardiovascular stamina, muscular strength and endurance, flexibility, and body composition are the aspects of physical fitness that are most closely related to health. Each of these characteristics is directly related to good health and to your risk of developing certain types of disease—notably those that are associated with inactivity.

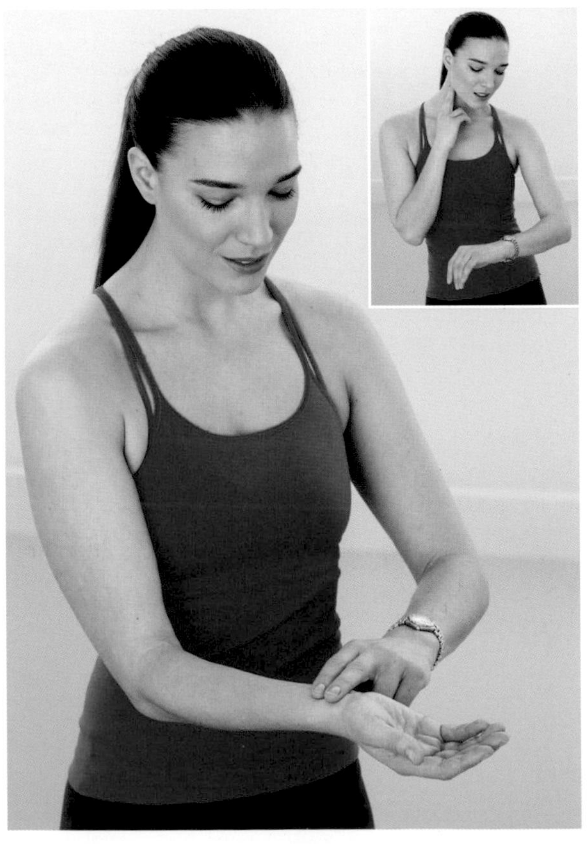

Benefits of cardiovascular fitness

A fit cardiovascular system is associated with a stronger heart muscle, slower heart rate, decreased chance of heart attack, and a greater chance of surviving if you do suffer a heart attack. Regular aerobic exercise can reduce your blood pressure and blood fats, including low-density lipids (LDL), which can help you resist build up of plaque in the arteries (atherosclerosis). It can also increase the protective high-density lipids (HDL) and improve circulation and the capacity of the blood to carry oxygen throughout your body. Improving cardiovascular fitness also decreases your risk of some cancers and of obesity, diabetes, osteoporosis, depression, and anxiety.

With training, your heart gets stronger and can pump more blood with each beat, resulting in a lower heart rate during exercise and at rest. The average resting rate is 60 to 80 beats per minute. Take your resting heart rate when you start your program and then eight weeks later and compare the numbers. Find your pulse (see left), count the first beat as "zero" and time yourself for 30 seconds. Multiply the score by two to arrive at the number of beats per minute.

Taking your pulse To take your pulse at the wrist (the "radial pulse") place your index and middle fingers on the palm side of the opposite wrist. Alternatively, you can take your pulse at the neck (the "carotid pulse"), just below the jaw bone to the side of the larynx.

Muscle strength and endurance

Muscular strength (the ability to exert force) and endurance (the ability of the muscles to exert themselves repeatedly) allow you to work more efficiently and to resist fatigue, muscle soreness, and back problems. Strengthening the muscles and joints allows you to increase the intensity and duration of your cardiovascular training. As you work the muscles, you simultaneously stimulate the bones to build and maintain density, decreasing the risk of developing osteoporosis.

Stretching and flexibility

Your ability to stretch out the muscles and maintain range of motion in the joints is another aspect of muscular fitness. Stretching helps improve posture by correcting the tendency of certain muscles to shorten and tighten; it counteracts the physical stressors of our day-to-day activities and discharges tension from the muscles.

Frequency and duration

For resistance training you need to do a minimum of two 15-minute sessions per week, and no muscle should be worked more than three times in one week. Allow a day of rest in between working each muscle group, since the repair and recovery of the muscle fibers is as important as the stress to the development of the muscle. The length of your session will vary from 15 to 60 minutes, depending on your initial fitness and available time.

Maintenance program

Periodically, you should vary the workouts you choose or the order you perform them in so that you keep your muscles "alert." You may also want to increase your weights (see pp122–123 for equipment), but be aware that this may trigger problems in the neck, shoulder, elbow, low back, or knee. You may be able to handle heavier weights in some muscle groups, but not in others, so experiment carefully. Posture and alignment, and core conditioning are also important aspects of your training (see pp118–121).

>> **myths** about weight training

- **Myth 1**

  Lifting weights will make you bulk up.

  Truth Only if you have high levels of testosterone and use very heavy weights. Most women lack the necessary hormones and strength to build significant muscle mass.

- **Myth 2**

  You shouldn't lift weights if you are an older adult, overweight, or out of shape.

  Truth Not so! Weight training can help you rejuvenate, lose weight, and shape up.

- **Myth 3**

  A thin person does not need to build lean body mass by lifting weights.

  Truth Appearances are deceiving when it comes to body composition, and being thin is no guarantee that you are lean. Without weight training, you steadily lose muscle and gain fat as you age.

- **Myth 4**

  Certain weight-training exercises can help you spot reduce.

  Truth You can spot strengthen and shape a body area, but fat belongs to the whole body and needs to be reduced all over, through expending more calories (aerobic exercise and weight training) than you consume.

- **Myth 5**

  Aerobic activities, not weight training, are the most efficient type of exercise to lose weight.

  Truth Losing weight requires a balanced exercise program of aerobic exercise to burn calories and weight training to speed up the metabolism.

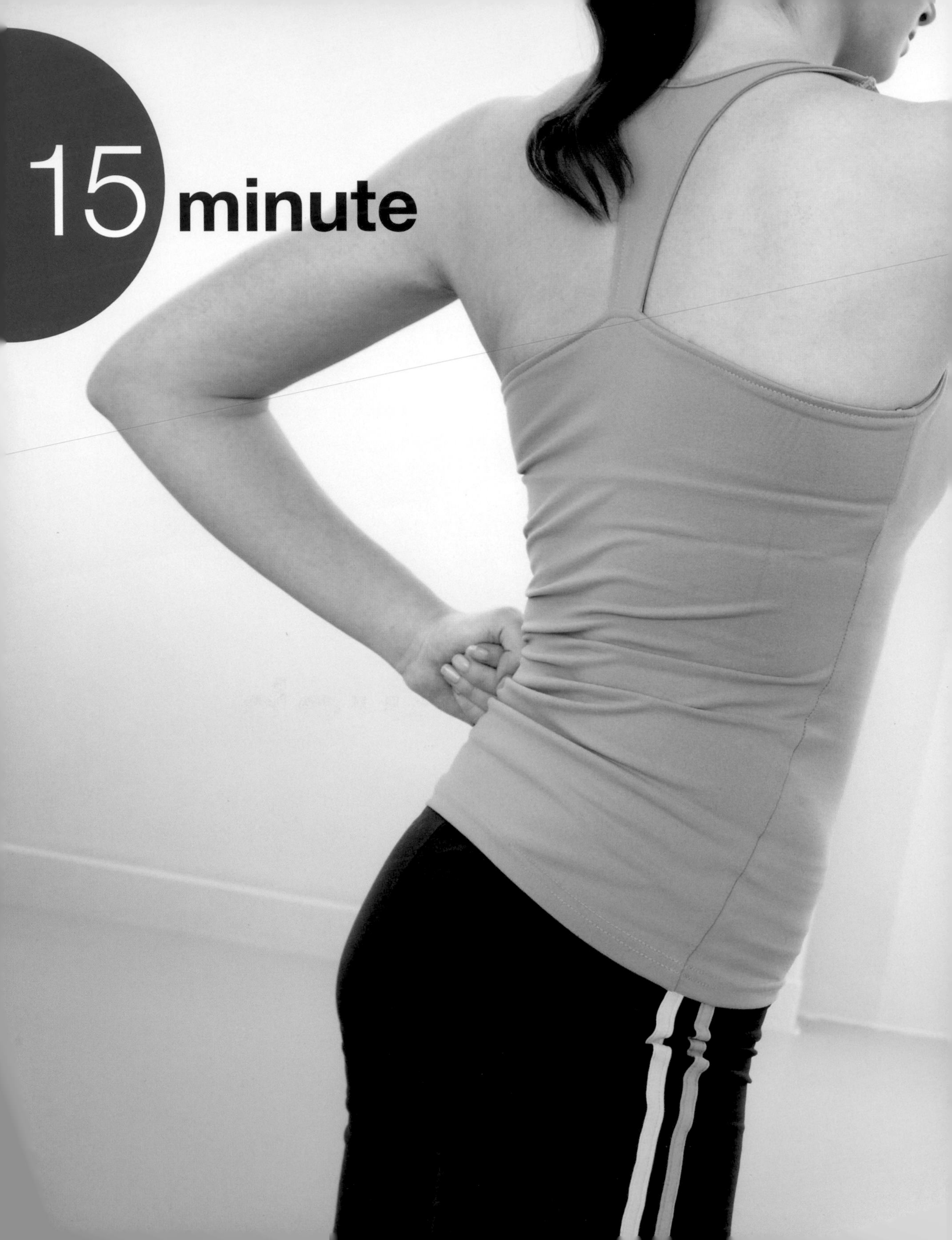
15 minute

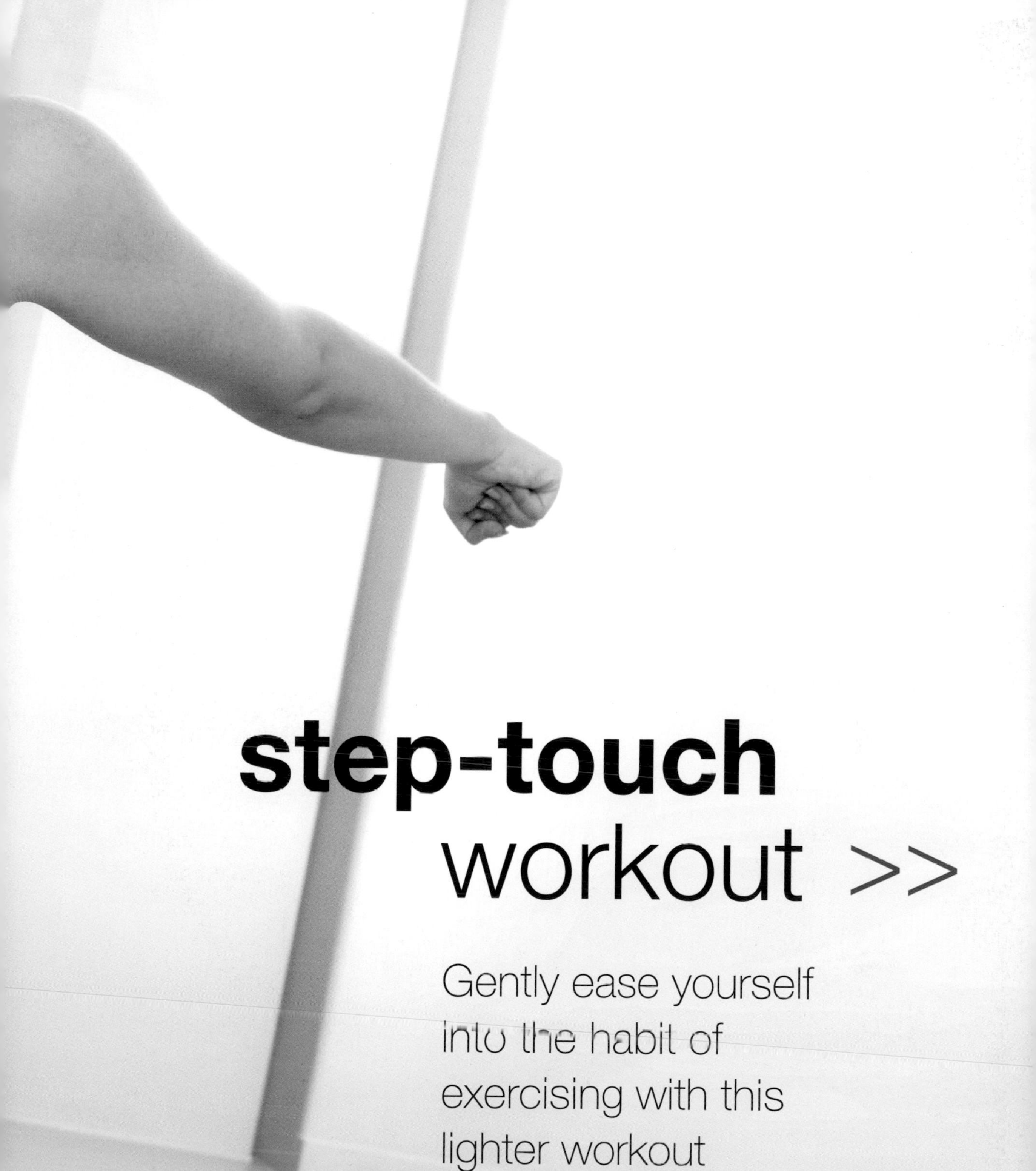

step-touch workout >>

Gently ease yourself into the habit of exercising with this lighter workout

>> **warm up** march/heel dig

1 **March** Stand with your feet parallel, hip width apart, knees soft, arms by your sides. Begin marching, bending one knee to bring the foot just off the floor and swinging the opposite arm forward and other arm back. Step down on the ball of your foot, rolling through to the heel. Continue marching, using opposite arm/leg action. Repeat for a total of 8 reps (1 rep = both sides).

2 **Heel Dig** Continuing to march, change the foot pattern to a heel dig to the front. Extend your leg to the front, knee straight, heel to the floor, toe to the ceiling. Continue to pump the arms in opposition as you march, with elbows bent close to your sides, raising the front fist to shoulder height. Remember to keep your abdominals pulled tight. Repeat for a total of 8 reps (1 rep = both sides).

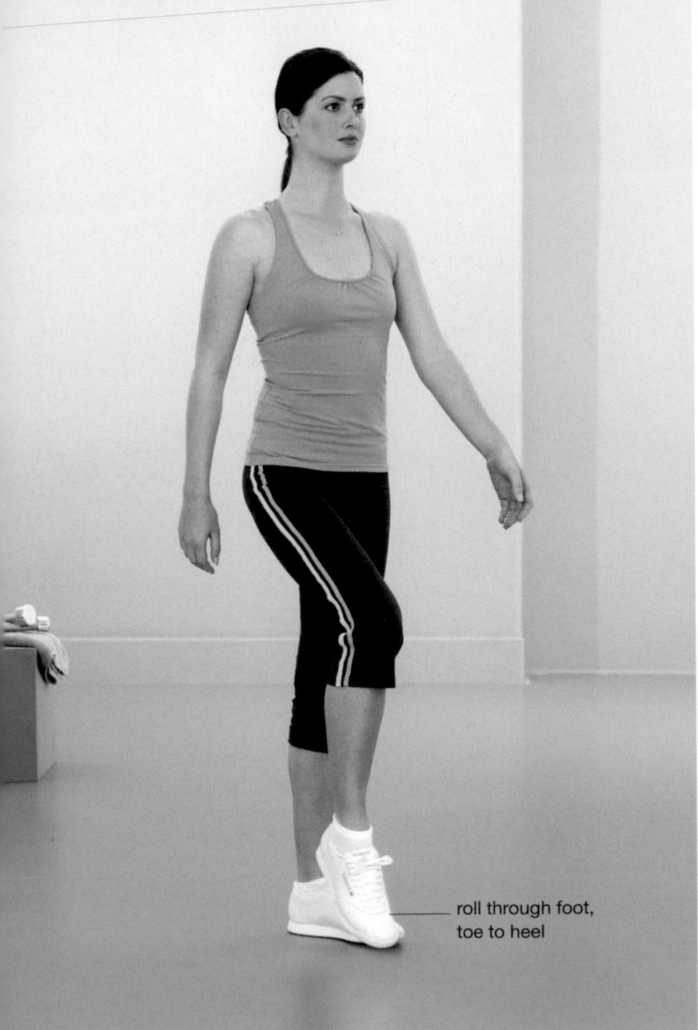

roll through foot, toe to heel

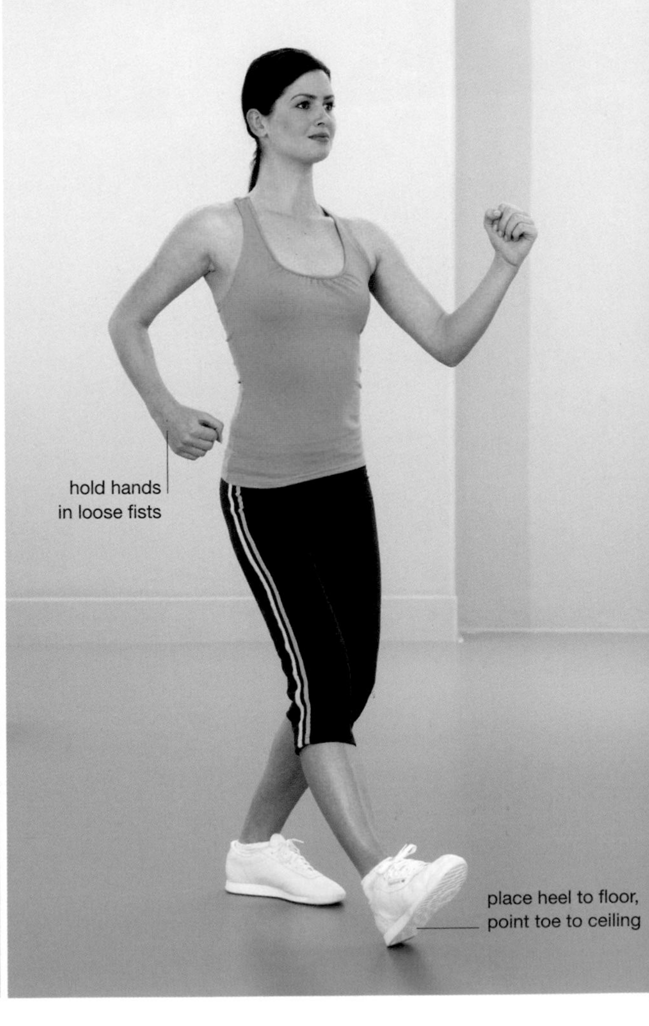

hold hands in loose fists

place heel to floor, point toe to ceiling

>> **warm up** toe reach/knee raise

3 **Toe Reach** Change the foot pattern to a toe reach to the front and continue marching, alternating feet and arms. As you extend your leg, point the foot, lengthening from toe to hip. Keep your arms straight as you swing them, raising the front hand to shoulder height. As you work, focus on your alignment. Stack your shoulders over your hips, over your ankles. Look straight ahead. Repeat the Toe Reach for a total of 8 reps (1 rep = both sides).

stack ribs over hips
keep toe pointed

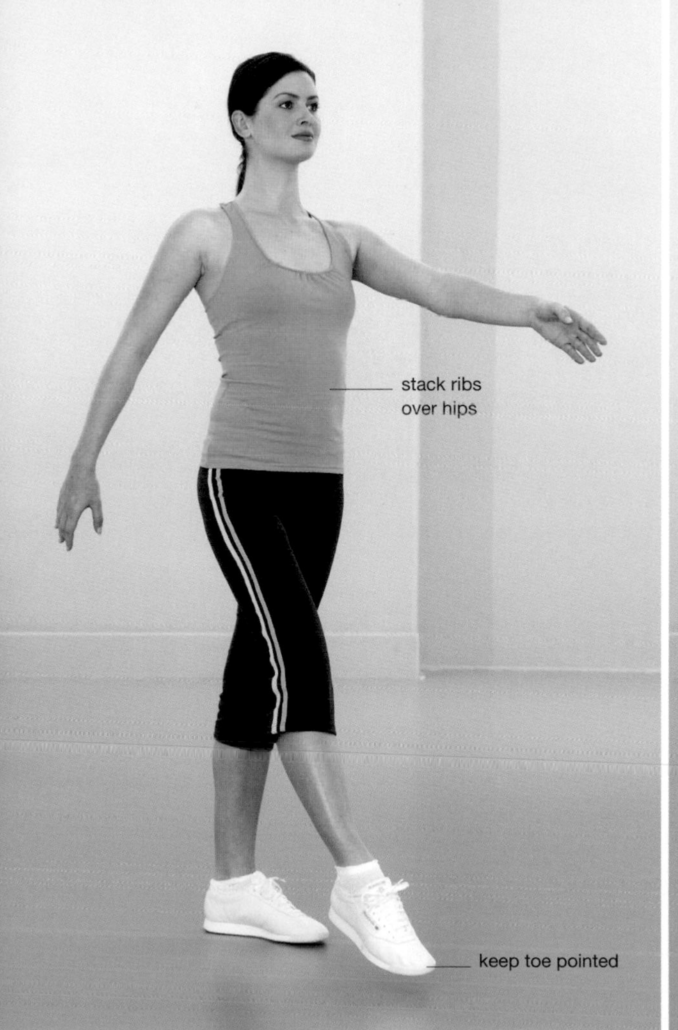

4 **Knee Raise** Step up the intensity by bending the front knee to hip height. If you are able to lift the knee higher than your hip, be sure to use your core muscles to maintain proper alignment. Continue to pump the arms in opposition, raising the front elbow to shoulder level. Repeat the Knee Raise for a total of 8 reps (1 rep = both sides).

bend elbows to 90°
keep body square to front
bend knee to 90°

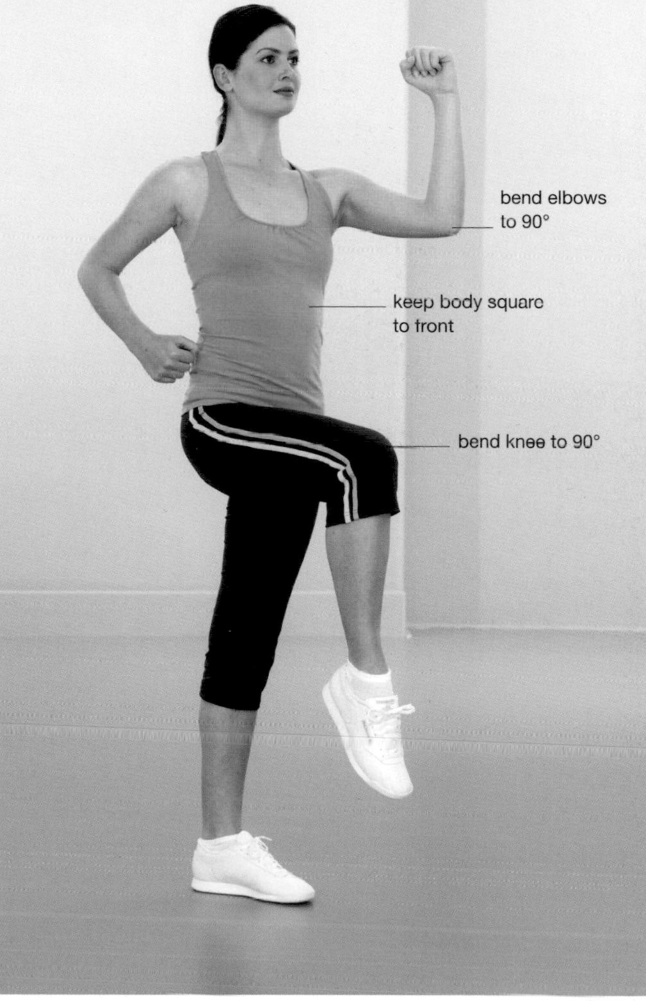

>> warm up reverse lunge/lateral lift

5 **Reverse Lunge** Maintaining the same rhythm, bend one leg and extend the the other leg behind, heel raised. Raise both arms to the front at shoulder height. Push off with the ball of your back foot to return to center, arms returning to your sides, then switch sides and repeat. Repeat the Reverse Lunge for a total of 8 reps (1 rep = both sides).

6 **Lateral Lift** Maintaining the same rhythm, bend both knees, arms by your sides. Then straighten both legs, lift one leg to the side and raise both arms to shoulder level. Return the raised leg to center, knees bent. Repeat, alternating sides, for 8 reps (1 rep = both sides). Now **reverse the warm up**, starting with Step 5, and working back through Steps 4, 3, and 2, and finishing with Step 1, marching in place.

raise arms to shoulders level
keep torso upright
position knee directly over ankle
push off with ball of foot

knees bend and straighten

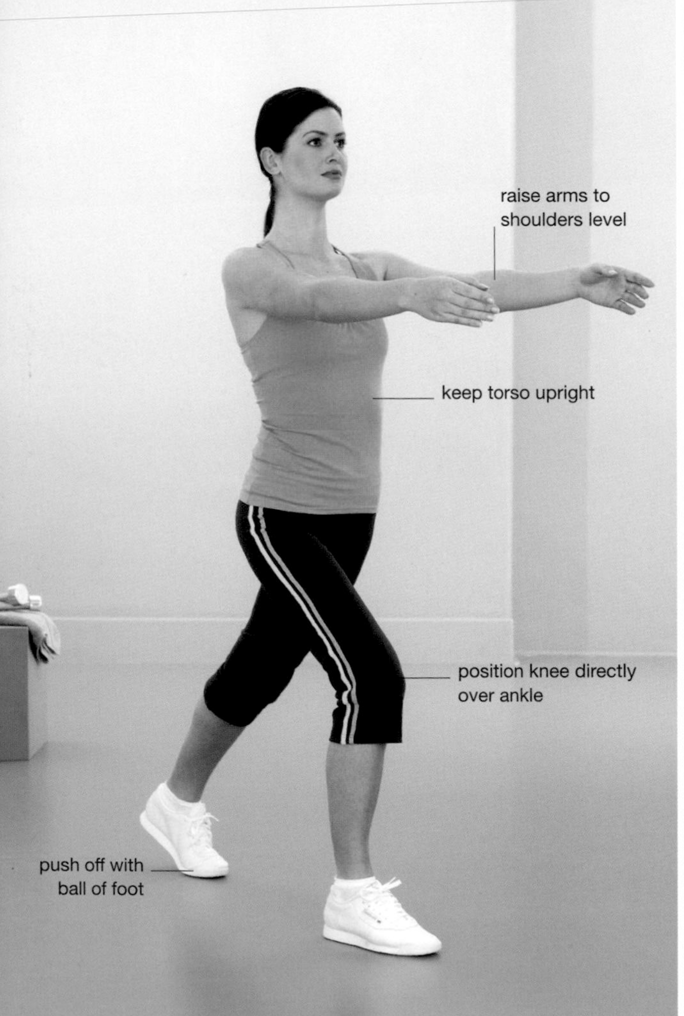

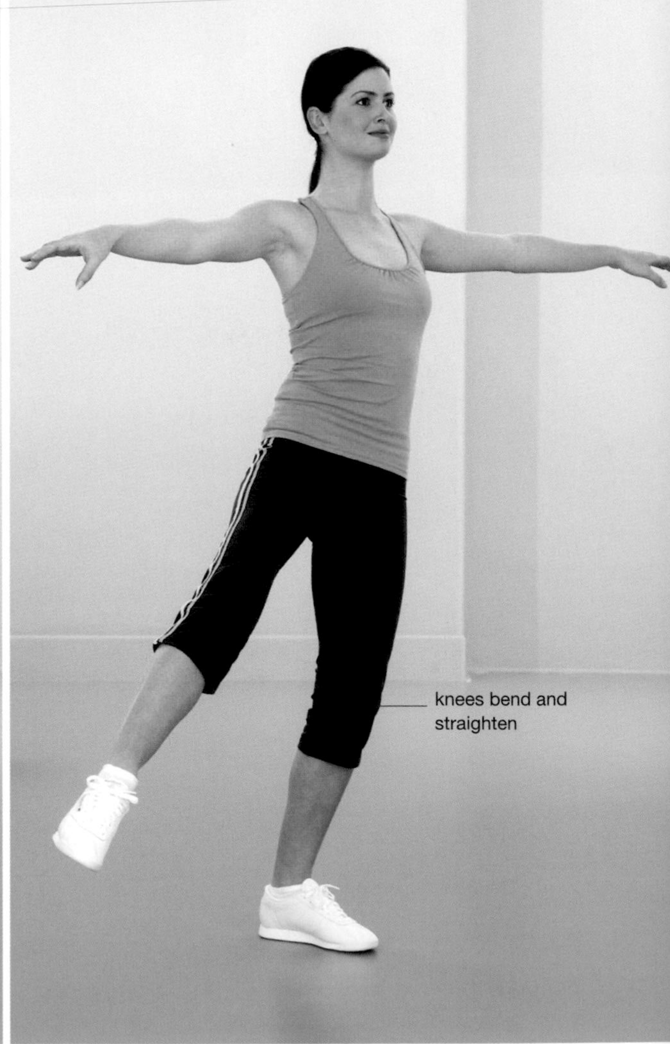

>> **resistance** plié with lateral raise

7a **Plié with Lateral Raise** Pick up two small free weights and stand with your feet in a wide stance. Shift your weight to your heels and turn your legs out from the hips as a unit until your feet are at 45° angles. Hold the free weights with palms facing in, arms straight by your sides. Remember to pull your abdominals tight and draw your shoulder blades down and together.

7b Inhale as you bend your knees in line with your feet, lifting your arms out to the sides to shoulder height, thumbs up to the ceiling. Angle your arms slightly forward of your body, directly above your thighs. Keep your elbows slightly rounded and your wrists straight. Exhale and press through your heels as you straighten your legs and lower your arms to return to the start position. As you move, imagine you are sliding up and down a wall. Repeat for a total of 12 reps.

keep chest lifted
turn legs out to 45°

keep elbows slightly rounded
bend knees in line with feet

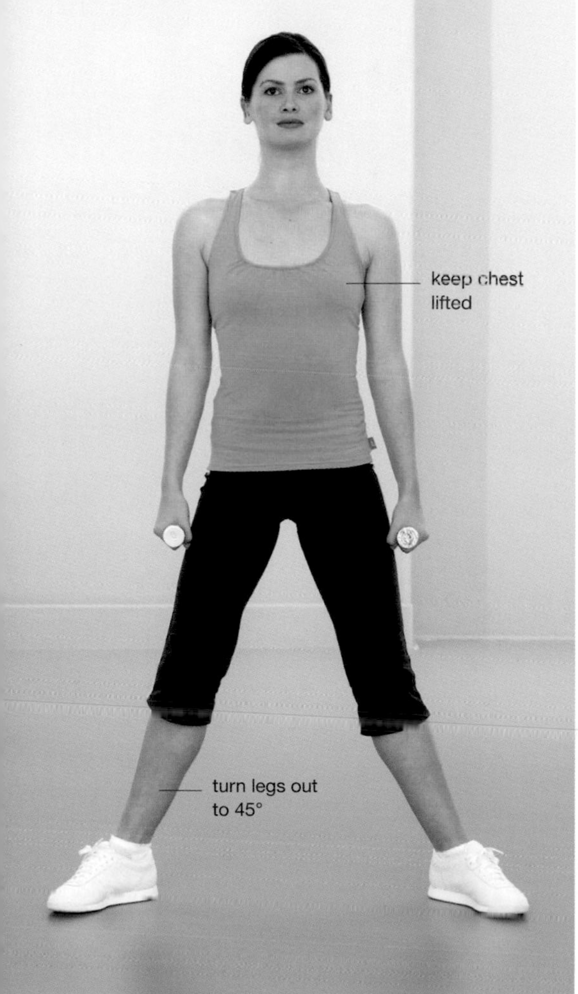

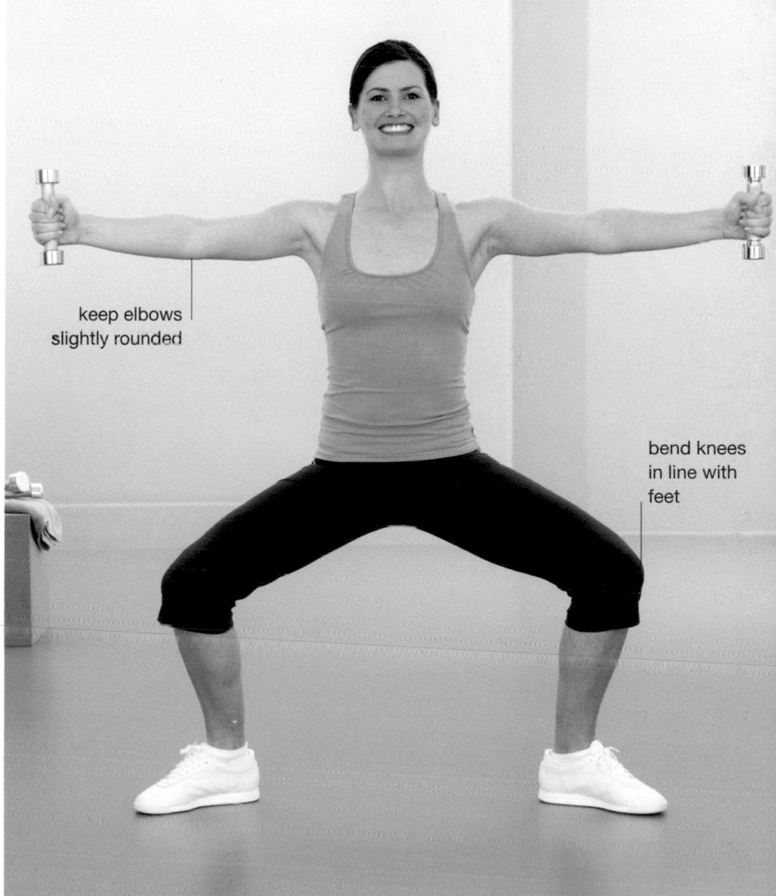

>> **cardio** step & punch

8a **Step & Punch** Put down the weights for the first cardio interval. Stand with your feet parallel, shoulder width apart, knees bent in a demi plié. Bend your arms and hold them at shoulder height, hands in loose fists. Check your alignment: keep your shoulder blades down, abdominals tight, chest lifted, and torso square to the front.

keep torso square to front
bend knees in demi plié

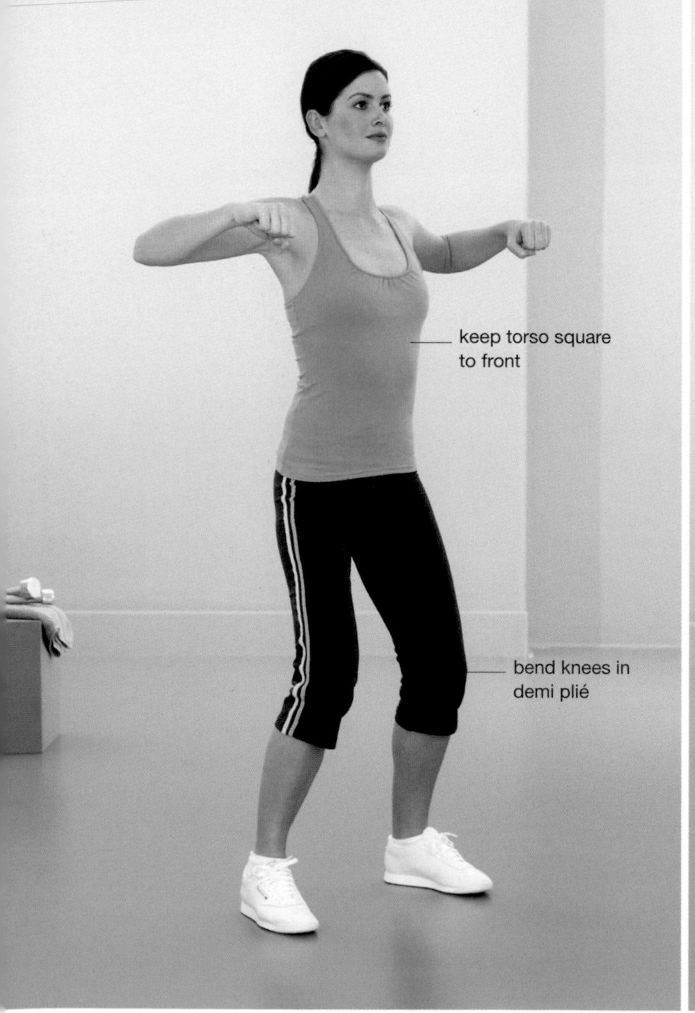

8b Breathe in, then exhale as you straighten your knees and extend one arm diagonally across your body (like a punch), at the same time lifting the heel of the same leg. Keep your other arm bent at shoulder height. Inhale as you return to the start position and repeat, alternating sides, for 12 reps (1 rep = both sides)

let your head follow action
twist the torso slightly
lift heel, toes on floor

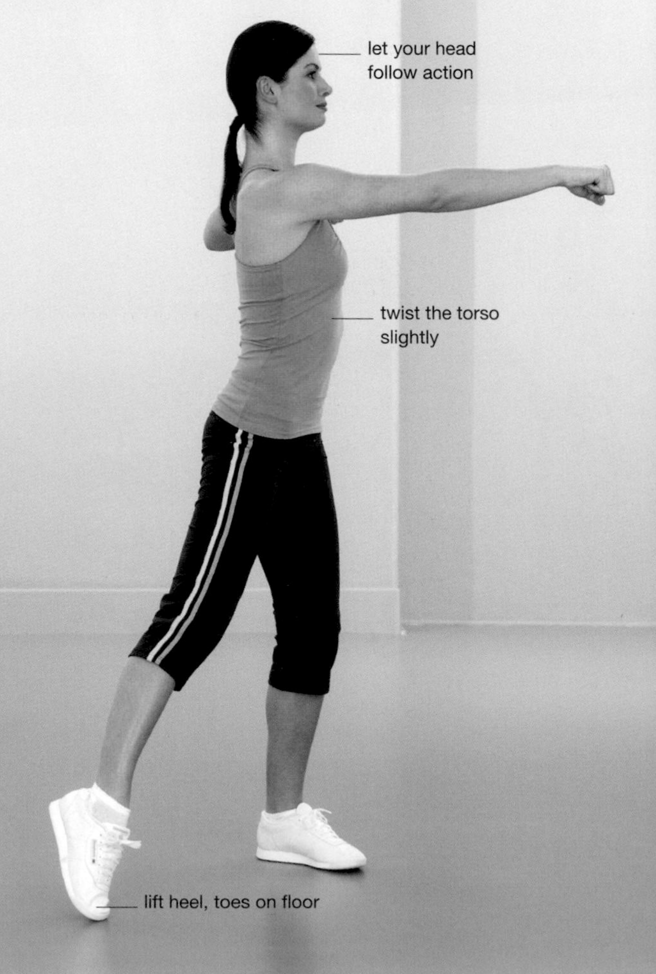

9a **Curl & Squeeze** Stand with your feet parallel, shoulder width apart, knees soft. Raise your arms to the front at shoulder level, shoulder width apart, hands in loose fists, palms down. Keep your knees soft. Use your core muscles to maintain neutral spine alignment, and lower your shoulder blades as you prepare to work the muscles of the mid-back.

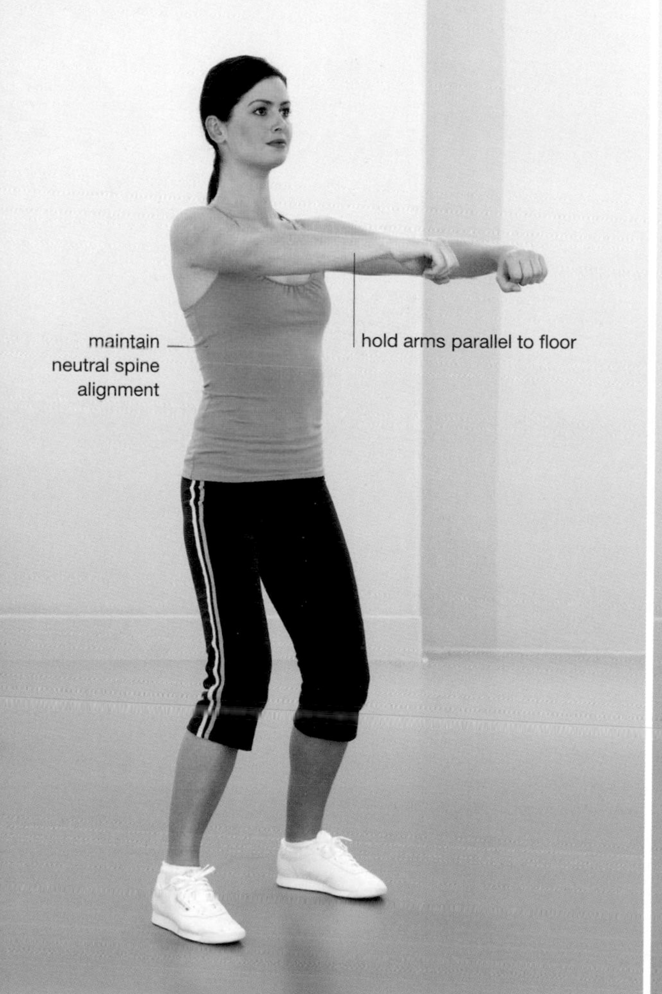

9b Breathing naturally throughout, shift your weight onto one leg and simultaneously bend the other leg back, heel toward your buttocks, in a hamstring curl. Keep your arms parallel to the floor, elbows bent at 90°, as you squeeze your shoulder blades together. Inhale as you return to the starting position. Repeat, alternating legs, for a total of 8 reps (1 rep = both sides).

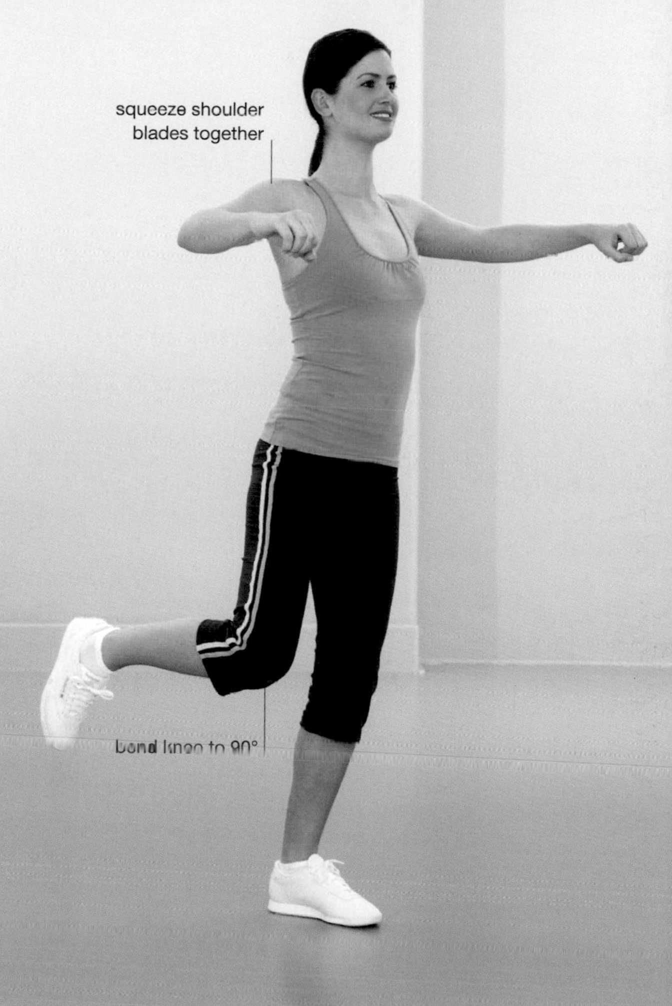

>> **cardio** twisting knee lift

10a **Twisting Knee Lift** Stand with your feet parallel, hip width apart, knees soft. Raise your arms out to the sides at shoulder height and bend your elbows to 90º; with palms facing forward, make your hands into loose fists. Remember to keep your shoulder blades down and abdominals pulled tight as you get ready to twist.

10b Keeping your back straight, bend your knee to hip height. Exhale and rotate your torso through the center to bring your elbow toward your raised knee. Inhale as you return to the center and repeat, alternating sides, for 8 reps (1 rep = both sides).

hold shoulder blades down and together

keep arms wide
hold torso upright

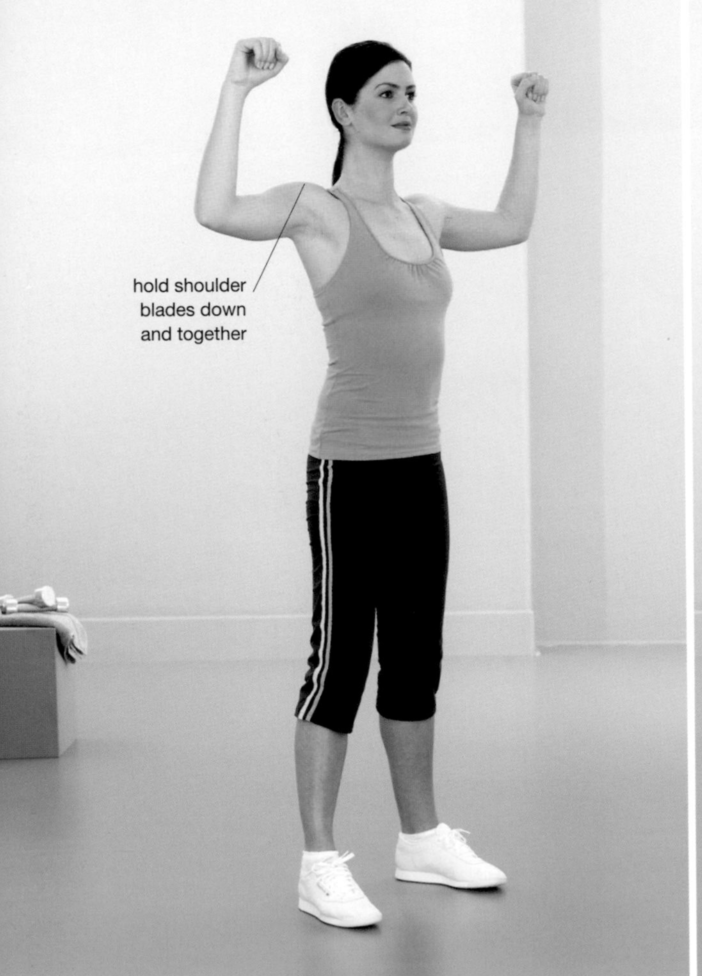

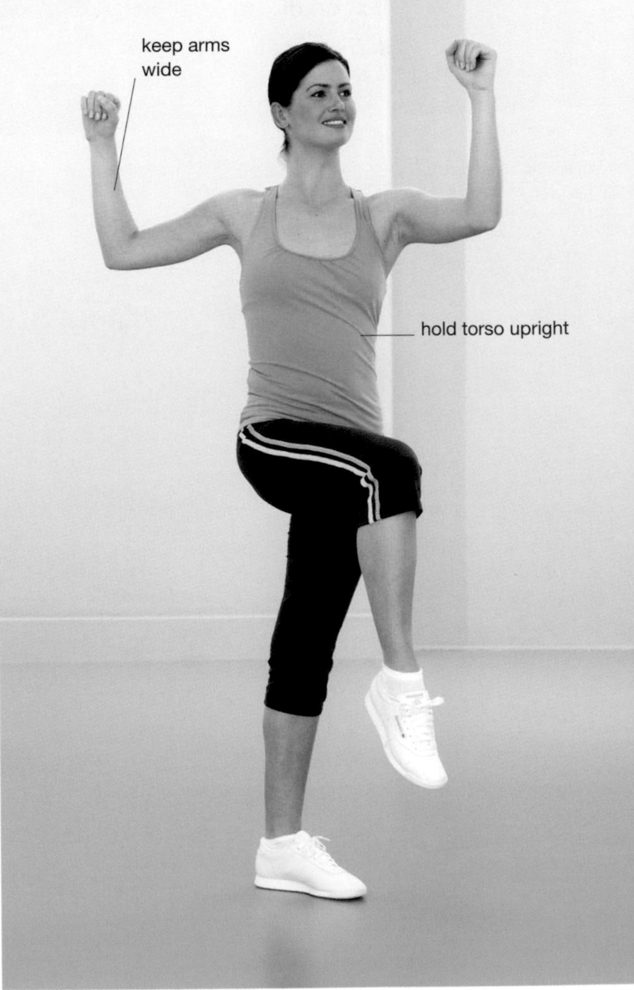

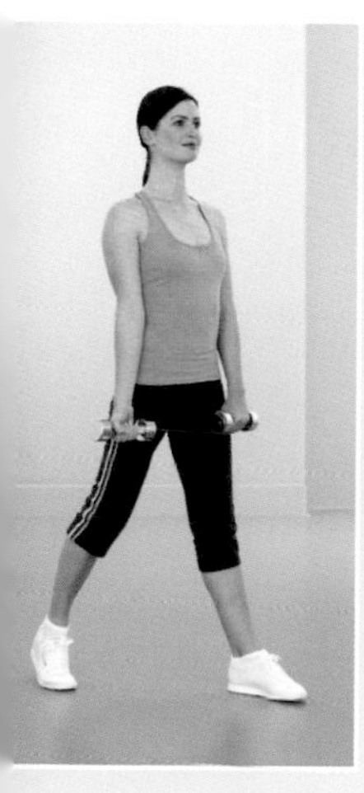

11 Lunge & Curl Pick up two large free weights. Stand in a staggered lunge position, one foot forward. Hold the weight in your opposite hand, palm forward. Inhale as you bend your knees into a lunge and bend one elbow to raise the weight to shoulder height. Exhale to return to center. Do 12 reps on each side (1 rep = both sides). **Do your next cardio interval, Steps 8–10 (pp24–26).**

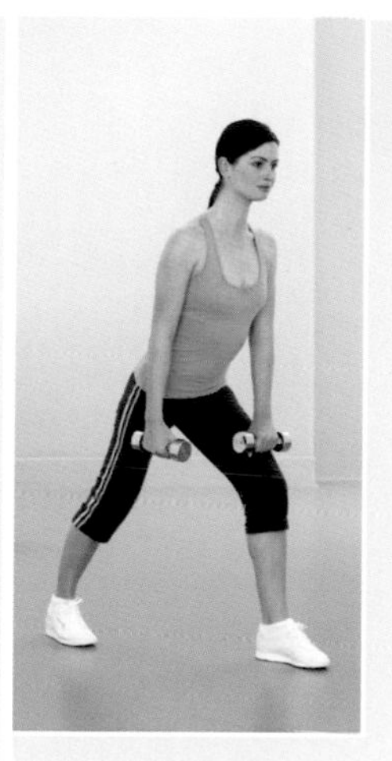

12 One-Arm Row Pick up two large free weights and step into a staggered lunge, bending from the hip to 45°. Inhale as you bend the opposite elbow behind you to 90°, lifting the weight to waist height. Do 12 reps on both sides. **Now do your next cardio interval, Steps 8–10 (pp24–26).**

keep elbow close to your side
rest supporting arm weight on thigh
press ball of foot into floor

draw shoulder blades in toward spine
press back heel to floor

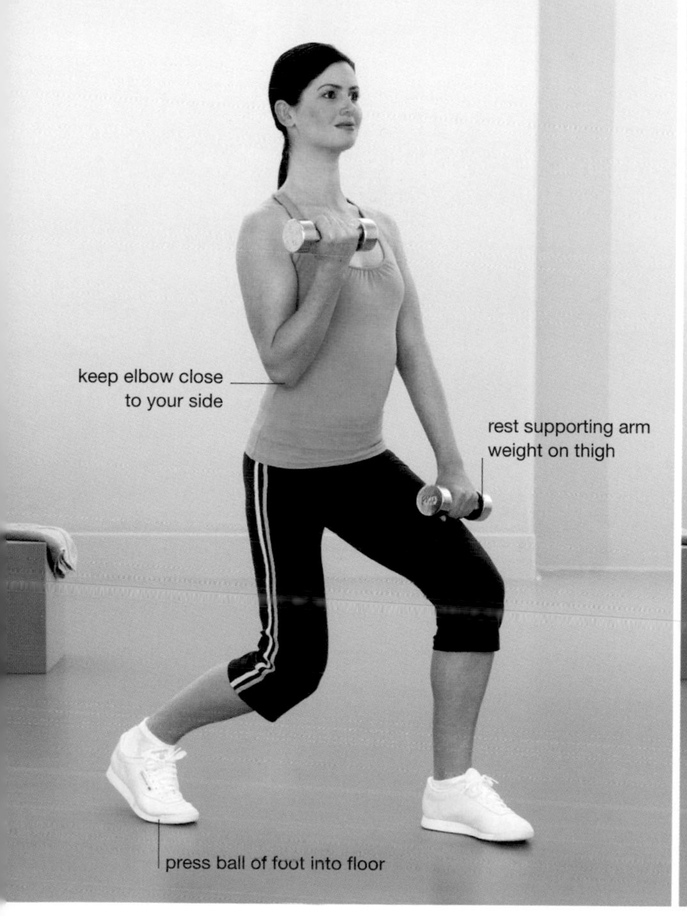

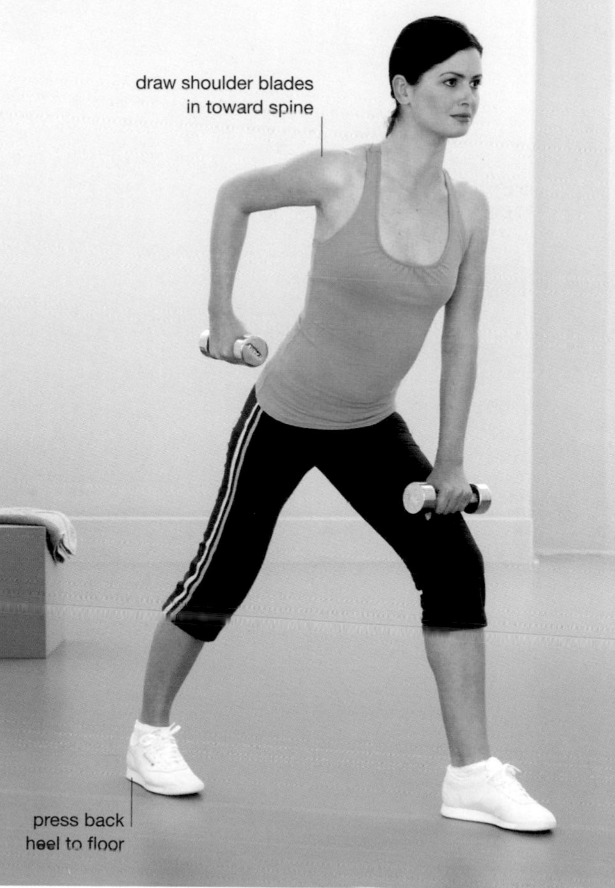

>> **resistance** squat/triceps kick back

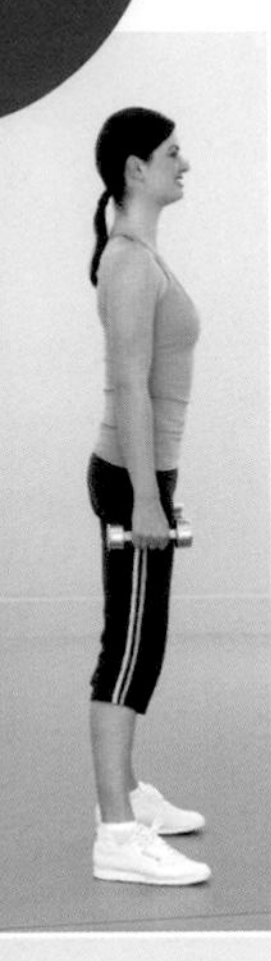

13 **Squat** Pick up two large free weights and stand with your feet parallel, shoulder width apart, knees soft. Hold the weights palms facing in. Shift your weight back onto your heels and as you inhale, bend your knees and reach back with your hips. Exhale and return to center, tightening your buttocks as you straighten your legs. Repeat for 12 reps. **Do your next cardio interval, Steps 8–10 (pp24–26).**

reach back
with your hips
shift weight
onto heels

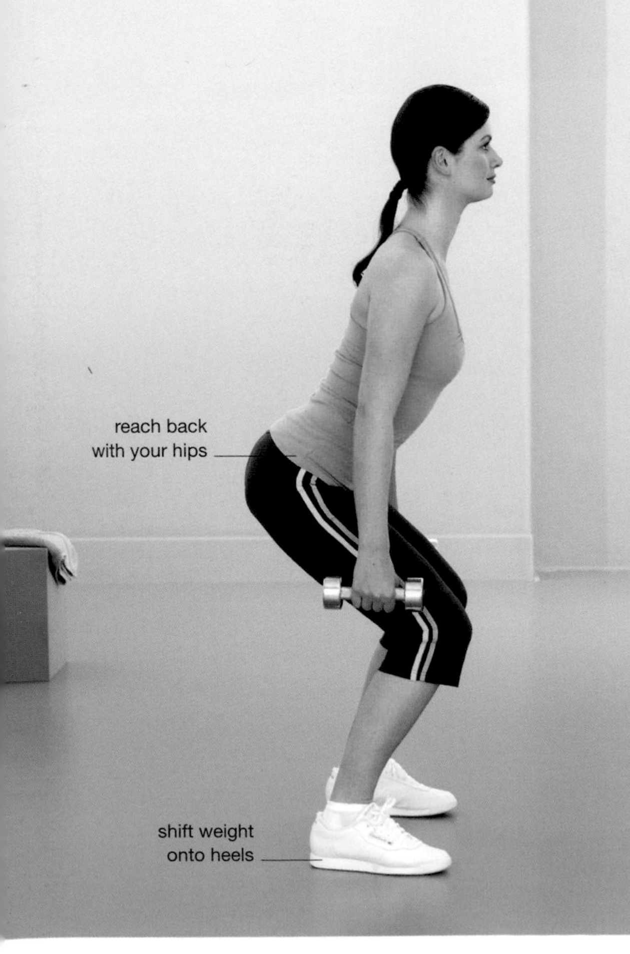

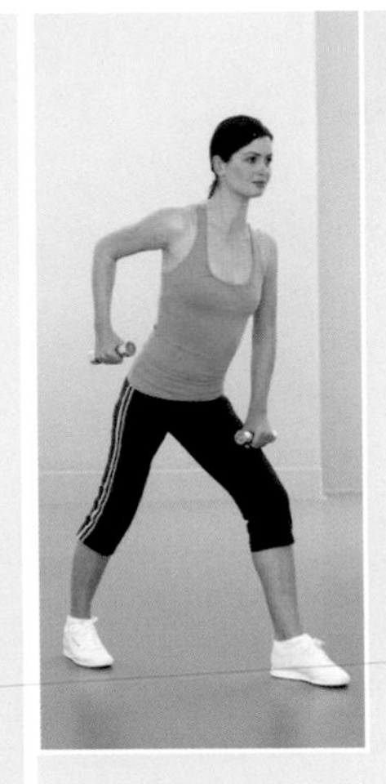

14 **Triceps Kick Back** Pick up two small free weights and stand in staggered lunge position, one foot back, leaning forward. Bend the elbow on the same side to 90° and raise the upper arm as parallel to the floor as possible. Breathe in, then exhale as you extend the forearm behind you. Do 12 reps on each side. **Do your next cardio interval, Steps 8–10 (pp24–26).**

keep spine
straight
keep back
heel down

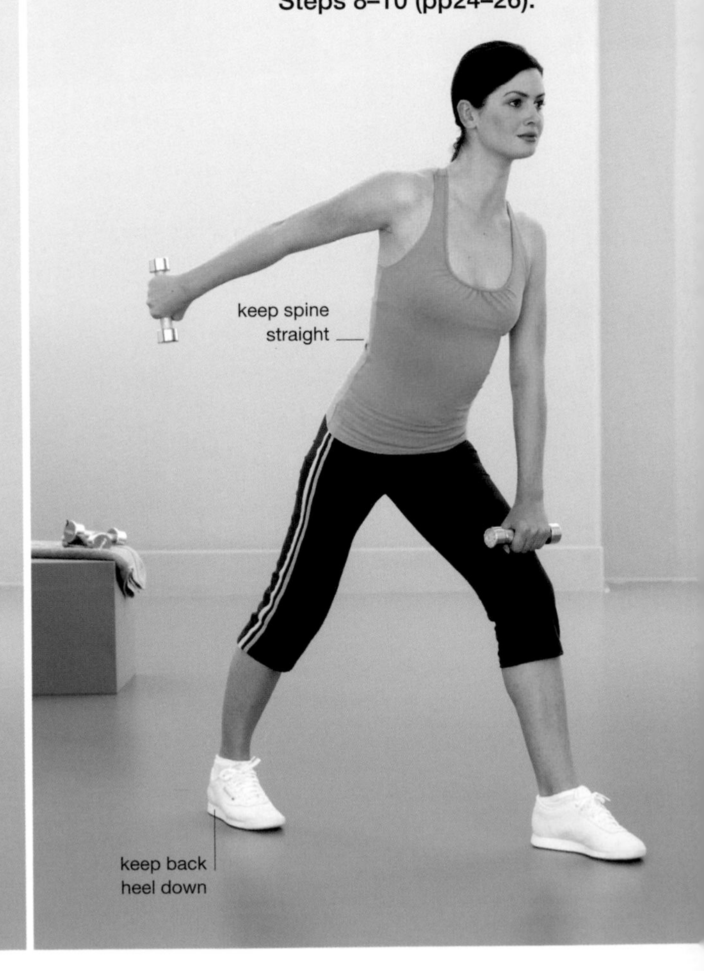

>> **cool down** lat stretch/sun salute

15 **Lat Stretch** Stand with your feet parallel, hip width apart, knees soft. Draw your shoulder blades down and reach both arms up. Interlock your thumbs and center your head between your elbows. Take a few deep breaths to lengthen the spine, lifting the top of your head toward the ceiling, separating your ribs from your hips.

lift ribs up from hips
place feet parallel, hip-width apart

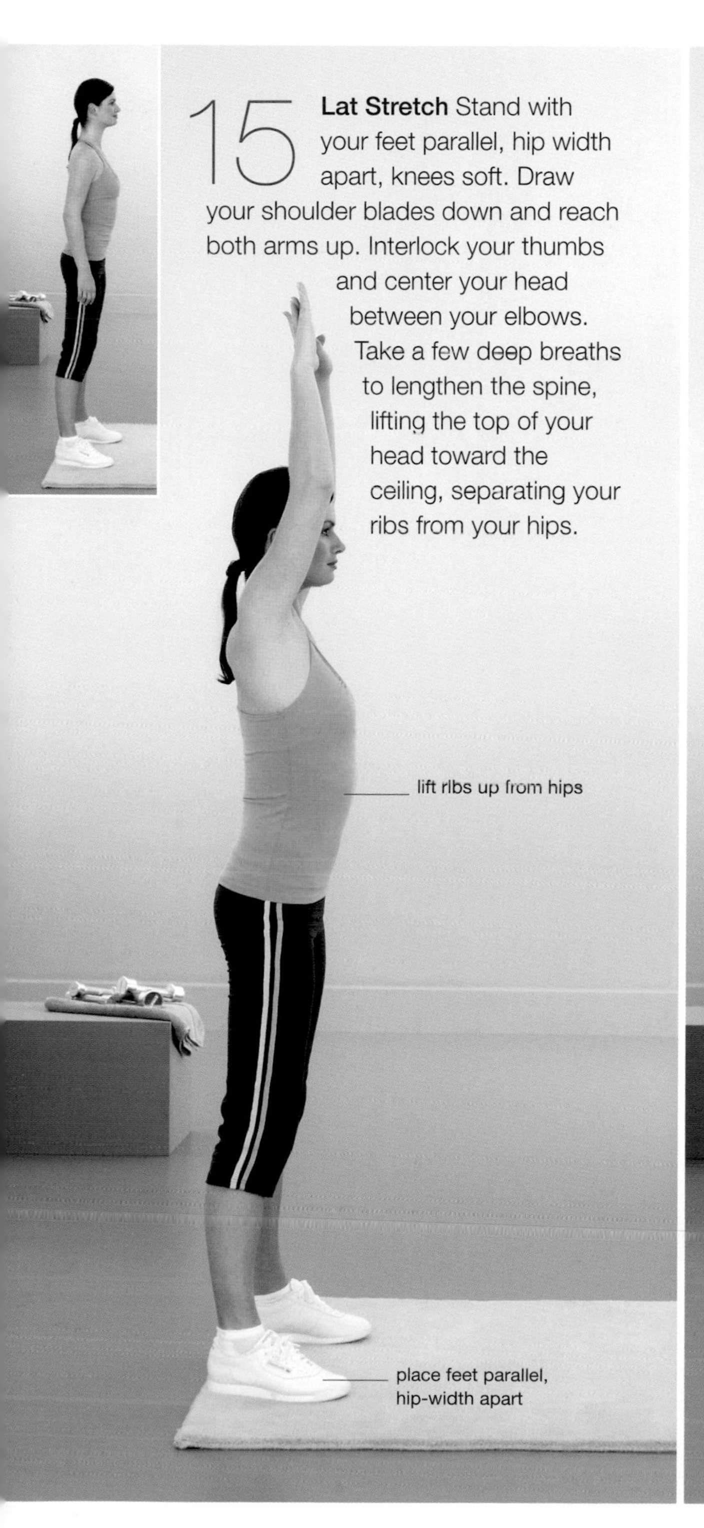

16 **Sun Salute** Maintaining length in the spine, tighten the hips, thighs, and buttocks. Reach up and out of the low back as you go into a mild back bend. Look up to the ceiling, keeping your head centered between your elbows. Return to center and lower your arms to your sides. Breathe naturally throughout.

look up to ceiling

lengthen the torso

>> **cool down** spinal roll-down/plank

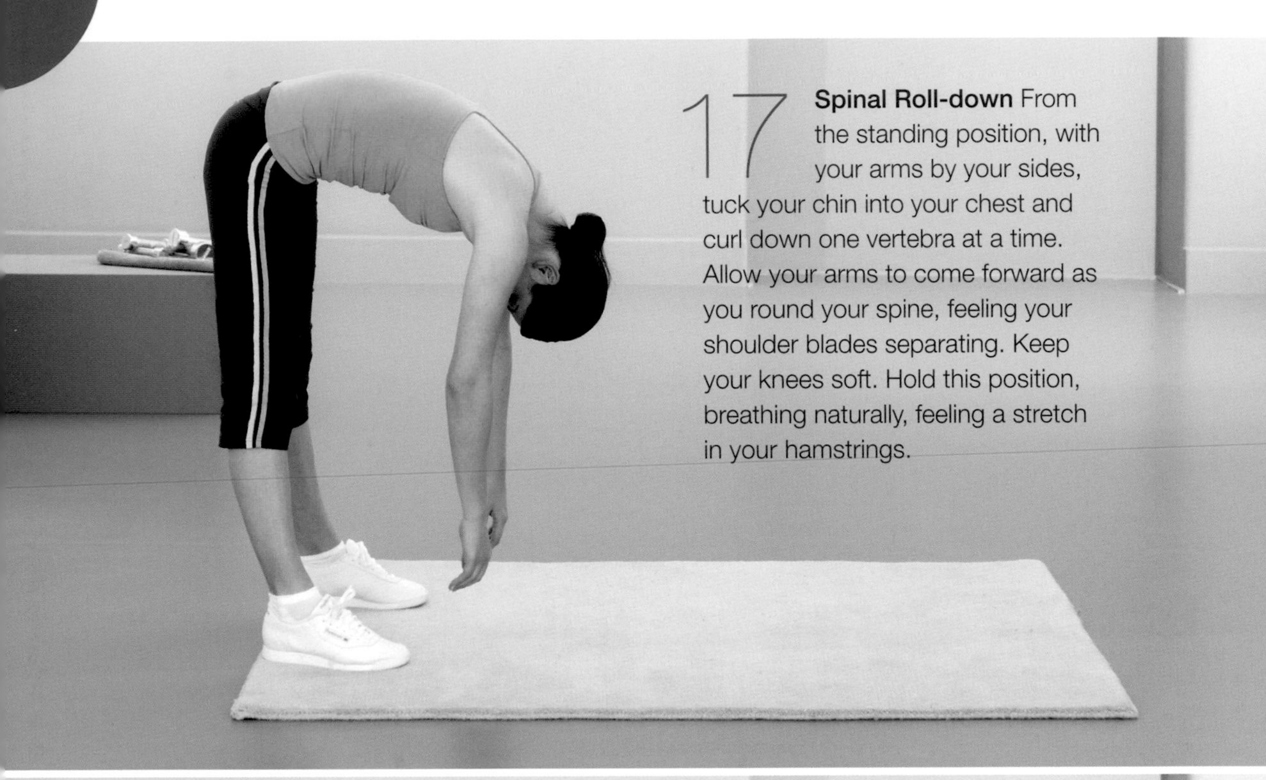

17 **Spinal Roll-down** From the standing position, with your arms by your sides, tuck your chin into your chest and curl down one vertebra at a time. Allow your arms to come forward as you round your spine, feeling your shoulder blades separating. Keep your knees soft. Hold this position, breathing naturally, feeling a stretch in your hamstrings.

maintain a straight line from head to heels
position wrists under shoulders, hands forward

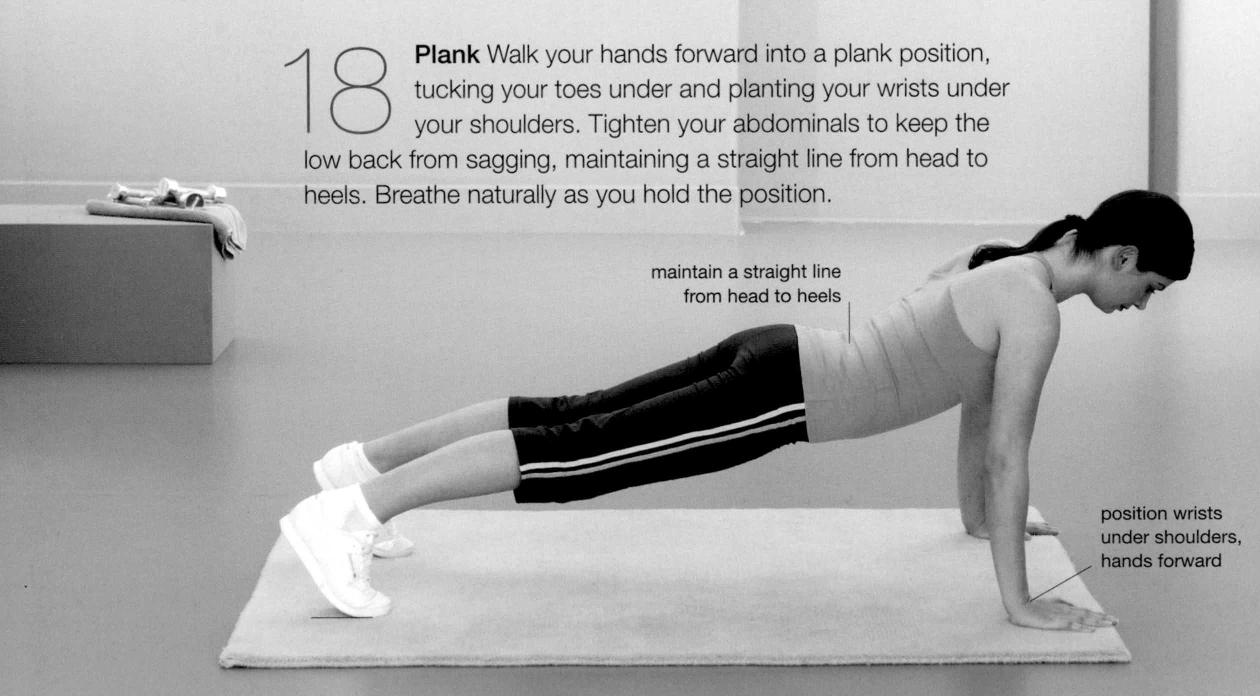

18 **Plank** Walk your hands forward into a plank position, tucking your toes under and planting your wrists under your shoulders. Tighten your abdominals to keep the low back from sagging, maintaining a straight line from head to heels. Breathe naturally as you hold the position.

>> **resistance** bicycle crunch

19a

Bicycle Crunch Turn onto your back with knees bent over your hips, calves parallel to the floor, feet relaxed. Be sure to keep a right angle at your knees and hips. Rest your head lightly on your fingertips, thumbs by your ears.

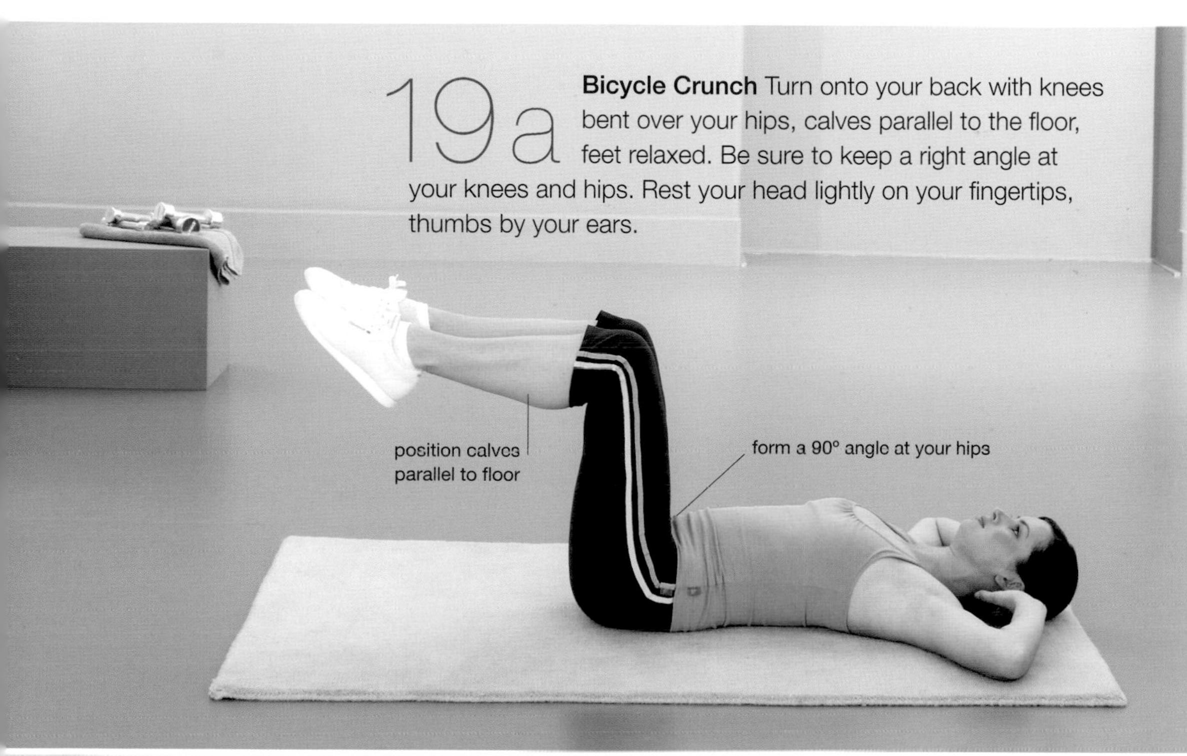

19b

Tighten your abdominals. Inhale, then exhale as you lift your shoulders off the floor, twisting your right shoulder toward your left knee as you extend your right leg. Return to center. Inhale, then exhale as you twist to the other side. Repeat, alternating sides, for 10 reps. (1 rep = both sides).

extend leg at 45° angle
feel it here
keep head and shoulders
lifted throughout
keep abdominals tight
feel it here

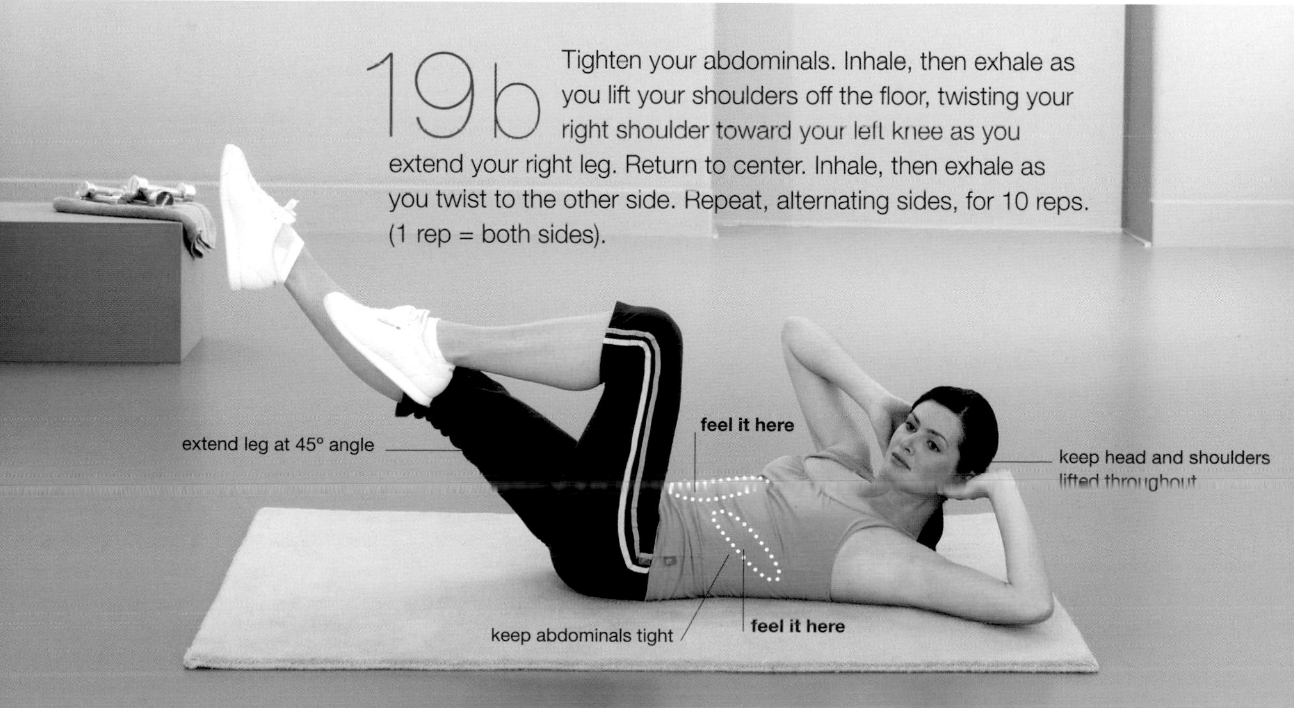

>> **cool down** spinal twist/quad stretch

drop knees to floor
turn head in opposite direction to knees

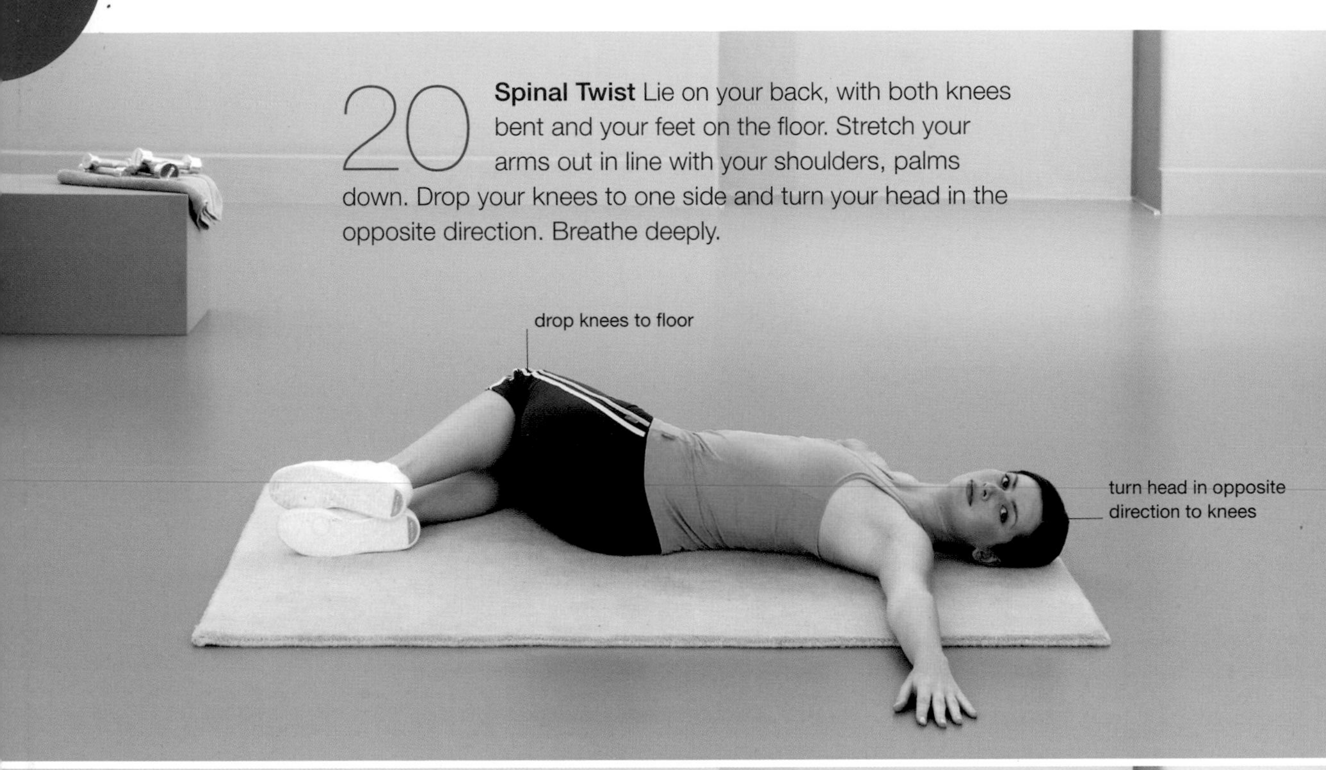

20 **Spinal Twist** Lie on your back, with both knees bent and your feet on the floor. Stretch your arms out in line with your shoulders, palms down. Drop your knees to one side and turn your head in the opposite direction. Breathe deeply.

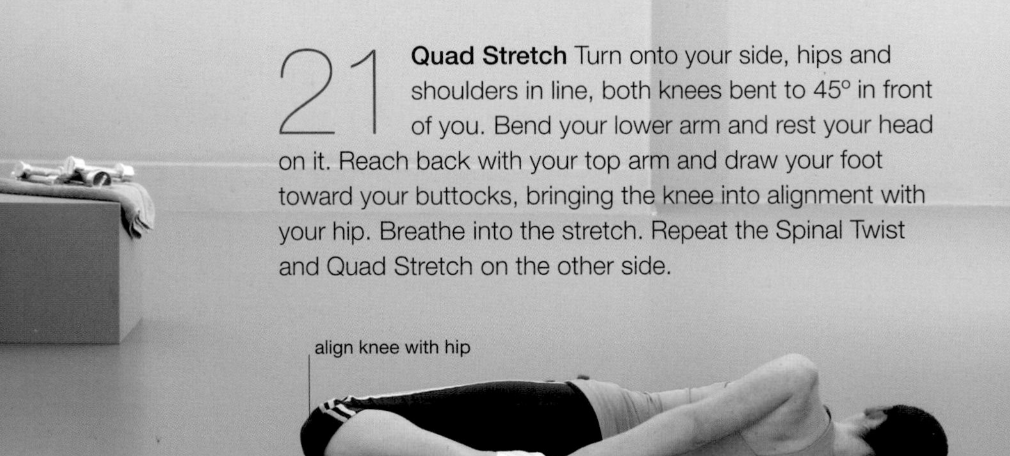

21 **Quad Stretch** Turn onto your side, hips and shoulders in line, both knees bent to 45° in front of you. Bend your lower arm and rest your head on it. Reach back with your top arm and draw your foot toward your buttocks, bringing the knee into alignment with your hip. Breathe into the stretch. Repeat the Spinal Twist and Quad Stretch on the other side.

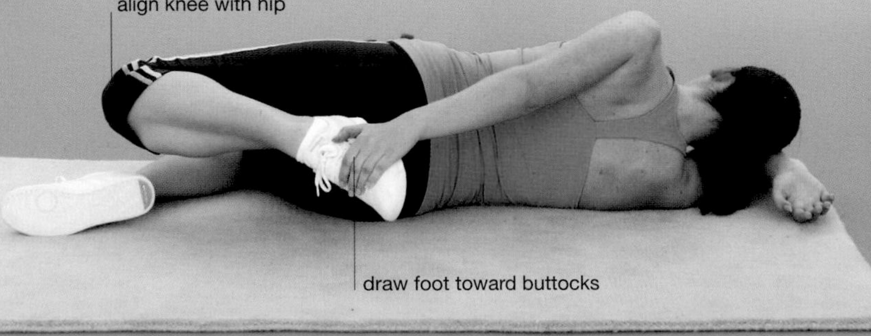

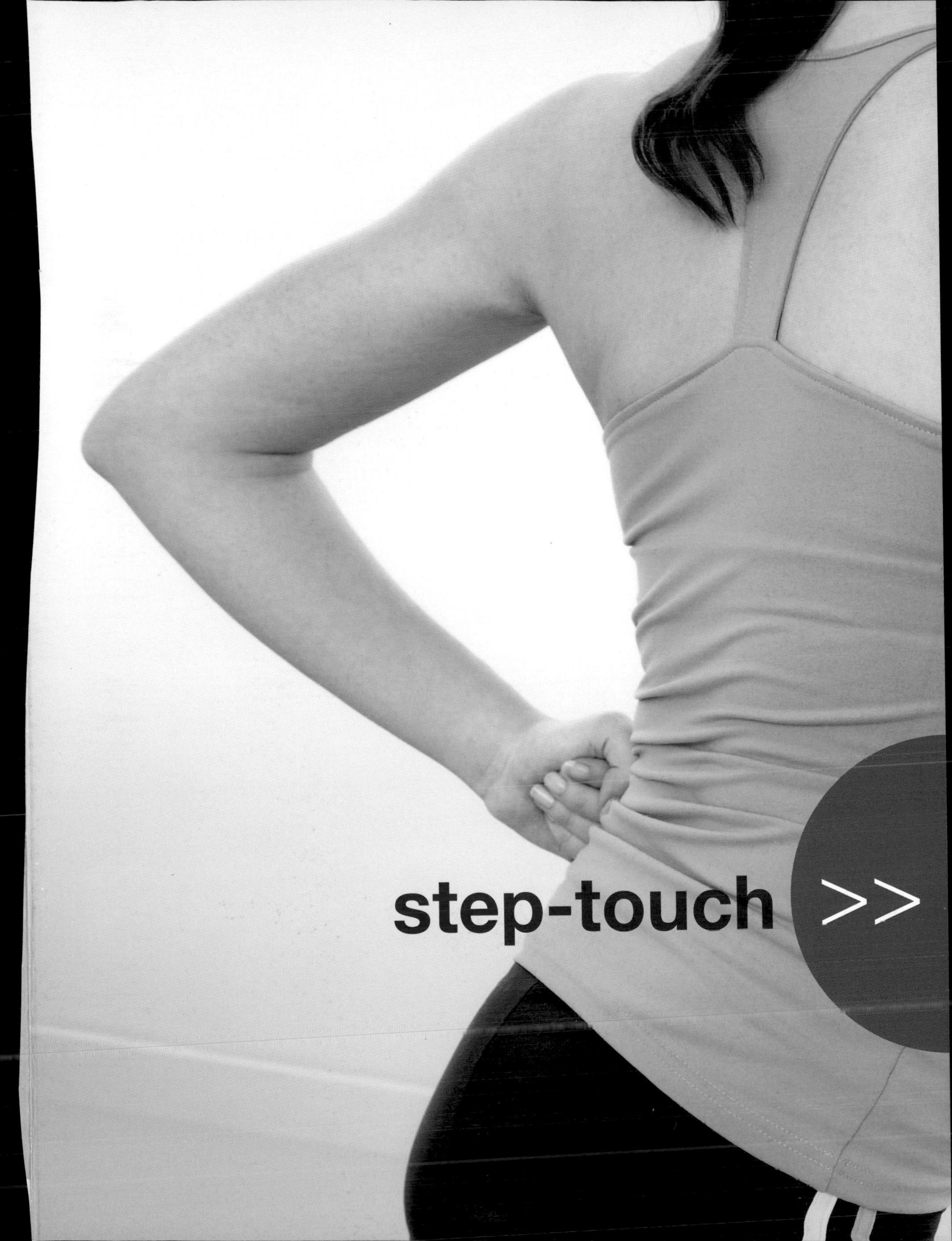

step-touch >>

step-touch at a glance

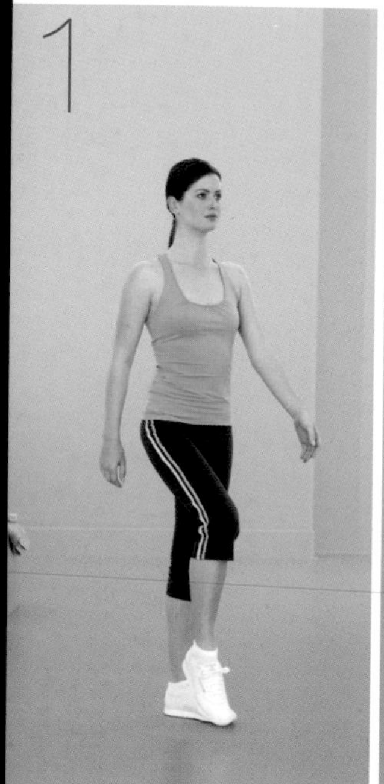

▲ **Warm up,** March, page 20

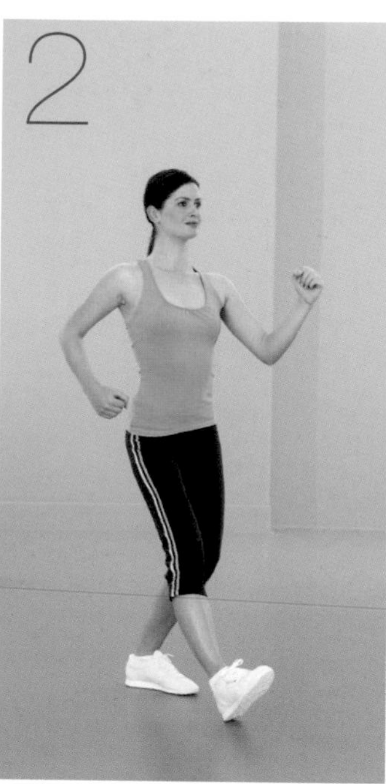

▲ **Warm up,** Heel Dig, page 20

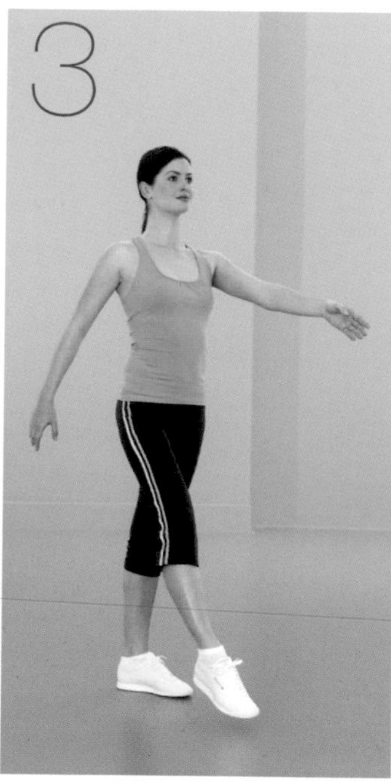

▲ **Warm up,** Toe Reach, page 21

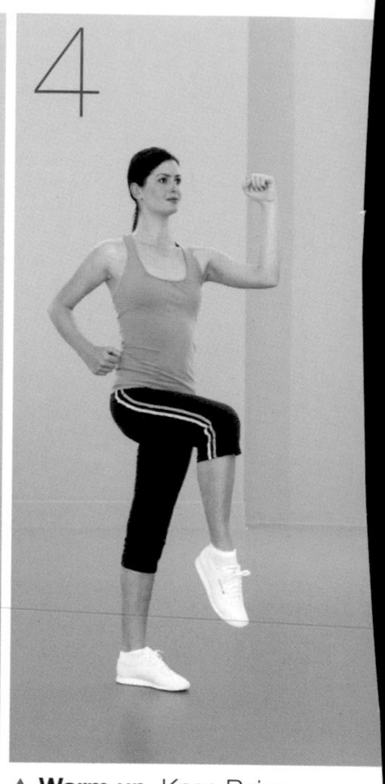

▲ **Warm up,** Knee Raise, page 21

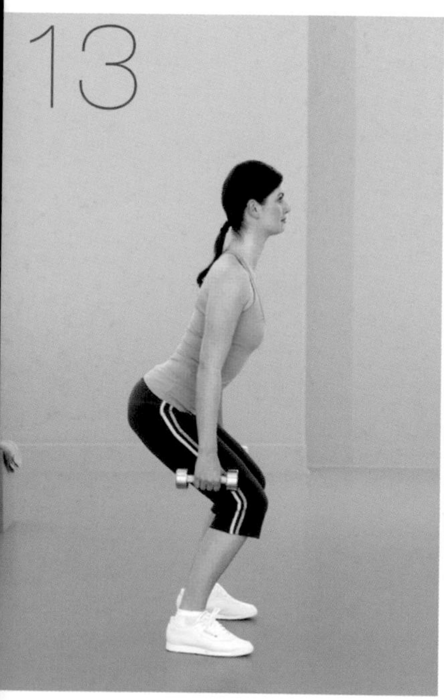

▲ **Resistance,** Squat, page 28. Repeat Steps 8–10

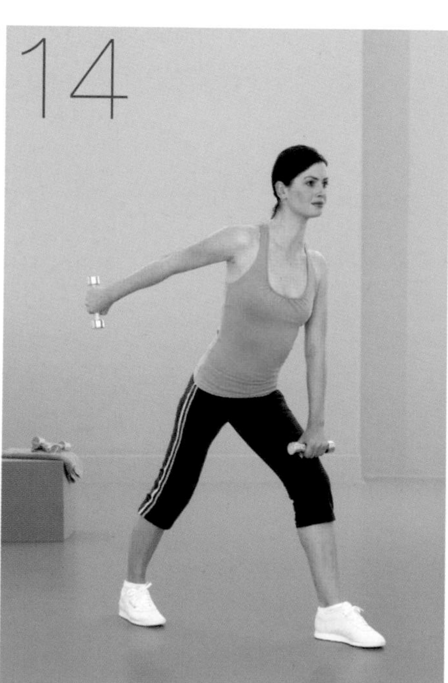

▲ **Resistance,** Triceps Kick Back, page 28. Repeat Steps 8–10

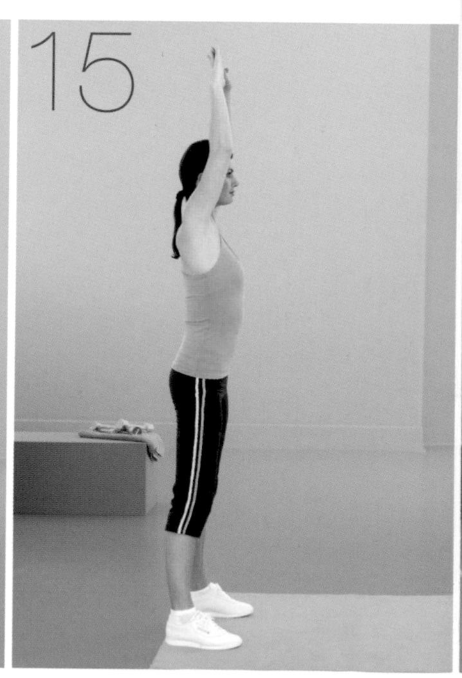

▲ **Cool down,** Lat Stretch, page 29

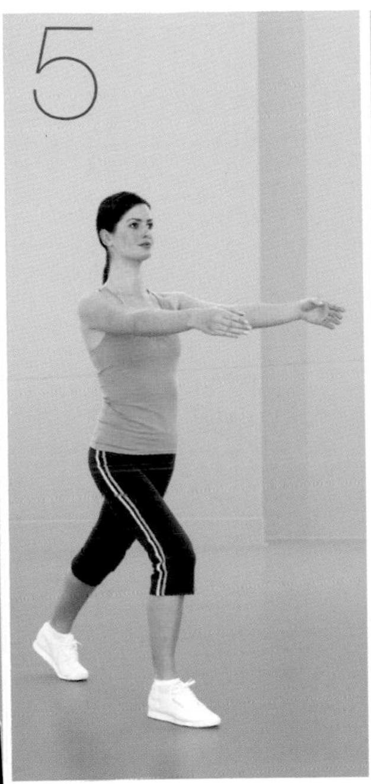

▲ **Warm up,** Reverse Lunge, page 22

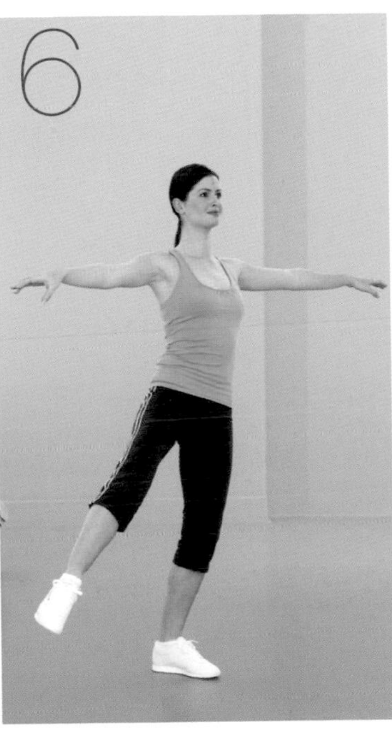

▲ **Warm up,** Lateral Lift, page 22. Repeat Steps 5–1

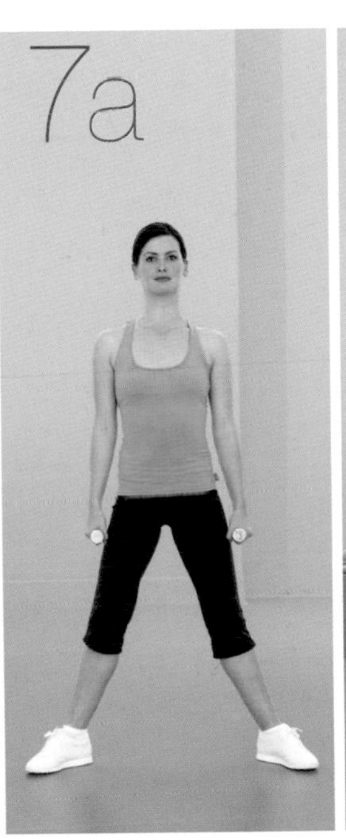

▲ **Resistance,** Plié with Lateral Raise, page 23

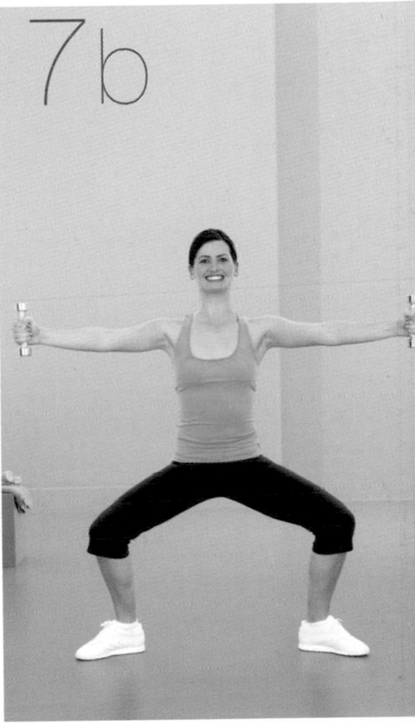

▲ **Resistance,** Plié with Lateral Raise, page 23

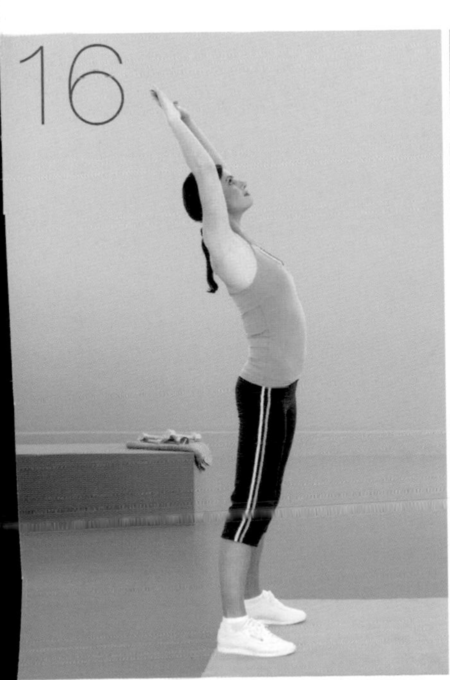

▲ **Cool down,** Sun Salute, page 29

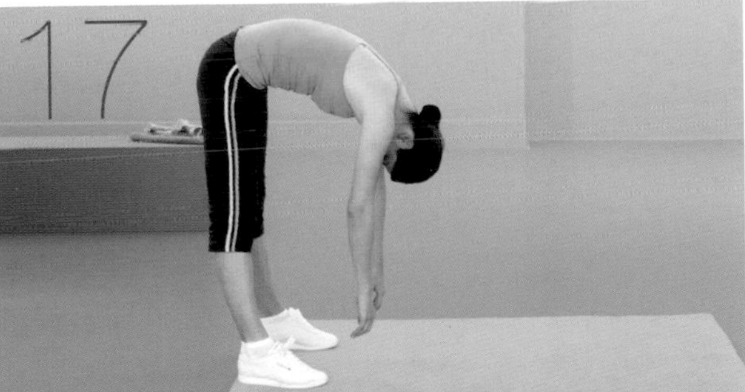

▲ **Cool down,** Spinal Roll-down, page 30

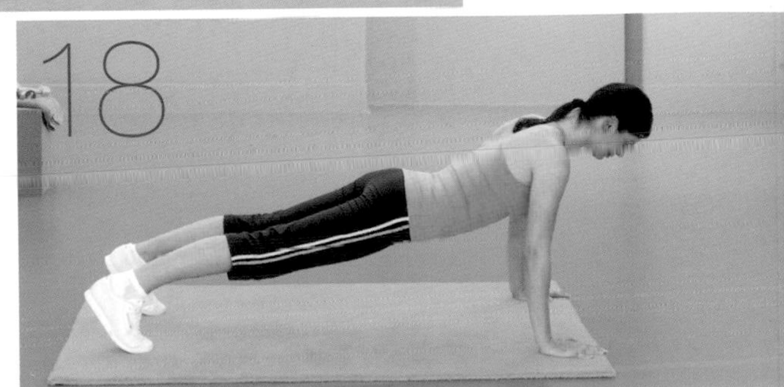

▲ **Cool down,** Plank, page 30

>> **cool down** sphinx/child's pose

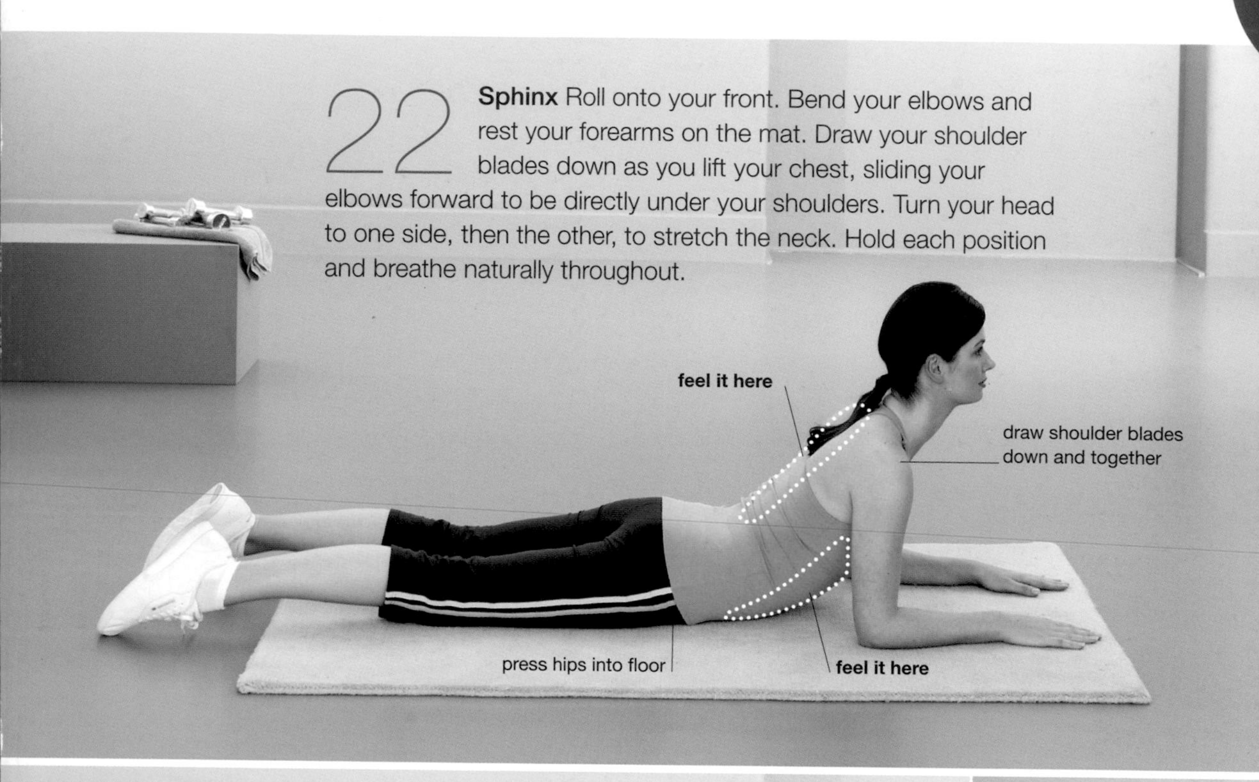

22 **Sphinx** Roll onto your front. Bend your elbows and rest your forearms on the mat. Draw your shoulder blades down as you lift your chest, sliding your elbows forward to be directly under your shoulders. Turn your head to one side, then the other, to stretch the neck. Hold each position and breathe naturally throughout.

23 **Child's Pose** Sit back on your heels and bend forward, forehead reaching to mat, arms stretching center. Walk your hands to one side, keeping your head centered between your elbows, then stretch to the other side. With every exhale, let your body sink deeper into the position.

feel it here
position head centered between elbows
reach arms forward

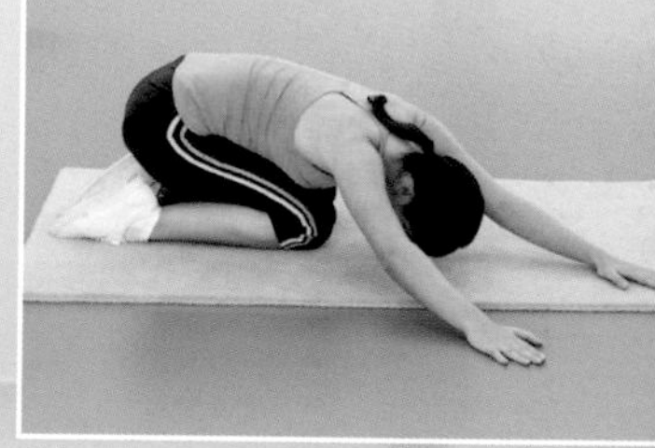

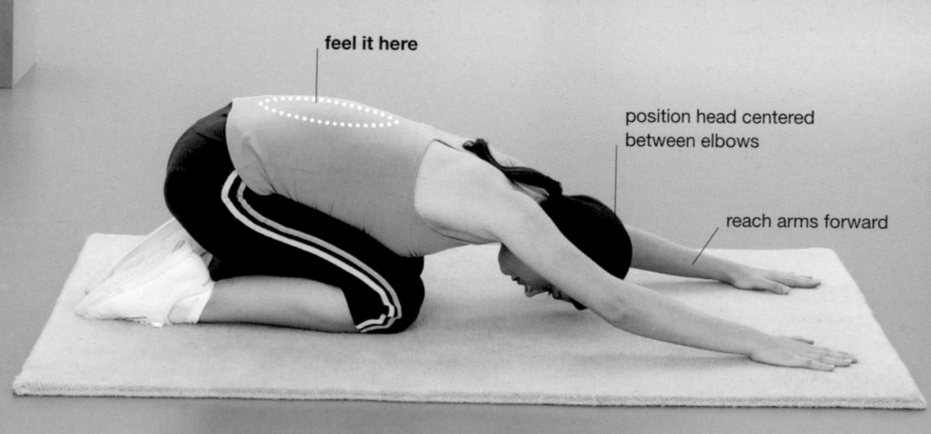

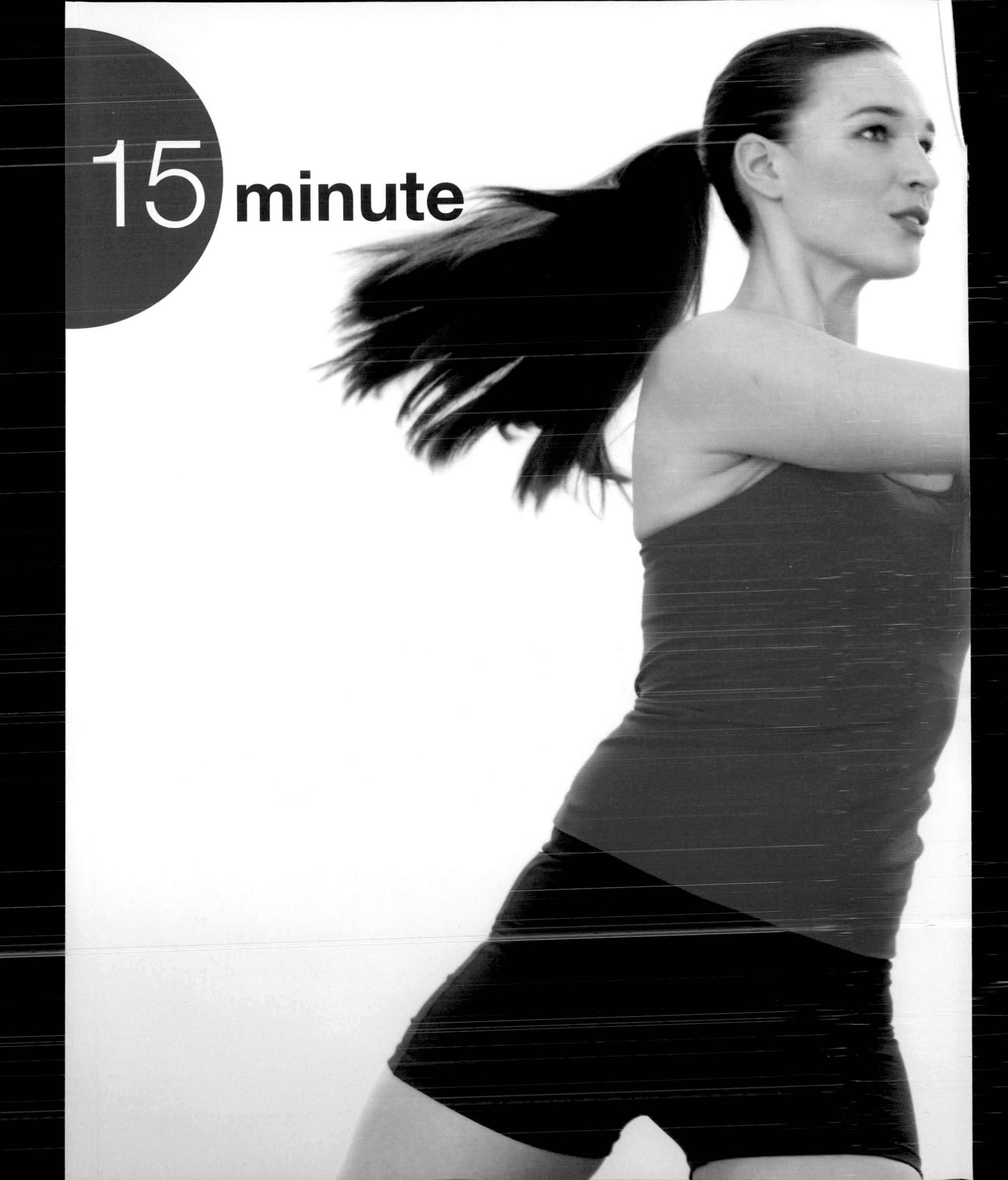
15 minute

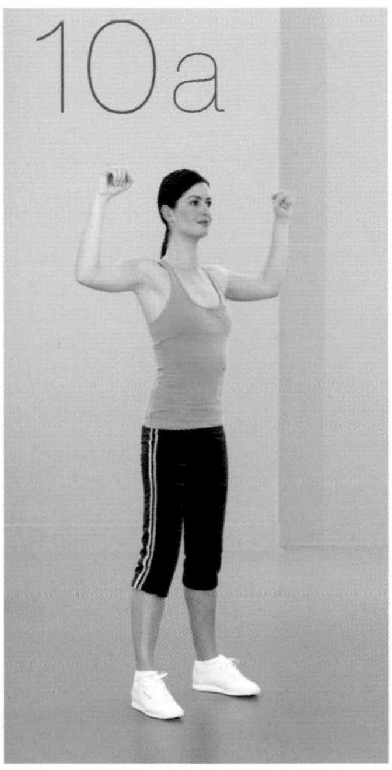

▲ **Cardio,** Twisting Knee Lift, page 26

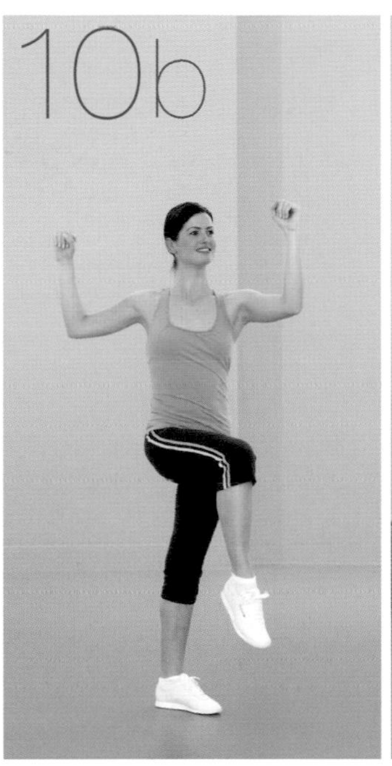

▲ **Cardio,** Twisting Knee Lift, page 26

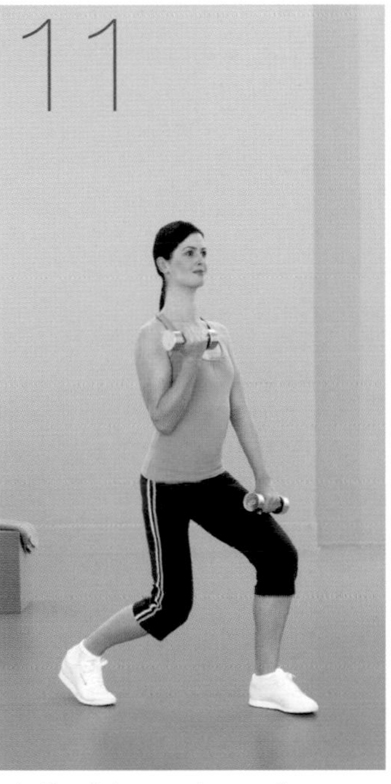

▲ **Resistance,** Lunge & Curl, page 27. Repeat Steps 8–10

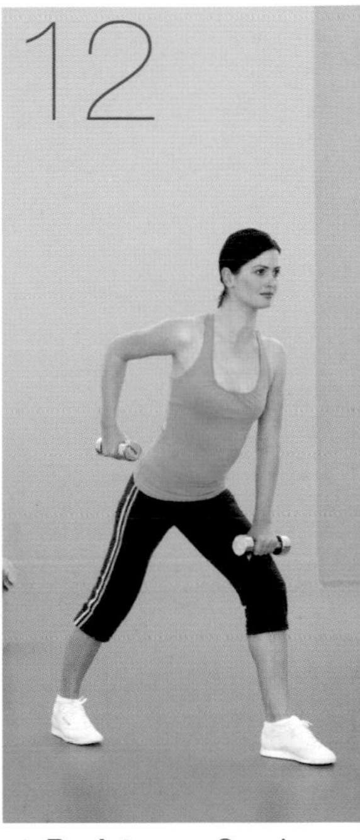

▲ **Resistance,** One Arm Row, page 27. Repeat Steps 8–10

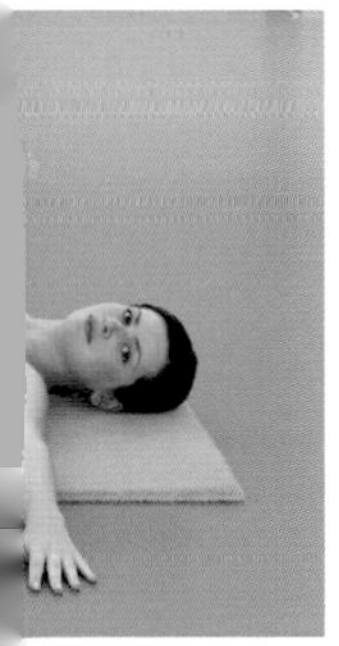

Quad Stretch, page 32

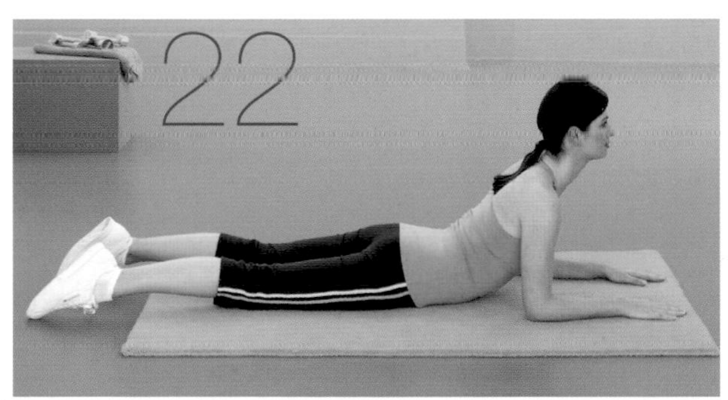

▲ **Cool down,** Sphinx, page 33

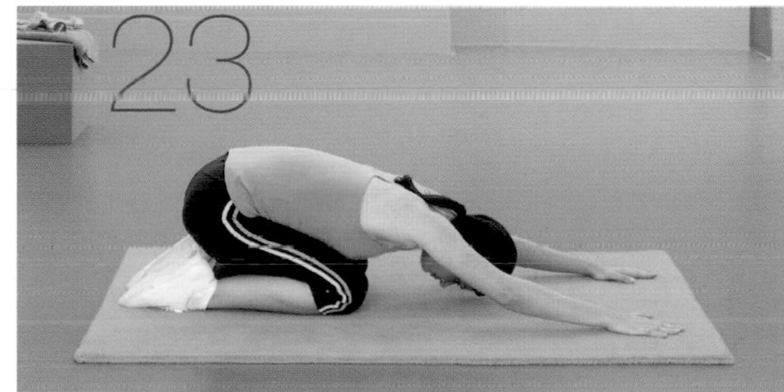

▲ **Cool down,** Child's Pose, page 33

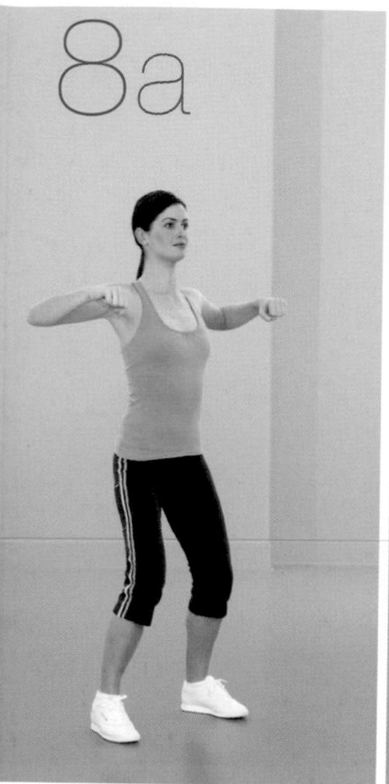

▲ **Cardio,** Step & Punch, page 24

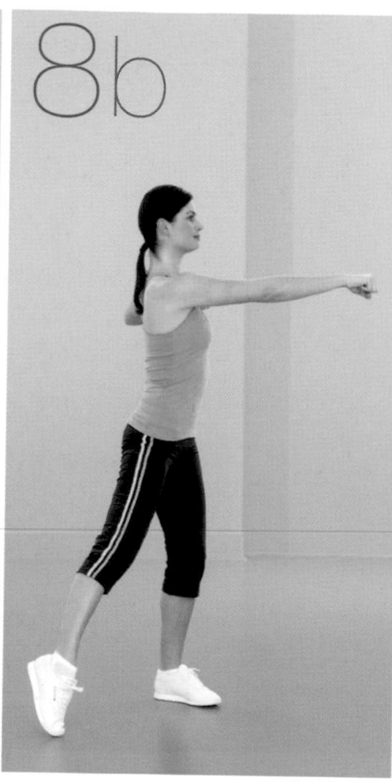

▲ **Cardio,** Step & Punch, page 24

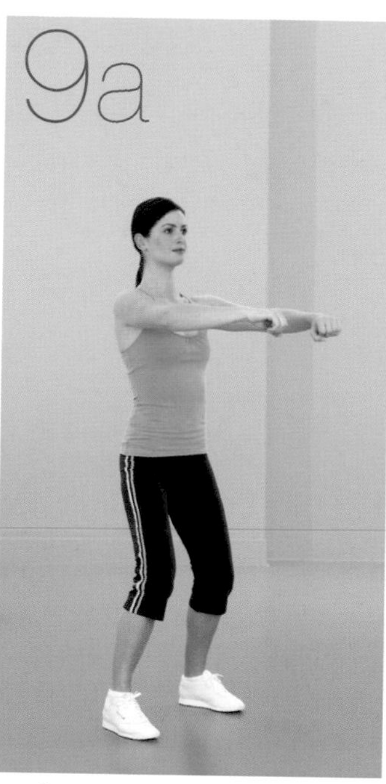

▲ **Cardio,** Curl & Squeeze, page 25

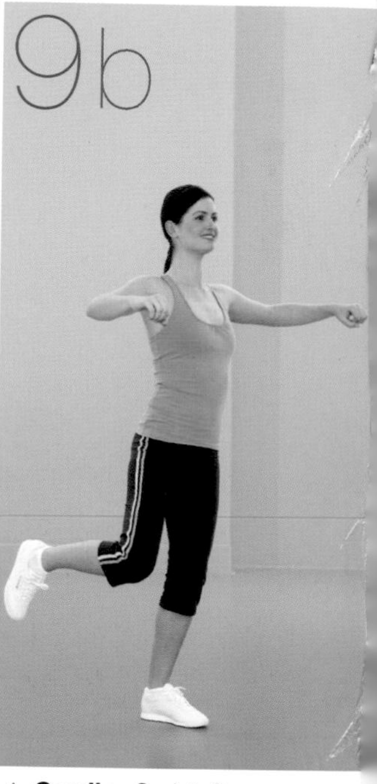

▲ **Cardio,** Curl & Squeeze, page 25

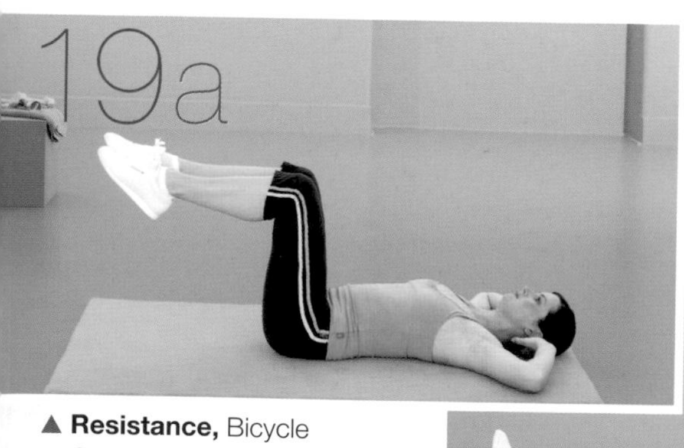

▲ **Resistance,** Bicycle Crunch, page 31

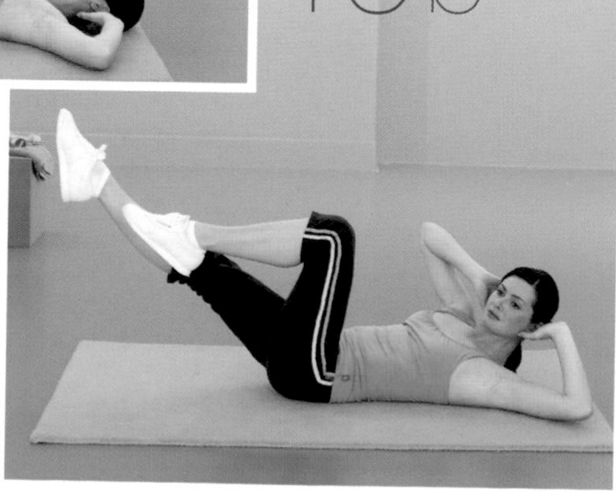

▲ **Resistance,** Bicycle Crunch, page 31

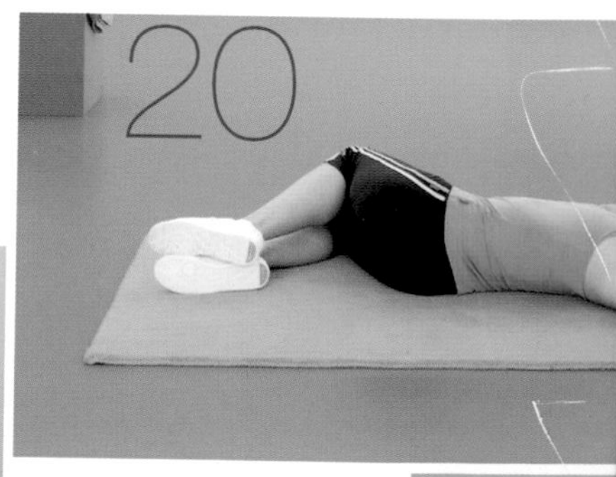

▲ **Cool down,** Spinal Twist, page 32

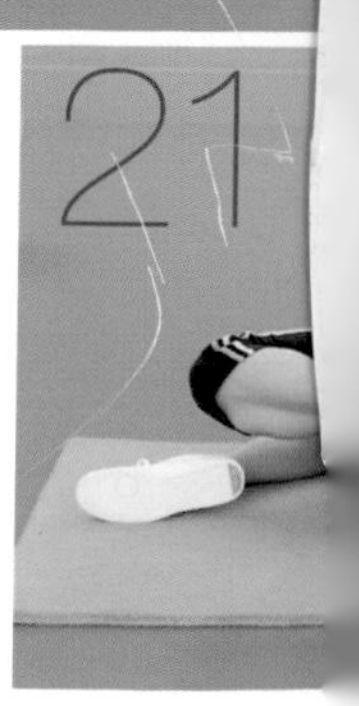

▲ **Cool down,**

>> **frequently** asked questions

When you first start training, you may find that there are various questions you want to ask. The selection listed below focuses on issues that may come to mind in your first exercise sessions, such as how often to work out, how your weight may be affected, and how to find the time in your busy schedule to exercise.

>> How can I lose as much weight as possible, as fast as I can?

First of all, don't be tempted to try a crash diet; it won't work! Dieting on its own works against healthy weight loss because it can lower the metabolism, increase the appetite, and reduce lean body mass. Conversely, exercise can increase metabolism, suppress appetite, and conserve muscle tissue. Weight loss from exercise is primarily fat loss. You need to eat and exercise In such a way that you can do it again tomorrow, and for the long term.

>> My schedule is so full that I can't find the time to exercise. What should I do?

Your health is getting shortchanged. Exercise can save your life! Doing cardio and strength training regularly reduces your risk of heart disease, diabetes, and endometrial, colon, and breast cancers. Figure out the best times for exercise and schedule your workouts into your weekly planner. Then be flexible and modify the plan if something else comes up, finding an alternative time, not skipping your session altogether.

>> I've heard that metabolism slows in your 30s. Can exercise help?

As early as age 25, you may begin to lose muscle mass and strength without being aware of it. Subtle changes begin to occur in your body composition that aren't reflected on the scale. Even if you maintain your weight over time, if you do not lift weights your lean body mass begins to decline and your body fat increases. Lean body mass is metabolically more active than fat, revving up the metabolism.

>> I'm thin already. Why do I need to build lean body mass by lifting weights?

Just because you are thin does not mean that you have good muscle tone or that you are enjoying all the benefits associated with muscle strength. Lifting weights sculpts the contours of your body and strengthens your bones. By building lean body mass, weight (or resistance) training boosts your metabolism and your energy levels, making you resistant to the slow down that occurs with age. Stronger people are more active and independent.

>> Are long, slow, steady workouts good for burning fat?

Although it's true that low-intensity aerobic activities burn a slightly higher percentage of calories from fat (as opposed to carbohydrate), when it comes to shedding body fat it doesn't matter what form the calories are stored in; what counts is the total number of calories burned. Shorter, higher-intensity workouts can burn the same number of calories as longer, lower-intensity workouts.

>> I exercise three times a week. Is it enough?

You need to do a minimum of two weight-training sessions per week to achieve desired training effects, and no muscle should be worked more than three times in one week. Three times a week is perfect for the *Total Body Workout* programs because they are "full-body" routines, targeting all the major muscle groups. Muscles need a full day of rest in between strength training workouts, so alternate workouts with a day of rest. If you want to exercise on "off" days, do a cardio exercise, like walking, swimming, or stair climbing.

>> I'm enjoying the workout, but how can 15 minutes a day make a difference?

Studies show that the effects of exercise are cumulative and all add up to health benefits, weight loss, and general fitness. The key is consistency. Brief doses of exercise done consistently over time are effective at reducing risk of developing chronic diseases such as diabetes and hypertension. They also have a positive effect on appearance, reducing fat and increasing muscle tone and flexibility.

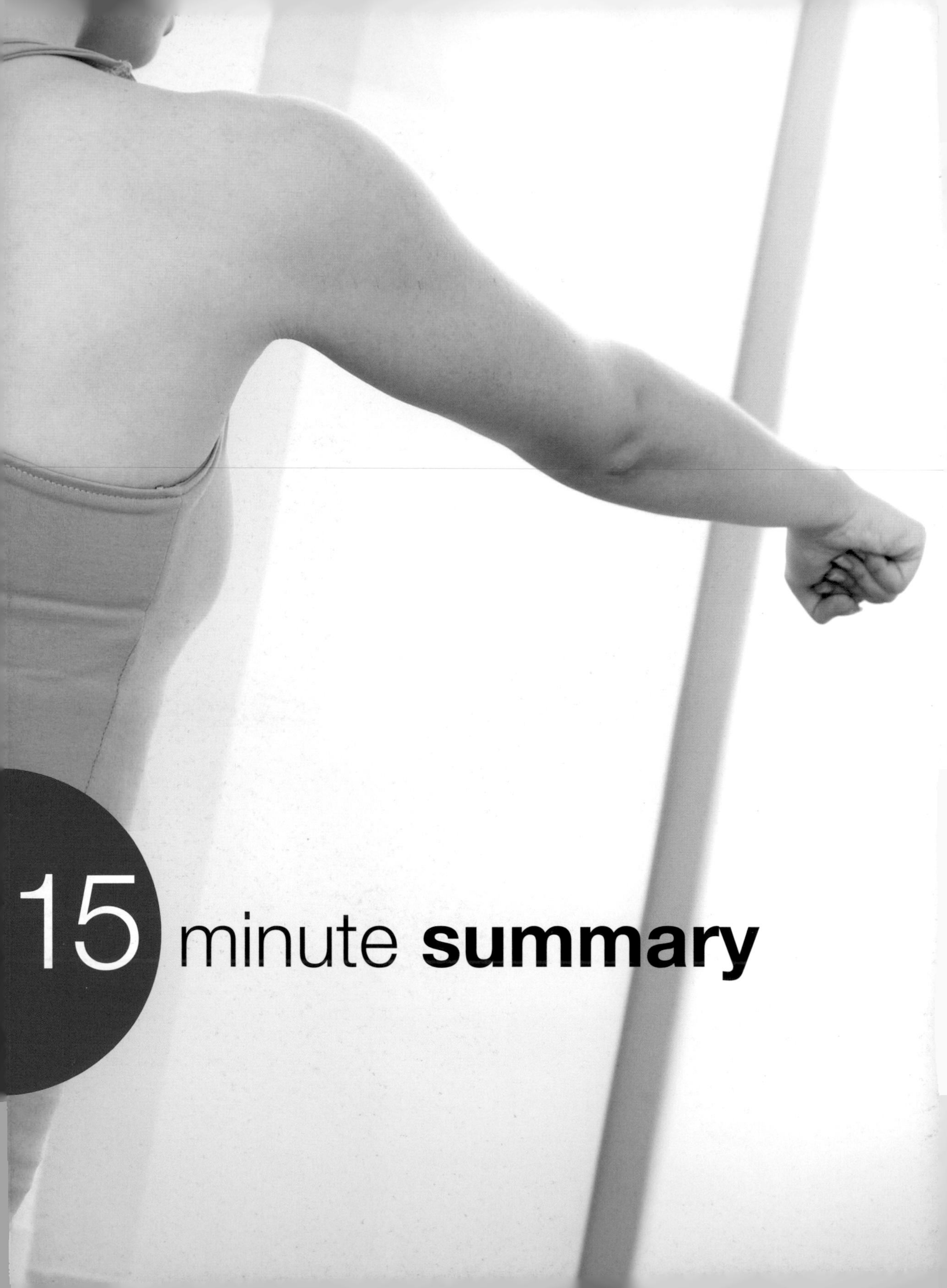

15 minute **summary**

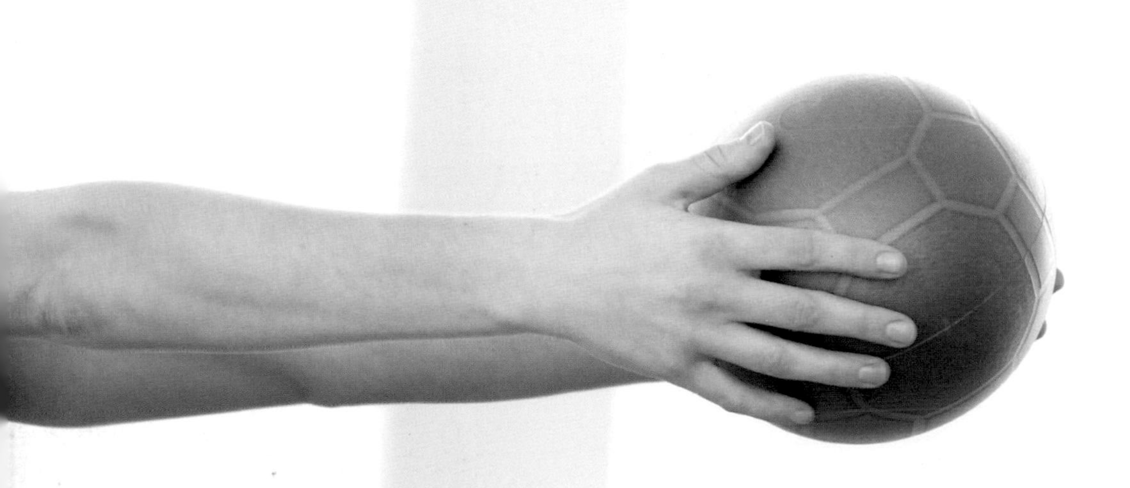

beach ball workout >>

Improve your coordination and balance while adding variety to your workout with a ball

>> **warm up** rock lunge/skater

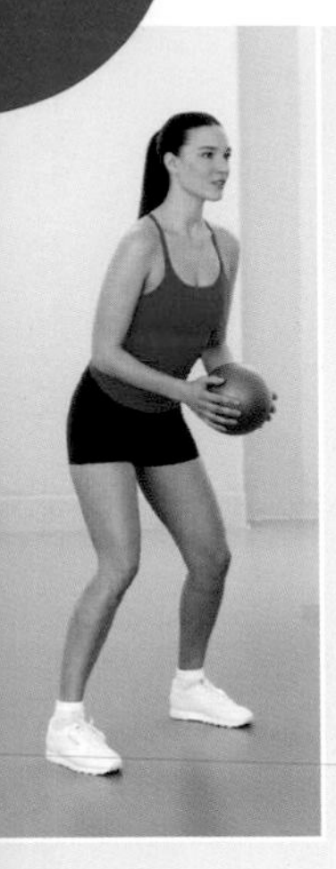

1 **Rock Lunge** Stand with your feet parallel, slightly wider than shoulder width apart, knees bent. Lean forward slightly and hold the ball in front of your hips. Straighten one leg and lunge the other way, moving the ball to your opposite hip. Repeat, alternating sides for a total of 8 reps (1 rep = both sides).

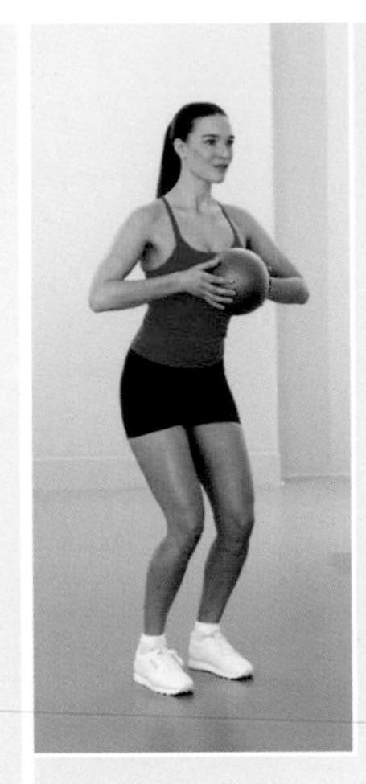

2 **Skater** Stand with your feet parallel, hip width apart, knees bent. Hold the ball in front of your chest. Keep one knee bent and shift your weight onto it as you extend the other leg out to the side, toe resting lightly on the floor. Stretch your arms out diagonally, pressing the ball away from your extended leg. Then return to the starting position and repeat, alternating sides, for a total of 8 reps (1 rep = both sides).

move ball from hip to hip
keep feet stationary as you lunge

let your head follow action
press ball away from extended leg
rest foot lightly on floor

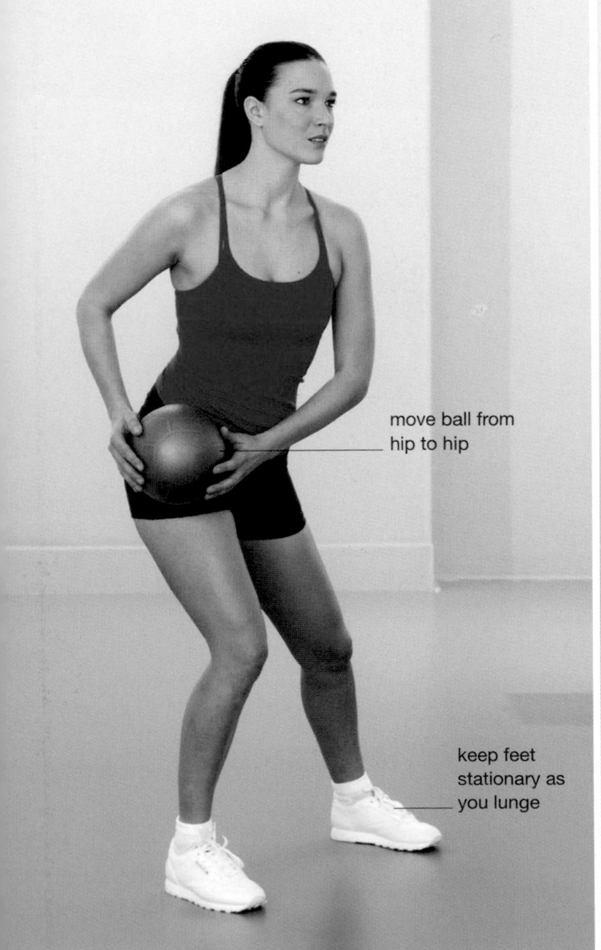

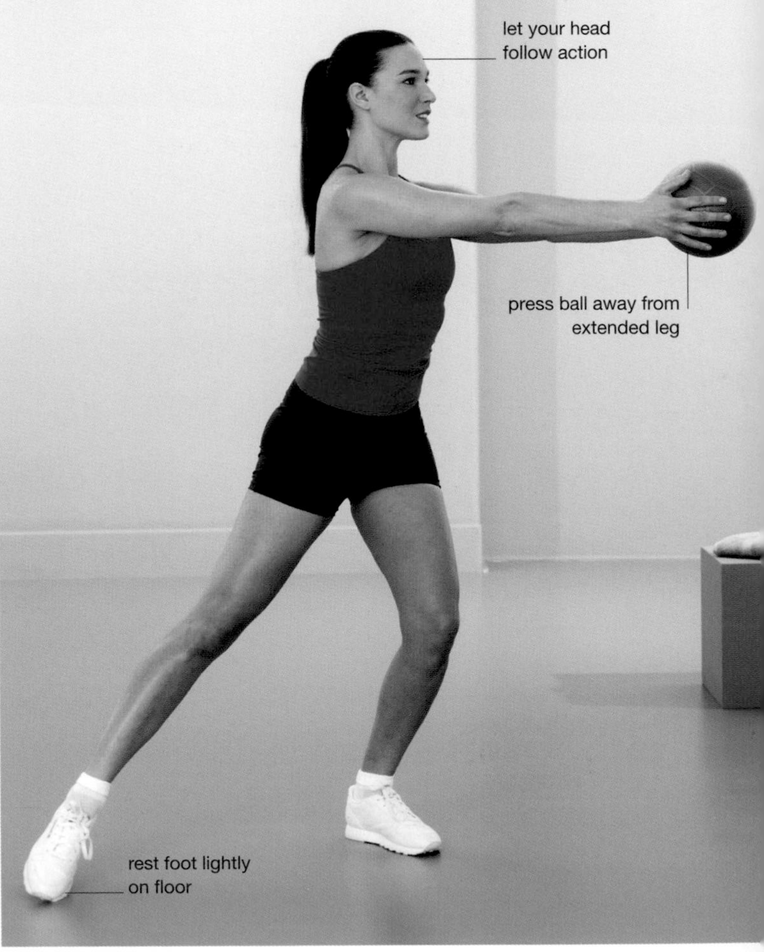

extend arms
to lift ball high
twist through
torso
lift heel
off floor

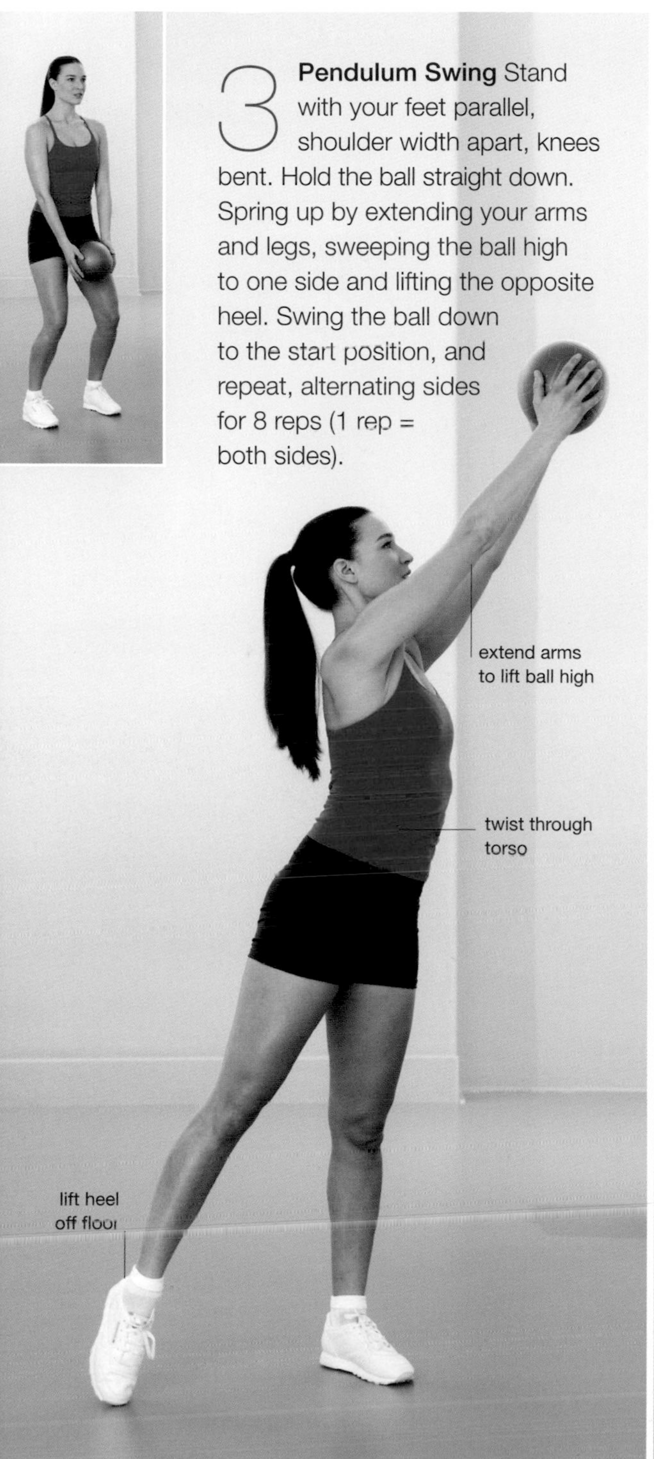

3 **Pendulum Swing** Stand with your feet parallel, shoulder width apart, knees bent. Hold the ball straight down. Spring up by extending your arms and legs, sweeping the ball high to one side and lifting the opposite heel. Swing the ball down to the start position, and repeat, alternating sides for 8 reps (1 rep = both sides).

draw shoulder
blades down
keep head
centered
as you step to the side,
touch your feet together

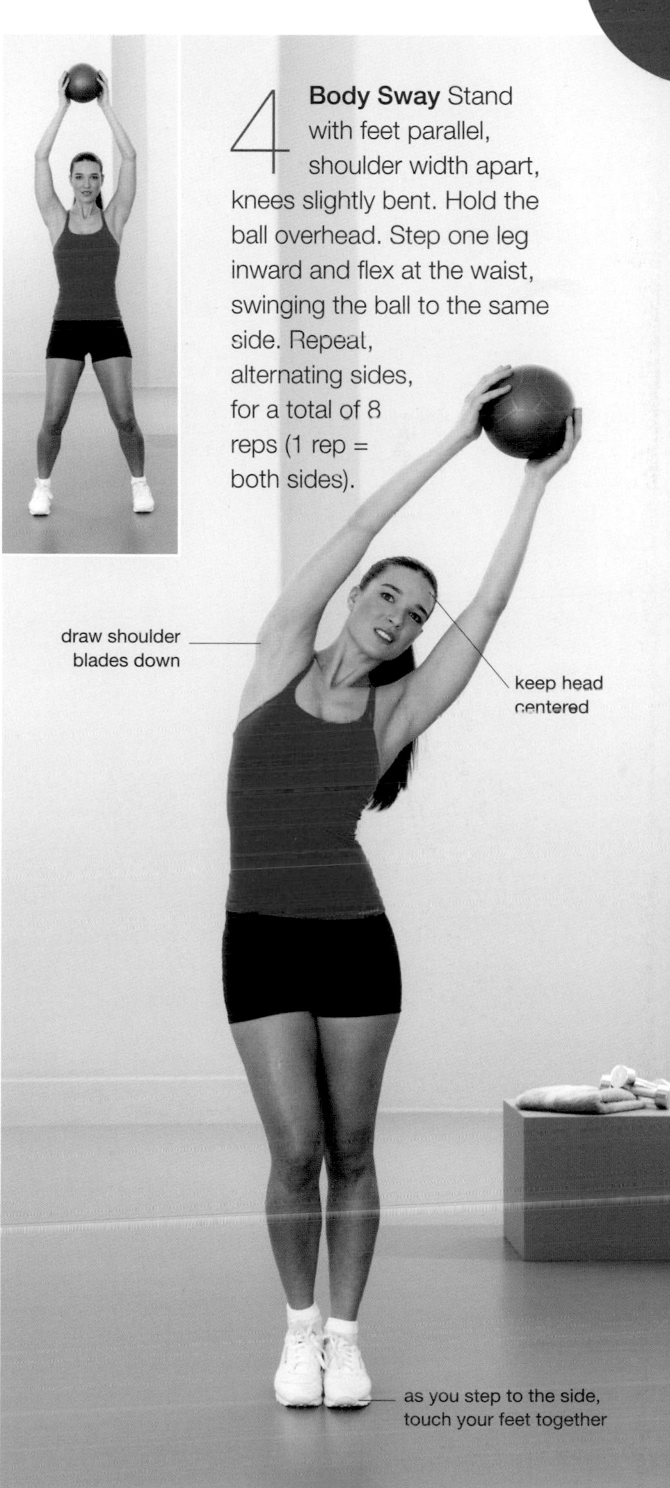

4 **Body Sway** Stand with feet parallel, shoulder width apart, knees slightly bent. Hold the ball overhead. Step one leg inward and flex at the waist, swinging the ball to the same side. Repeat, alternating sides, for a total of 8 reps (1 rep = both sides).

>> **warm up** wood-chop squat/curl & press

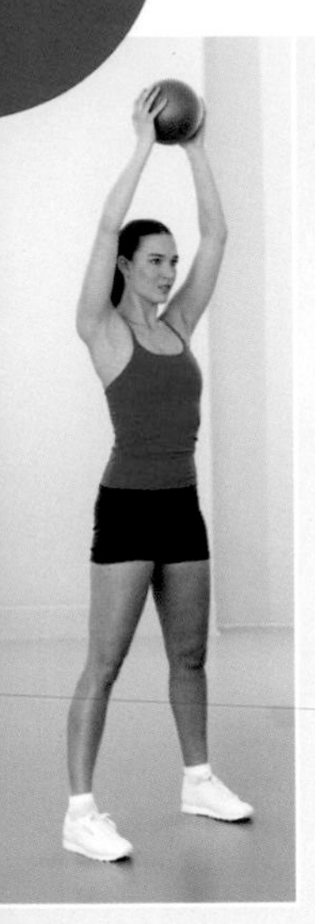

5 Wood-Chop Squat

Still holding the ball above your head, stand with your feet parallel, shoulder width apart, knees soft. Bend your knees into a squat, reaching back with your hips, keeping your heels pressed into the floor. With your arms straight, "chop" the ball down, lowering it to the knees. Repeat 8 times.

reach back with your hips
keep arms straight
keep heels down

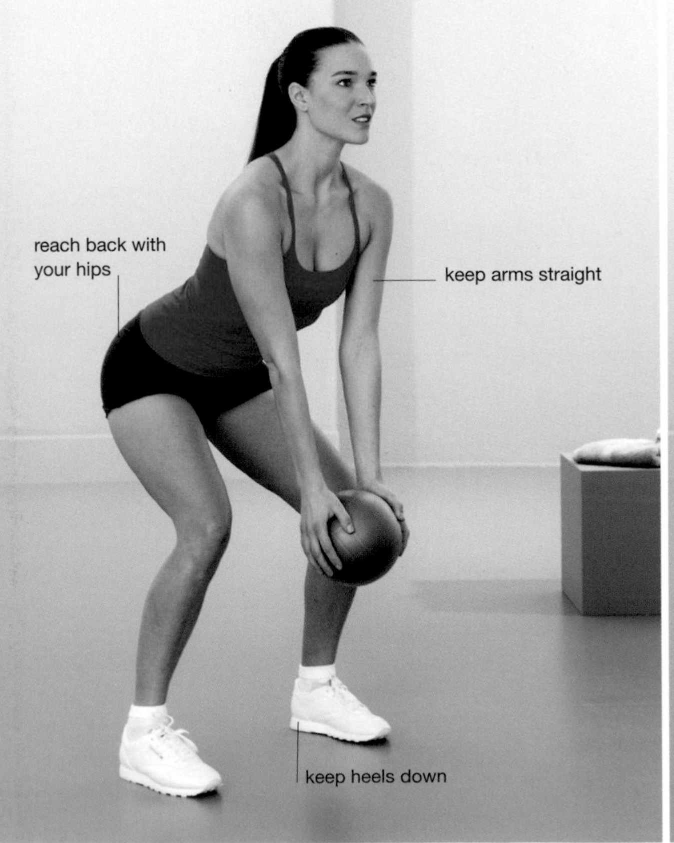

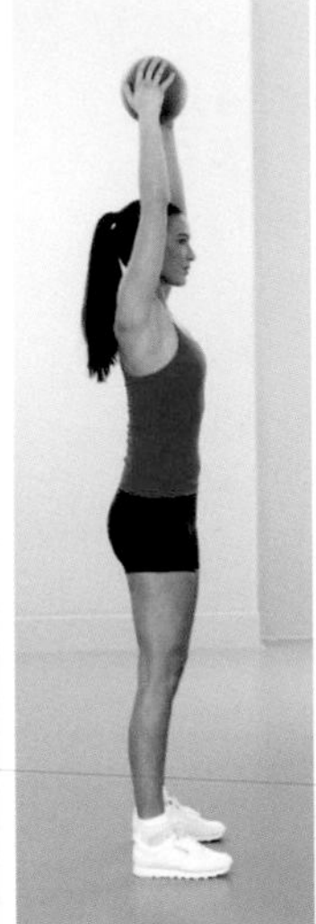

6 Curl & Press

Reach the ball toward the ceiling, then bend both elbows, lowering it behind your head. At the same time, bend one leg back, lifting your heel toward the buttocks. Repeat, alternating legs, for a total of 8 reps (1 rep = both sides). **Repeat Steps 5–1 (reverse order) to complete your warm up.**

maintain a straight line from elbow to knee
keep thighs aligned

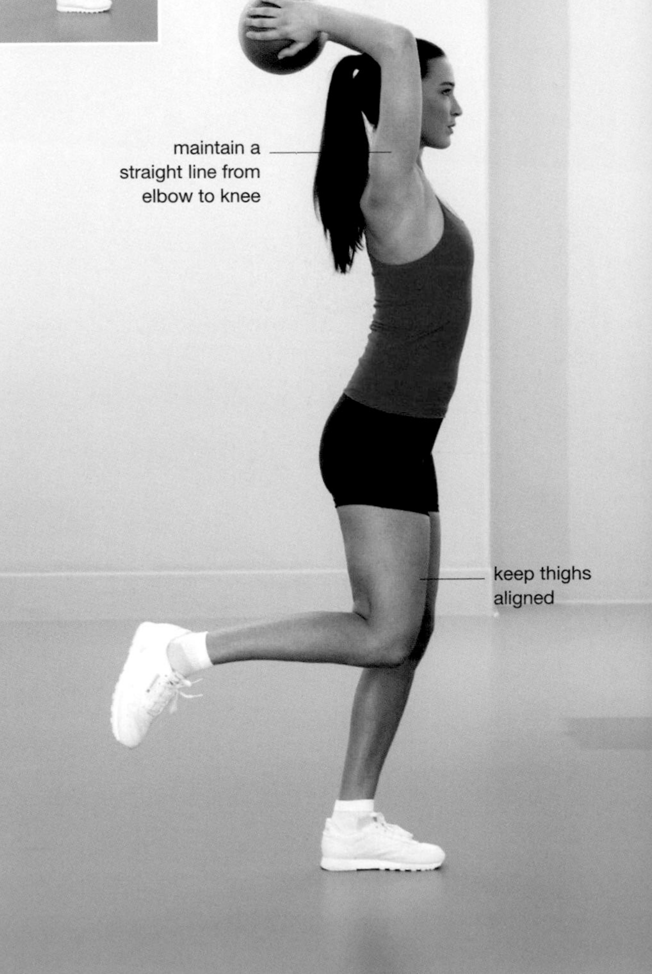

>> **resistance** plié with front raise

7a **Plié with Front Raise** Put down the ball and pick up one large weight for the first resistance exercise. Stand with your feet slightly wider than shoulder width apart, shift your weight to your heels, and turn your legs out from the hips until your feet are at 45° angles. Hold the weight horizontally with one hand at each end, your arms straight down in front.

7b As you inhale, bend your knees until your thighs are as parallel to the floor as possible; simultaneously lift the weight to shoulder height, keeping your arms straight. Exhale, press through your heels, and tighten your inner and outer thighs as you return to the starting position. Repeat 12 times.

turn legs
out to 45°

drop shoulder
blades down
feel it here
feel it here
keep torso
vertical
position
knees in line
with feet

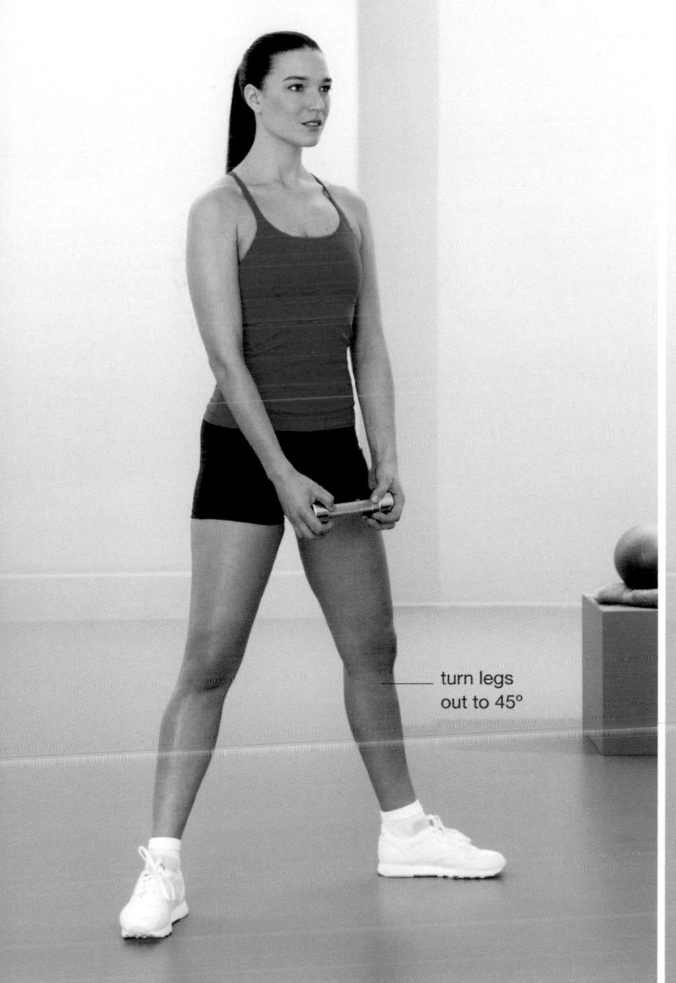

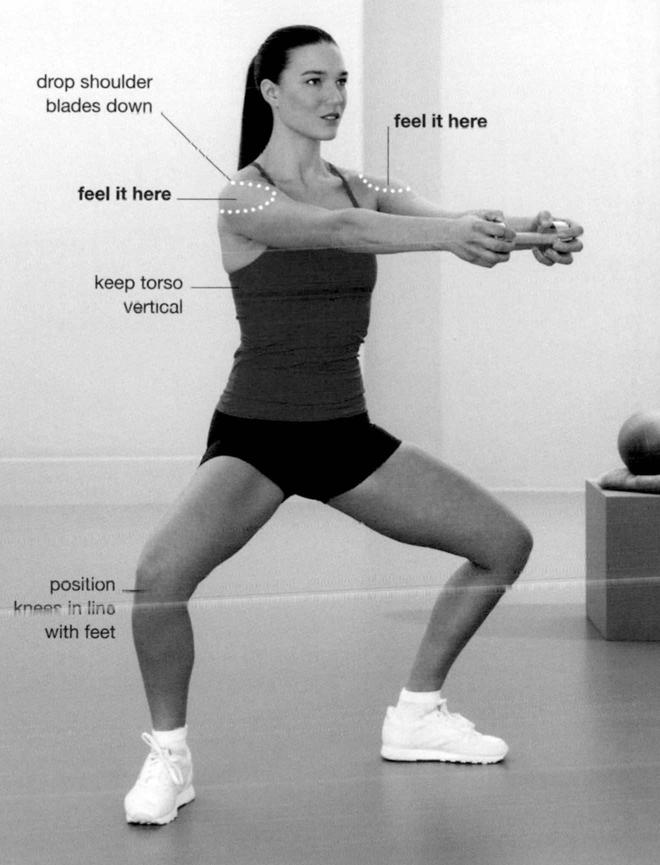

>> **cardio** step & dig/knee lift

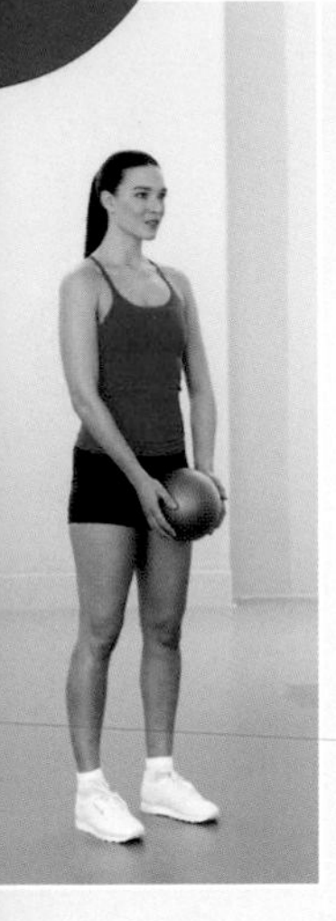

8 **Step & Dig** Start your first cardio interval. Stand with your feet hip width apart, knees soft, feet parallel or slightly turned out. Hold the ball with your arms straight down. Tap your heel to the front, pointing your toes to the ceiling, as you bring the ball up to shoulder height. Keep your arms straight but not stiff. Alternate legs for a total of 8 reps (1 rep = both sides). Breathe naturally throughout.

keep arms straight but not stiff
bend knee slightly
toes point to ceiling

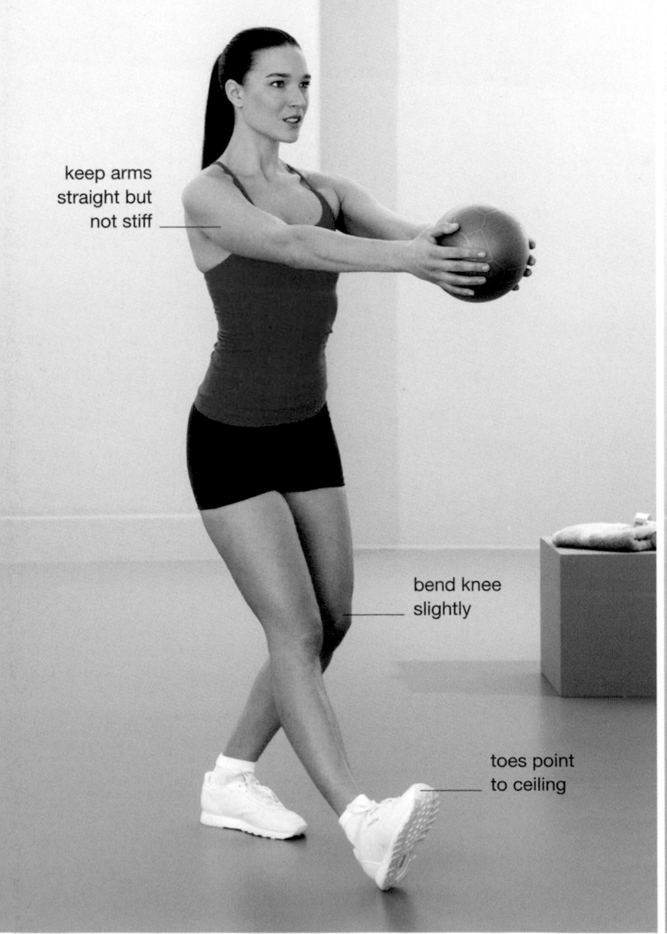

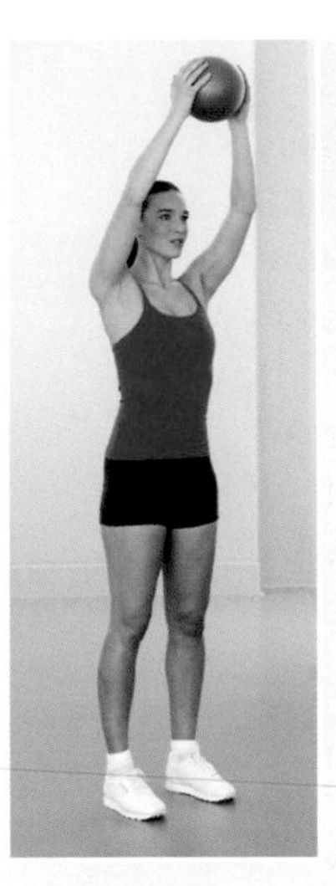

9 **Knee Lift** Stand with your feet parallel, hip width apart, knees slightly bent. Hold the ball above your head, with elbows slightly rounded. Bring your knee up to hip height as you lower the ball toward your knee. Repeat, alternating legs for 8 reps (1 rep = both sides). Breathe naturally throughout.

keep chest lifted
keep your back straight
thigh parallel to floor

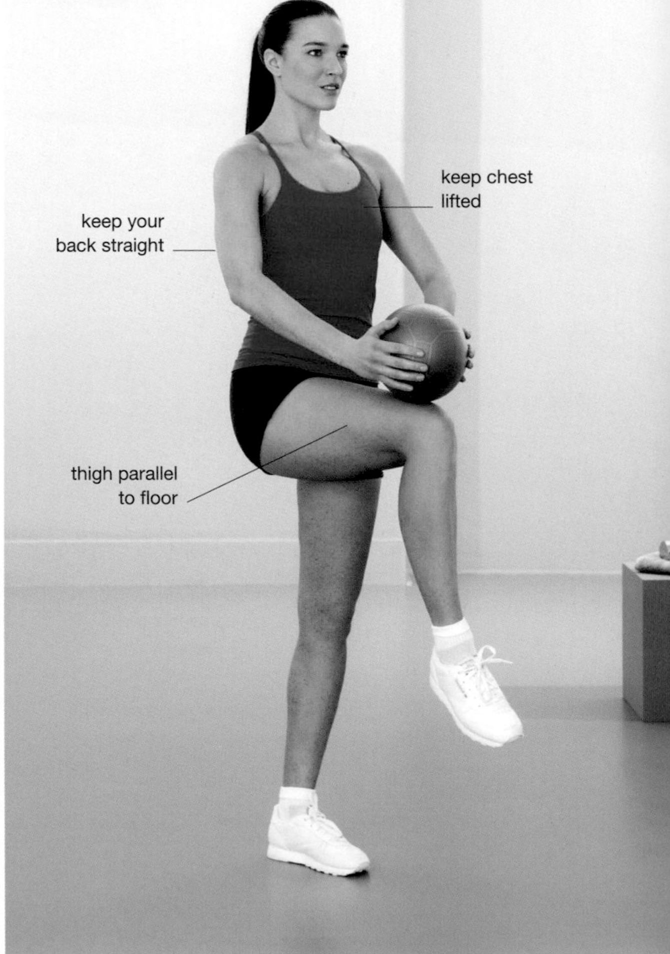

>> **cardio** squat plus

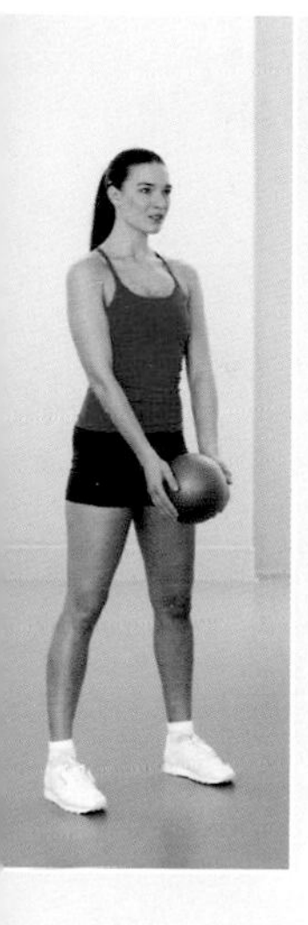

10a

Squat Plus Stand with your feet shoulder width apart, holding the ball with your arms straight down. Bend your knees into a squat, at the same time bending your elbows to lift the ball to your chest. Keep your weight centered, heels down. Reach back with your hips, keeping your knees behind your toes.

hold elbows close to sides
press down through your heels

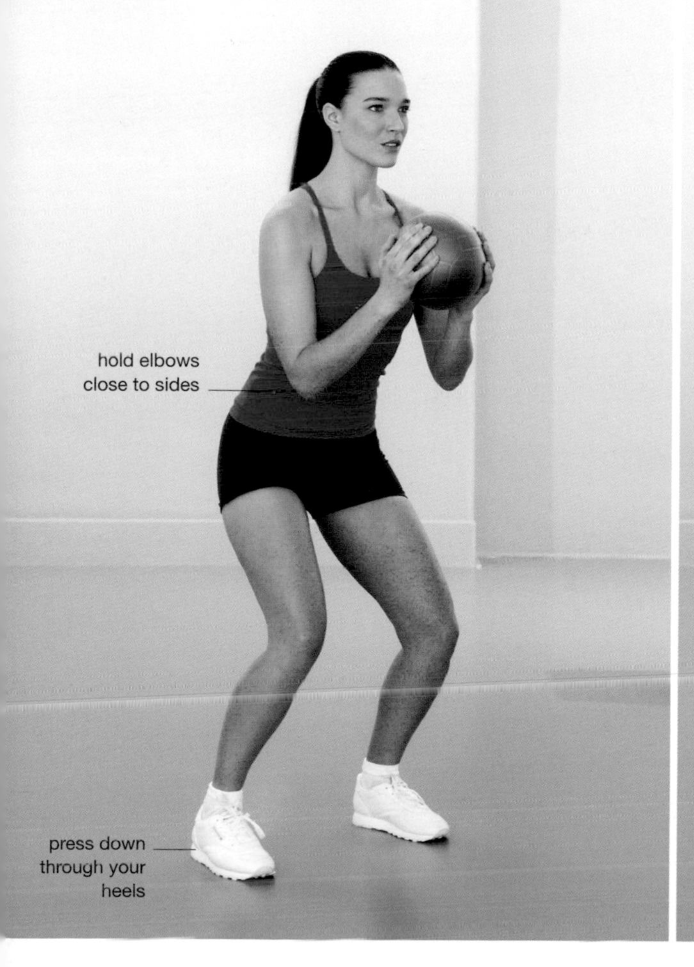

10b

Lift the ball up above your head as you straighten your legs. Then bend into the squat, ball to chest (10a), before returning to the starting position. Take full, deep breaths. Repeat the sequence 12 times. **Steps 8–10 complete the cardio interval.**

keep shoulders down

keep your back straight

straighten legs

>> **resistance** squat with knee lift

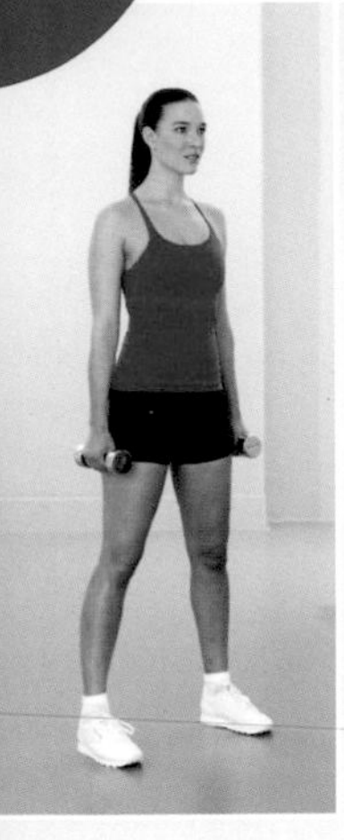

11a

Squat with Knee Lift Put down the beach ball and pick up two large free weights. Stand with your feet parallel, shoulder width apart, knees soft. Hold one weight in each hand, with your arms by your sides and palms facing in. Inhale as you squat: shift your weight back into your heels, reaching back with your hips and letting your torso lean forward. Release your pelvis to allow a natural curve in your back.

look straight ahead
keep chest lifted
keep knees aligned with toes

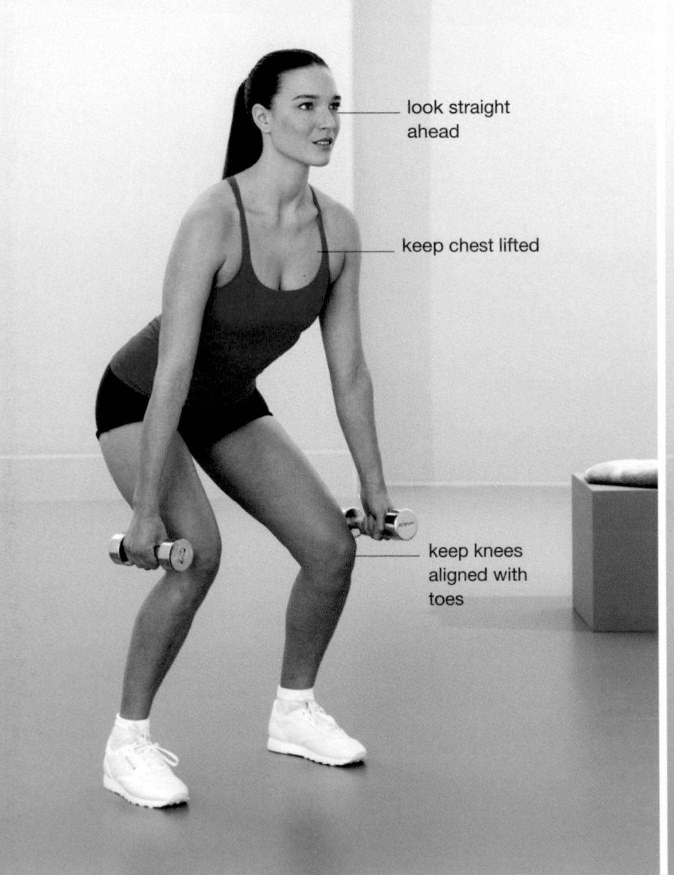

11b

Exhale and straighten your legs. Shift your weight to one side and bring the other knee up to hip height. Balance for a moment, then return to the starting position (see inset, left). Squat again (see left), straighten your legs, and change sides for the knee lift (as shown below). Keep your hips level, chest lifted, eyes forward throughout. Repeat for a total of 8 reps (1 rep = both sides). **Do your next cardio interval, Steps 8–10 (pp 48–49).**

stand tall

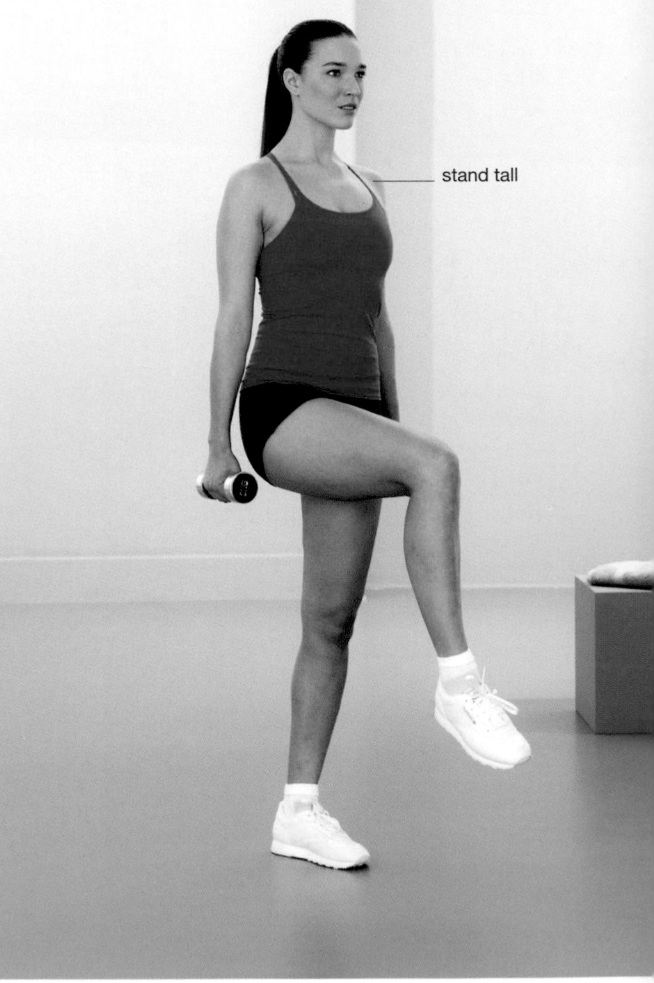

>> **resistance** lunge & row

12a

Lunge & Row Exchange the ball for two large free weights. Stand with your feet parallel, hip width apart, knees soft. Hold the weights at your hips, palms in, elbows bent at right angles and close to your sides. Stabilize your shoulder blades by drawing them down and together. Keep your wrists straight, in line with your forearms.

12b

Inhale as you step forward with one leg, bending both knees. At the same time, straighten your arms, lowering the weights toward your knee. Exhale as you spring back, pulling the weights to your hips. Alternate legs for 8 reps (1 rep = both sides). **Do the next cardio interval, Steps 8–10 (pp48–49).**

draw shoulder blades down and together

feel it here
position knee over ankle

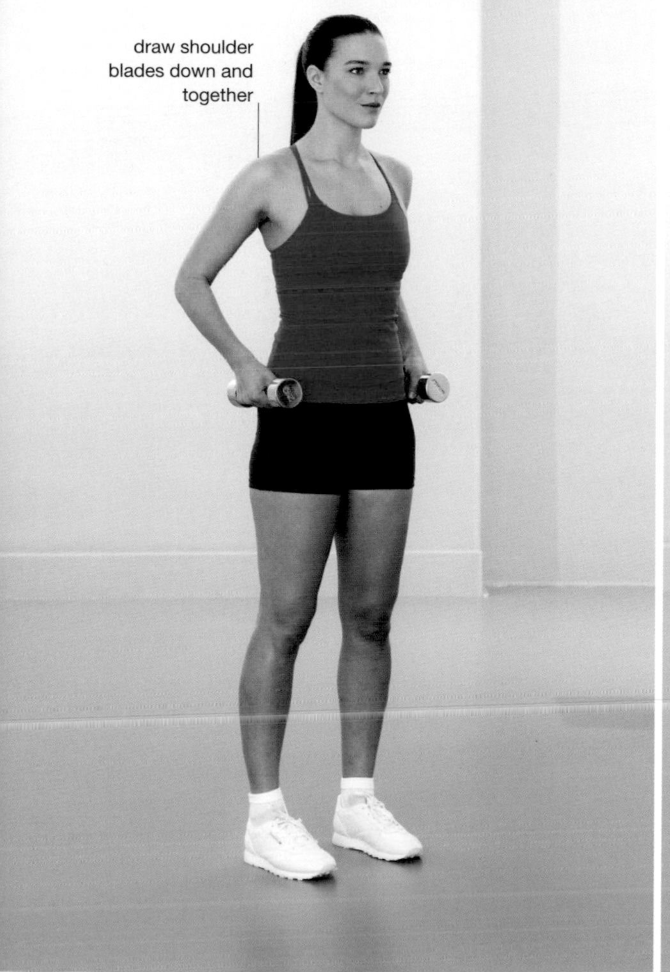

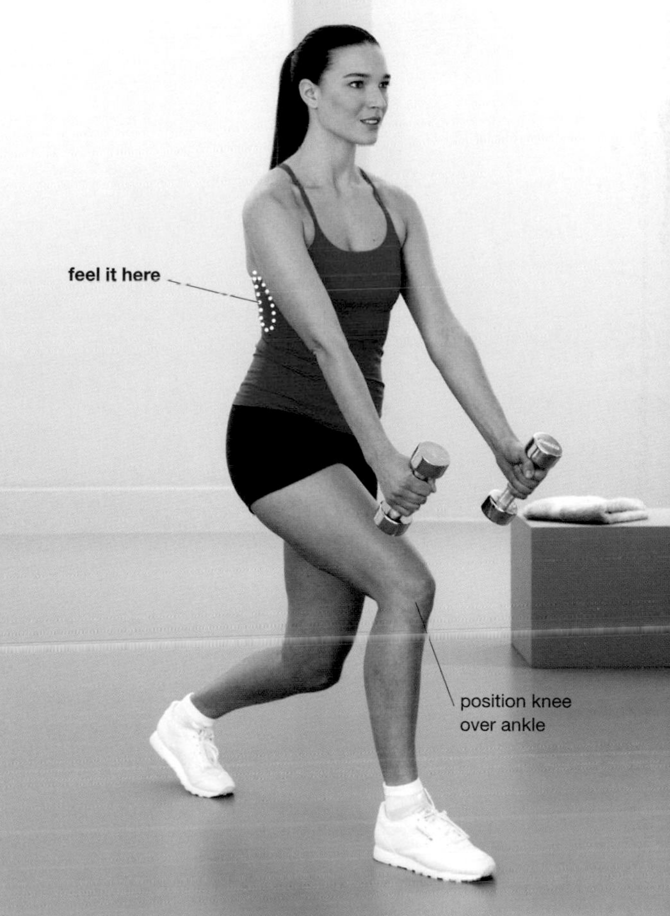

>> **resistance** squat with weight shift

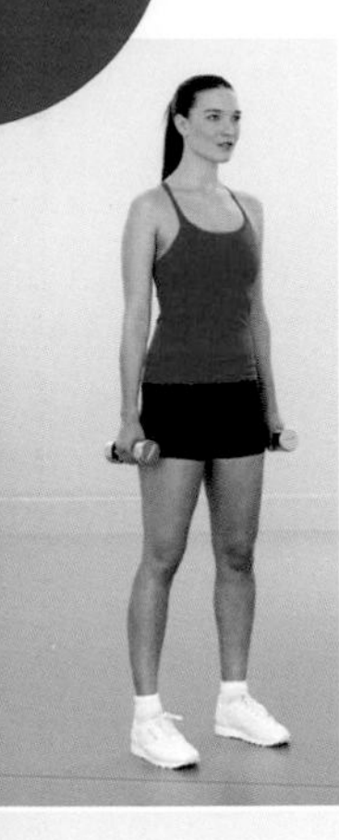

13a **Squat with Weight Shift** Pick up two large weights. Stand with your feet parallel, hip width apart. Hold the weights by your sides. Shifting your weight into your heels, inhale as you bend your knees into a squat; at the same time, bend your elbows, bringing the weights up toward your shoulders.

13b Exhale as you straighten your arms and legs to the starting position. Inhale again, then exhale as you shift your weight onto the balls of your feet and lift your heels high. Balance for a moment before lowering the heels onto the floor and preparing for the next squat. Do 8 reps, combining both moves. **Then do your next cardio interval, Steps 8–10 (pp 48–49).**

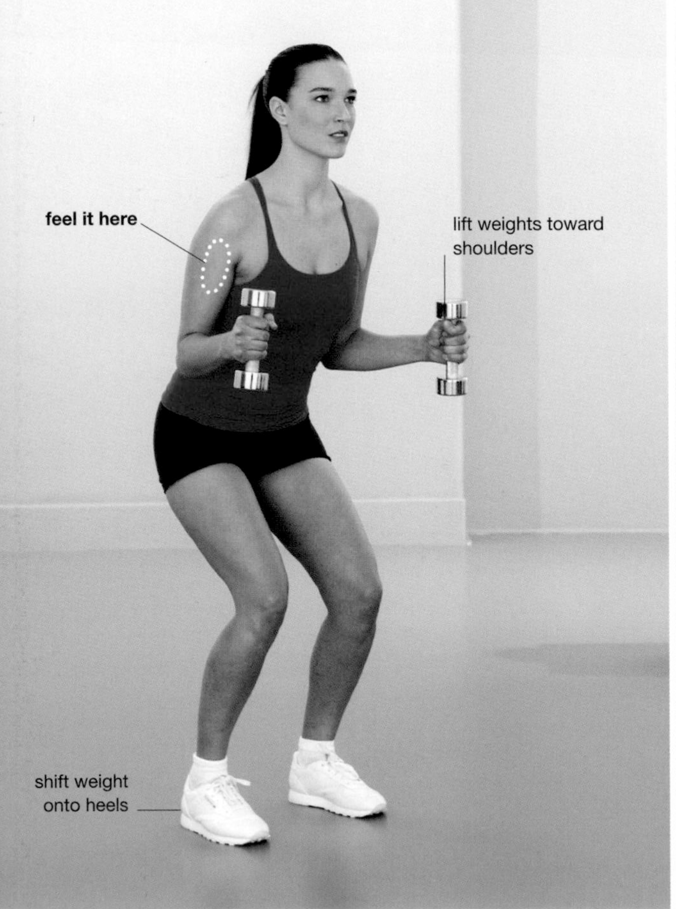

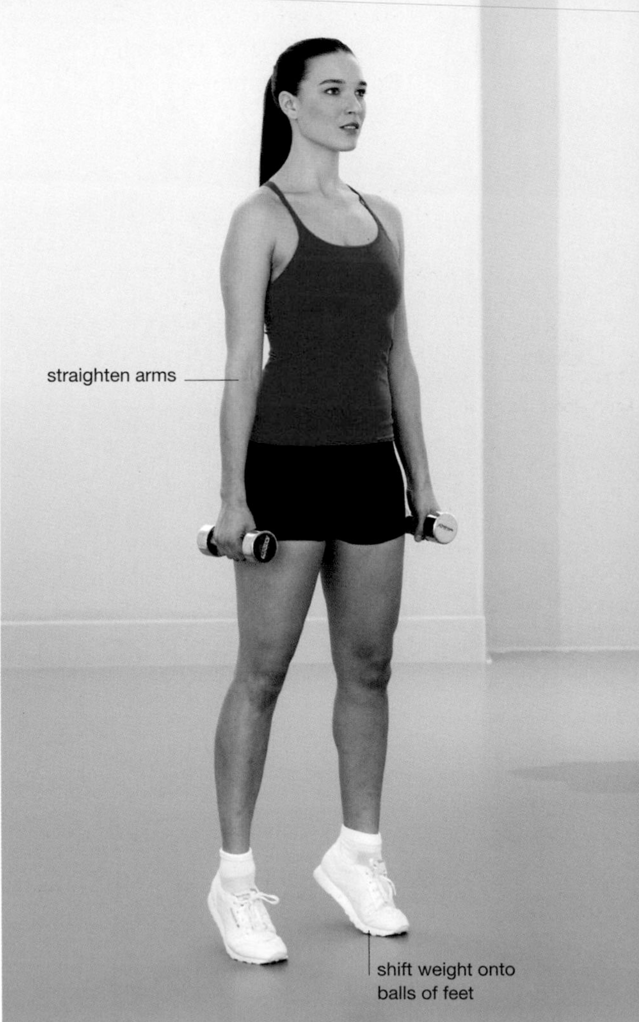

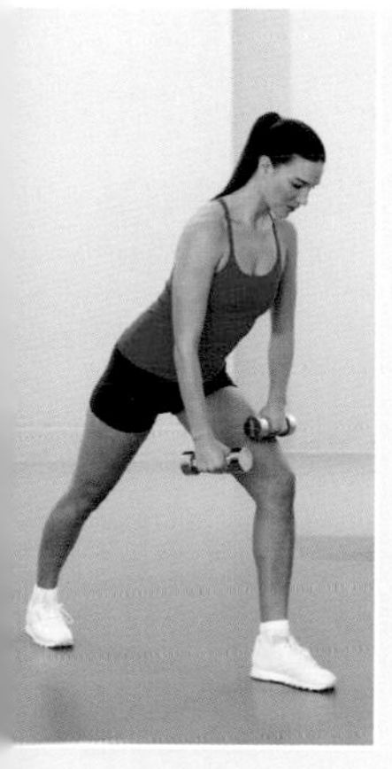

14 Reverse Fly

Exchange the ball for two large free weights. Stand in staggered lunge position, one foot forward and the arm on the same side resting on your thigh. Draw your shoulder blade in and exhale as you lift the other arm out to the side at shoulder height. Repeat 12 times, then switch sides. **Do your next cardio interval, Steps 8–10 (pp48–49).**

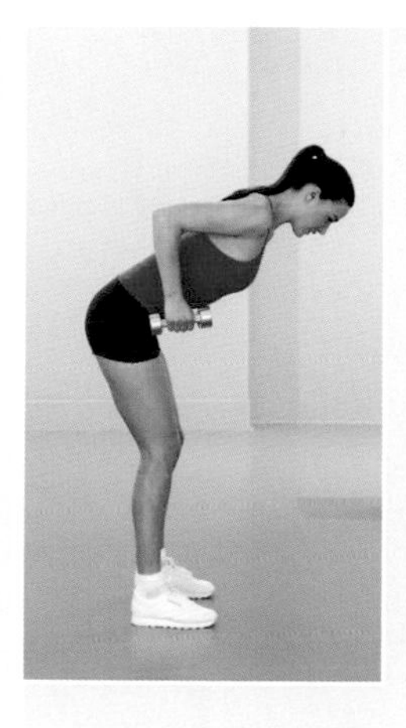

15 Triceps Kick Back

Exchange the ball for two large weights. Bend your knees and hinge forward. Bend your elbows to 90° and raise your upper arms parallel to the floor. Exhale, extending forearms behind. Inhale as you bend your elbows.

align head and neck with spine
feel it here
keep elbow rounded

feel it here
position upper arms parallel to floor
keep knees slightly bent

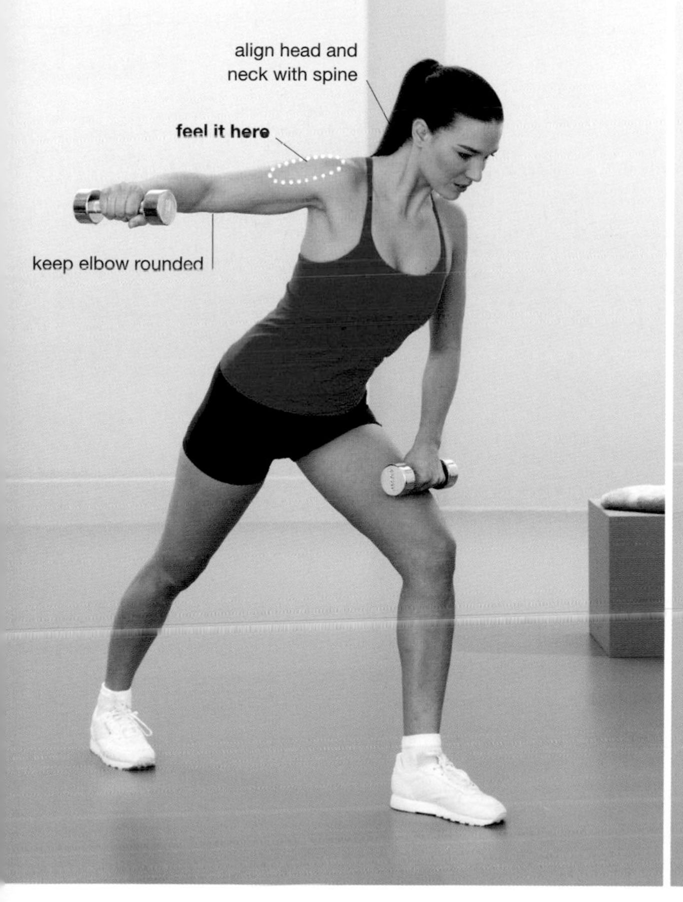

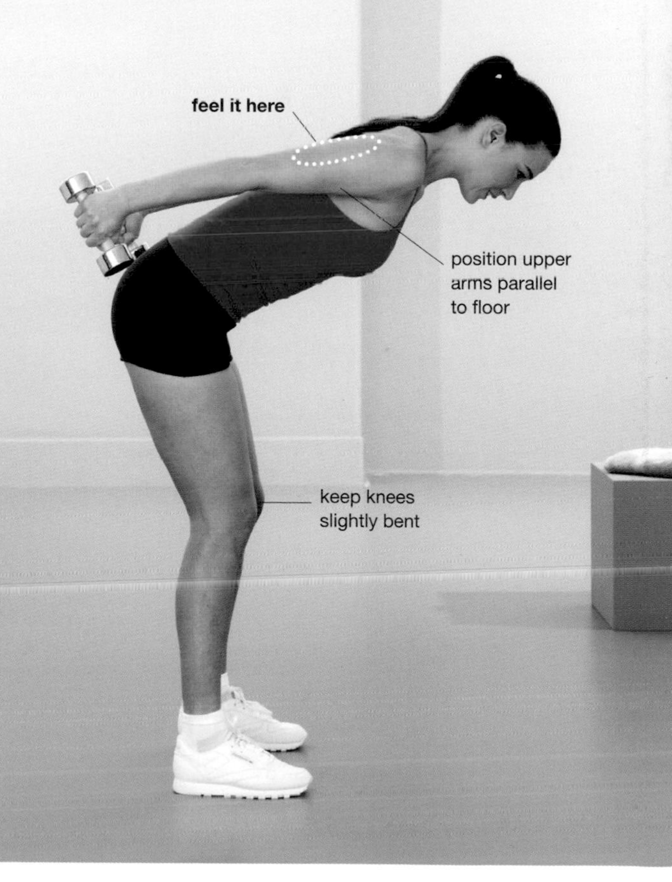

>> **floor** lat stretch/triceps stretch

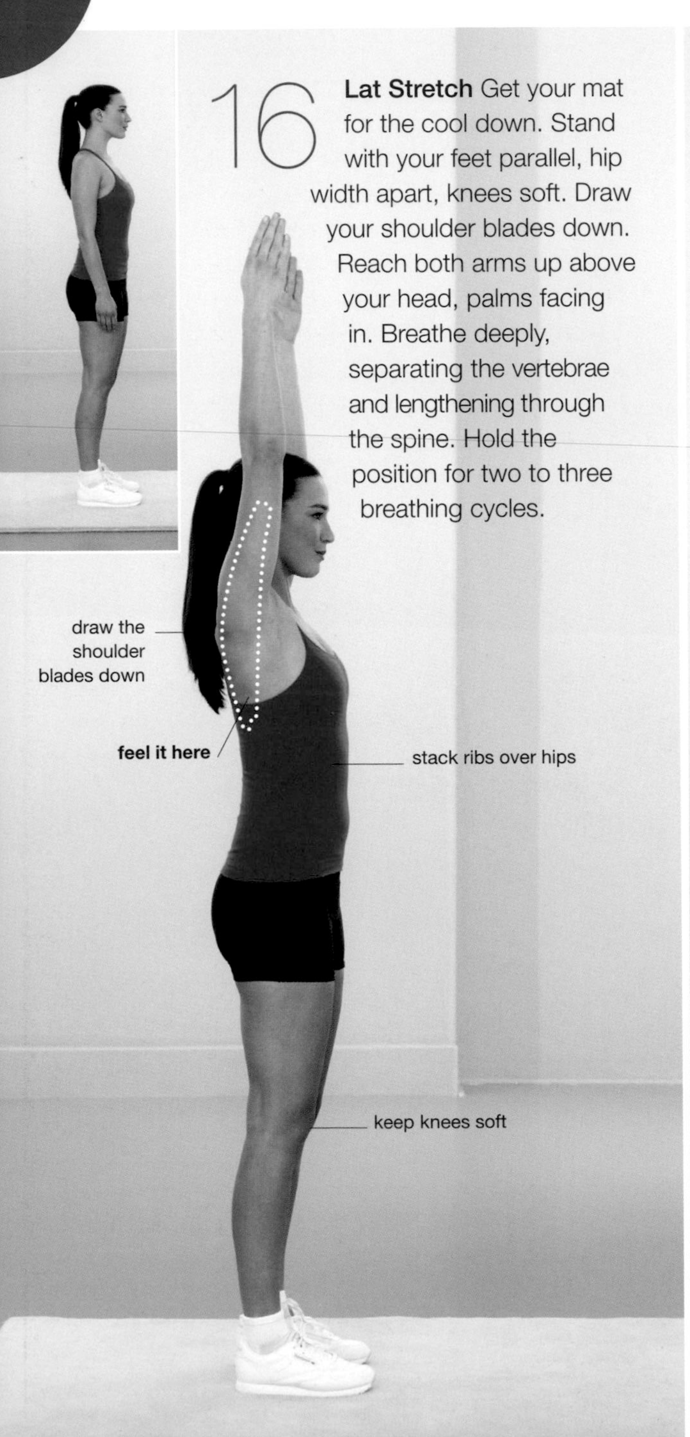

16 **Lat Stretch** Get your mat for the cool down. Stand with your feet parallel, hip width apart, knees soft. Draw your shoulder blades down. Reach both arms up above your head, palms facing in. Breathe deeply, separating the vertebrae and lengthening through the spine. Hold the position for two to three breathing cycles.

17 **Triceps Stretch** Cross your arms and take hold of your elbows. Keep your head centered. Gently pull your elbows back and hold. If this is too difficult, hold one elbow at a time. Use a steady stretch without bouncing to allow the muscle to lengthen gradually. Breathe deeply.

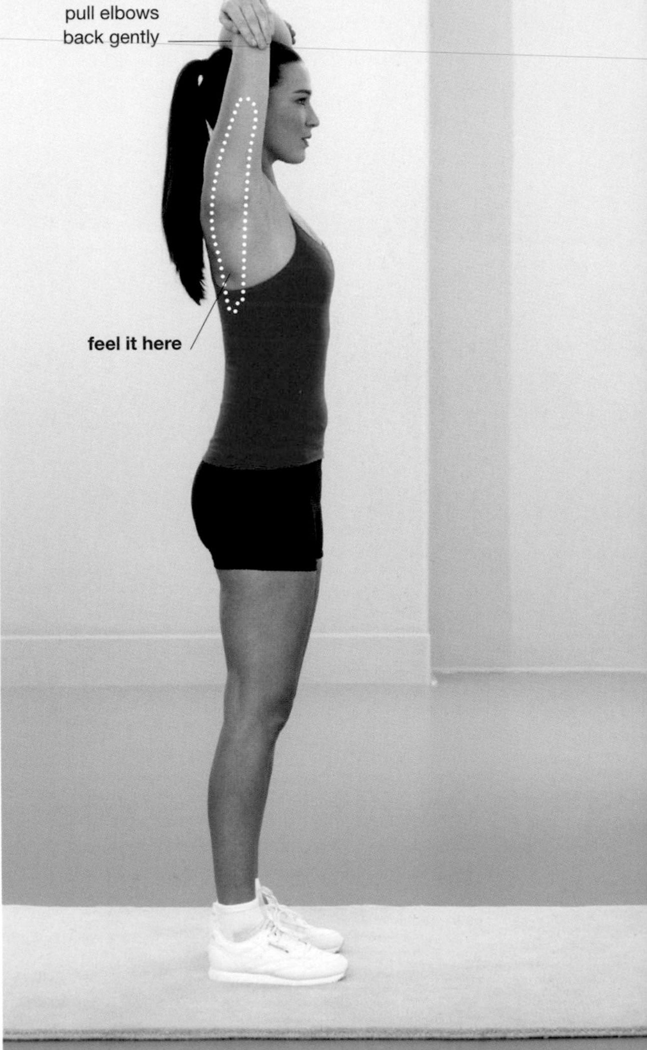

>> **floor** side bend/forward bend

18 **Side Bend** Still holding your elbows, and with your head centered, lift up from the waist and bend to one side, feeling a stretch all the way down your side to the hip. Hold, breathing into the stretch; then pass through the center and bend to the other side. Hold, take a deep breath and then return to center.

keep head centered between elbows
keep weight evenly distributed on your feet

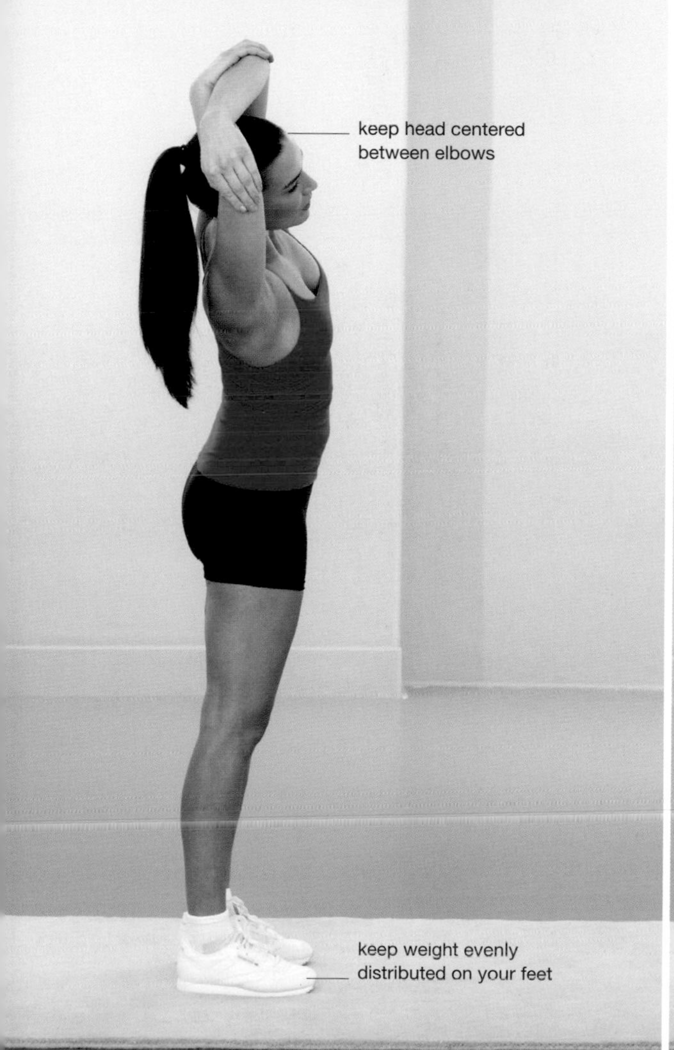

19 **Forward Bend** From the center position reach forward with your arms at shoulder height. Cross your wrists and turn your palms inward to bring them together, thumbs facing down. Round your upper back, head and neck aligned with your spine, ears between your upper arms. Separate your shoulder blades and reach as far forward as possible. Breathe and relax deeper into the stretch with each exhalation.

allow shoulder blades to separate
keep head and neck aligned with spine
feel it here

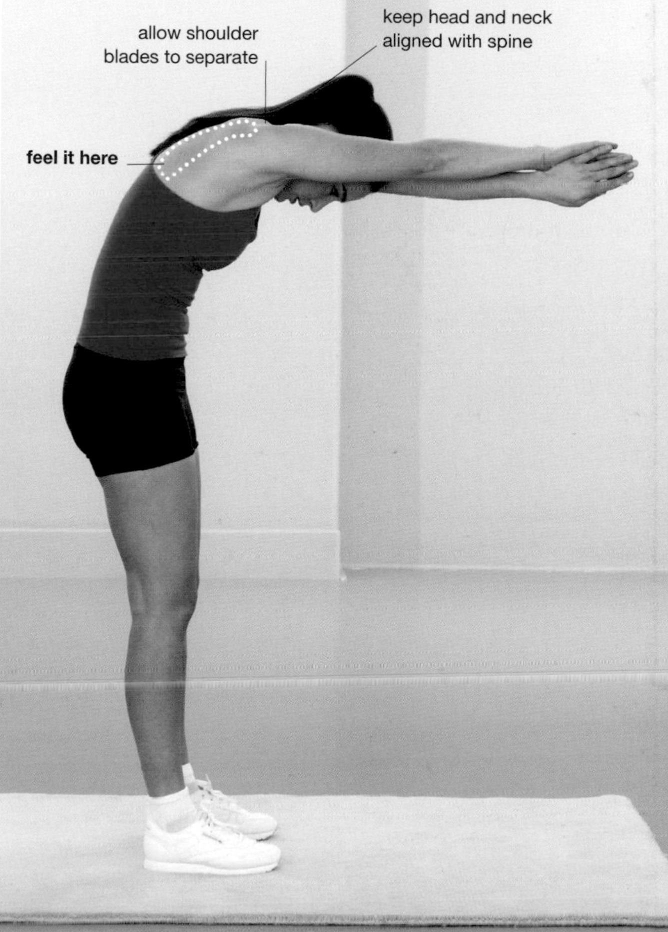

>> **floor** spinal roll-down/downward dog

keep chin
tucked in
keep knees
soft

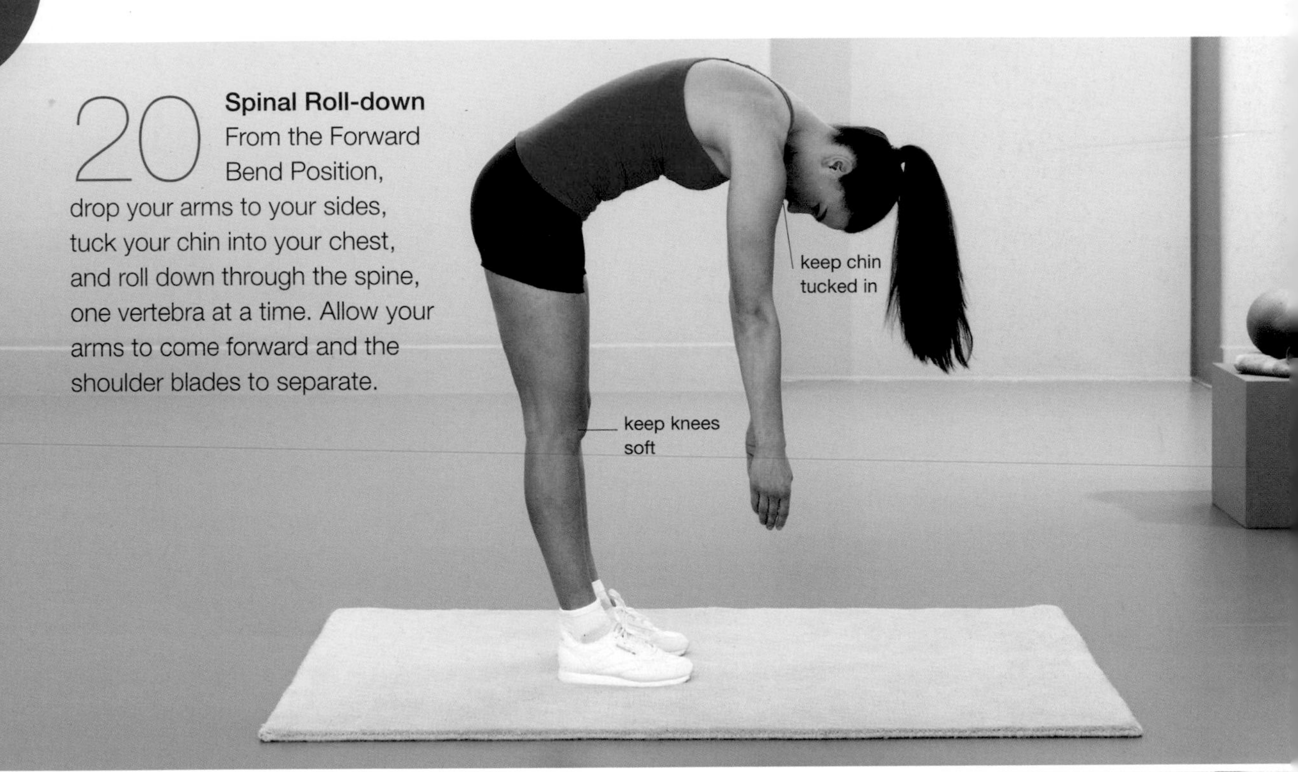

20 Spinal Roll-down

From the Forward Bend Position, drop your arms to your sides, tuck your chin into your chest, and roll down through the spine, one vertebra at a time. Allow your arms to come forward and the shoulder blades to separate.

reach up
with the hips
lengthen through
the spine

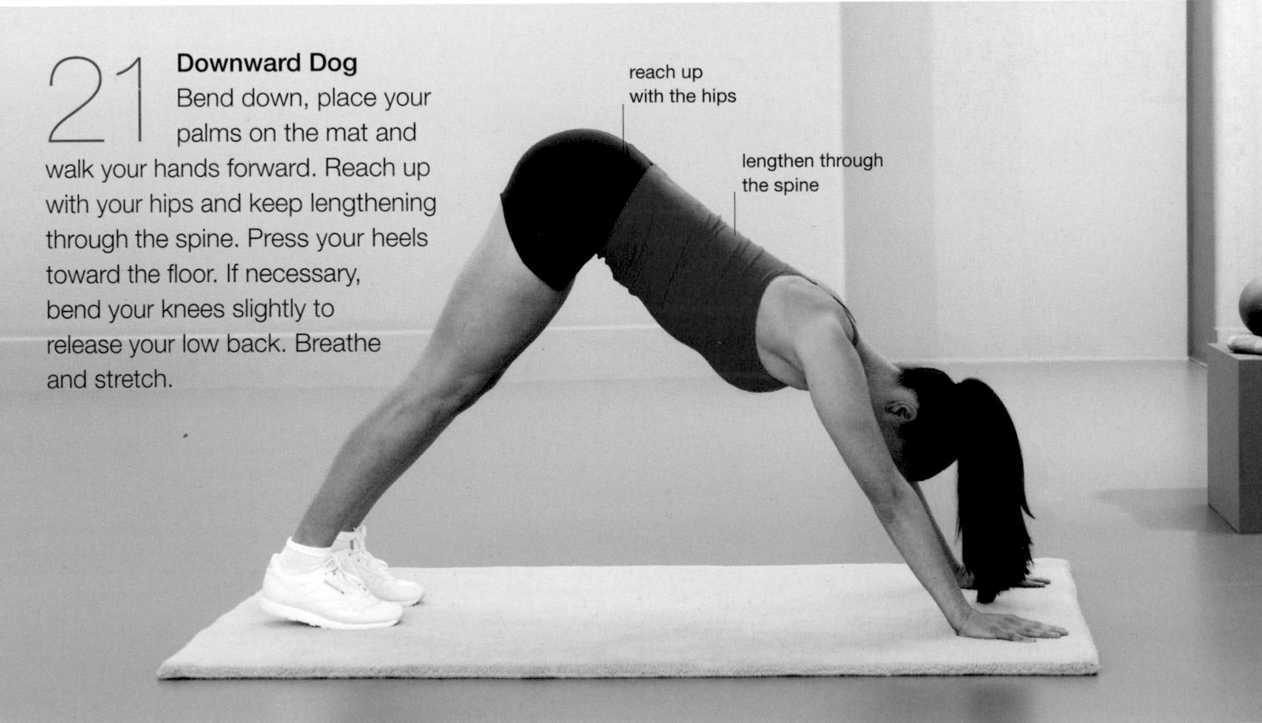

21 Downward Dog

Bend down, place your palms on the mat and walk your hands forward. Reach up with your hips and keep lengthening through the spine. Press your heels toward the floor. If necessary, bend your knees slightly to release your low back. Breathe and stretch.

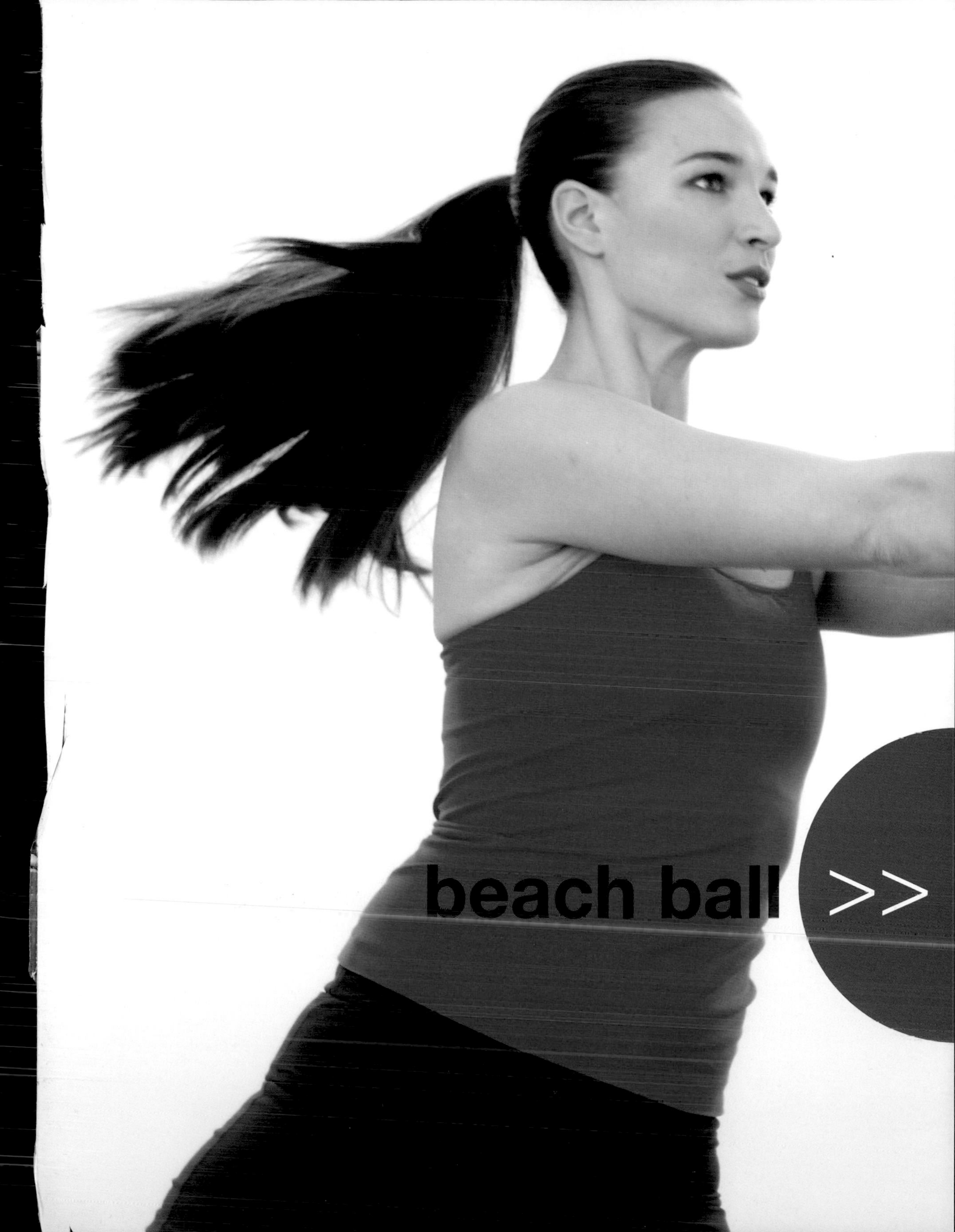
beach ball >>

beach ball at a glance

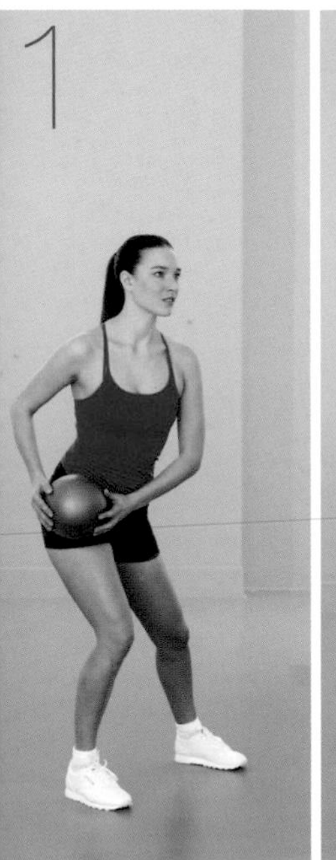

▲ **Warm up,** Rock Lunge, page 44

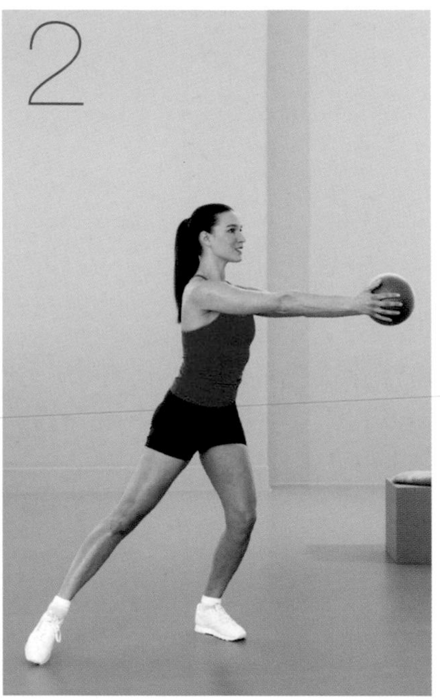

▲ **Warm up,** Skater, page 44

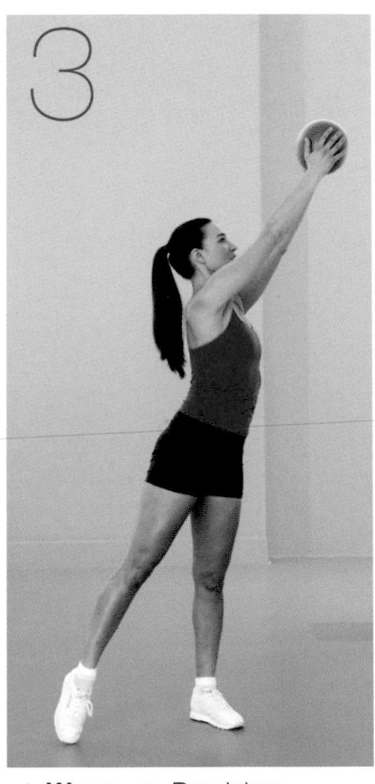

▲ **Warm up,** Pendulum Swing, page 45

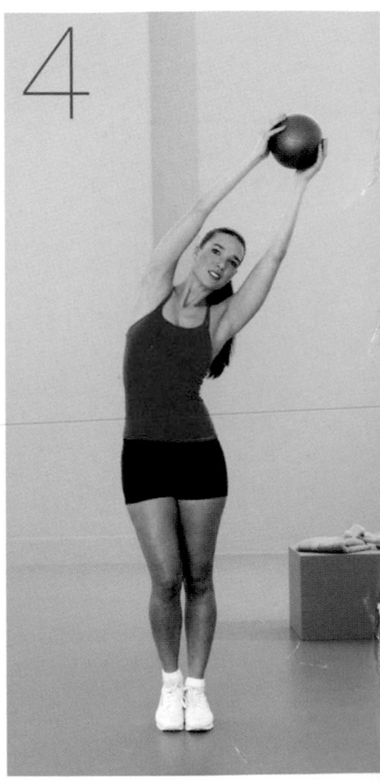

▲ **Warm up,** Body Sway, page 45

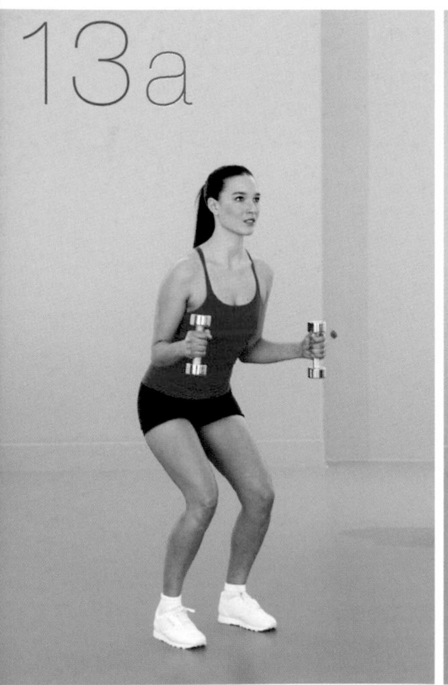

▲ **Resistance,** Squat with Weight Shift, page 52

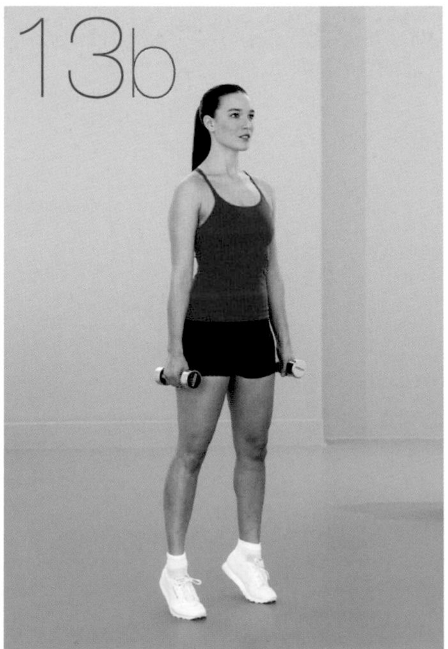

▲ **Resistance,** Squat with Weight Shift, page 52. Repeat Steps 8–10

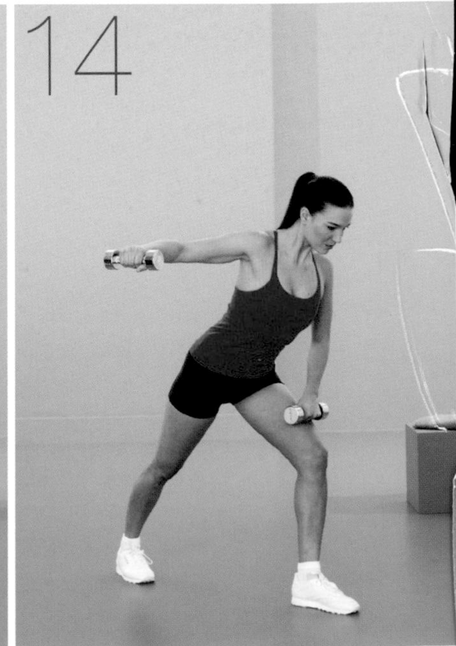

▲ **Resistance,** Reverse Fly, page 53. Repeat steps 8–10

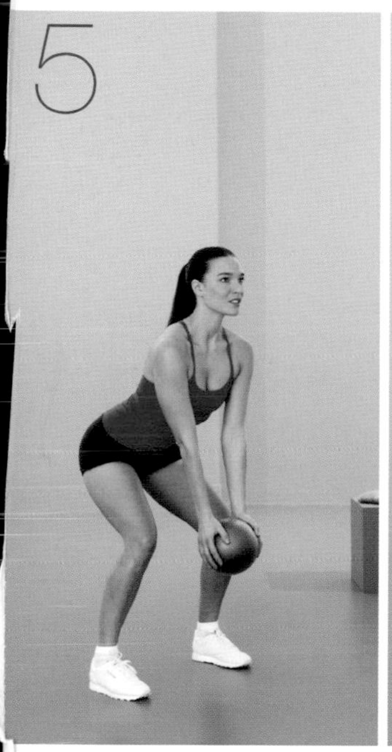

▲ **Warm up,** Wood-Chop Squat, page 46

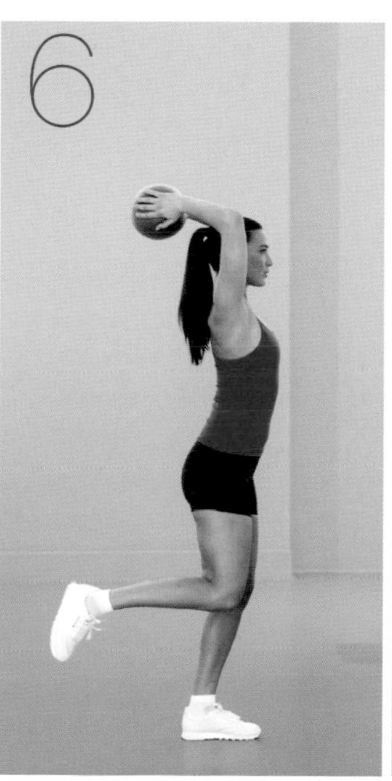

▲ **Warm up,** Curl & Press, page 46. Repeat Steps 5–1

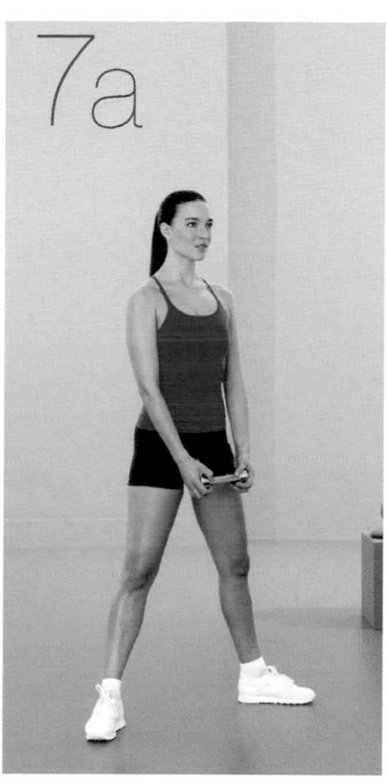

▲ **Resistance,** Plié with Front Raise, page 47

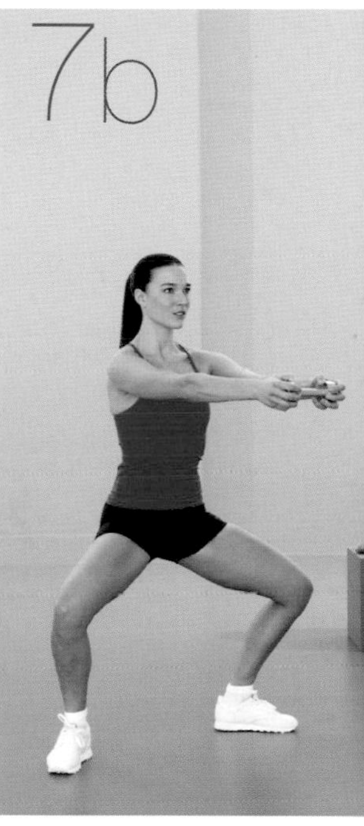

▲ **Resistance,** Plié with Front Raise, page 47

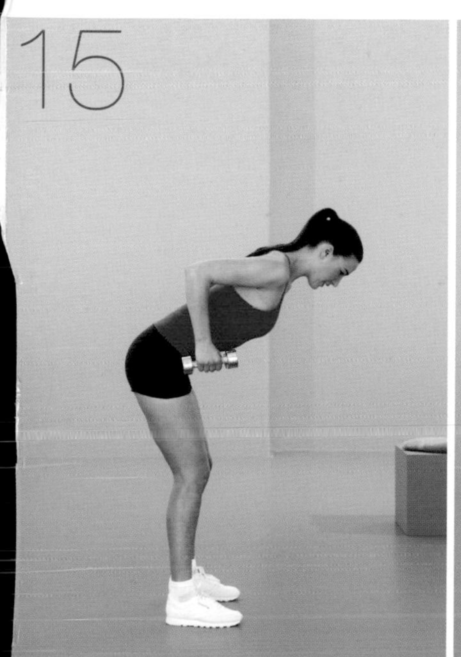

▲ **Resistance,** Triceps Kick Back, page 53. Repeat Steps 8–10

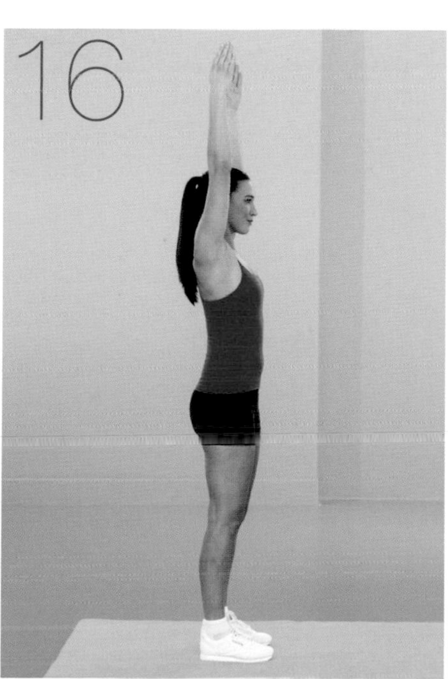

▲ **Cool down,** Lat Stretch, page 54

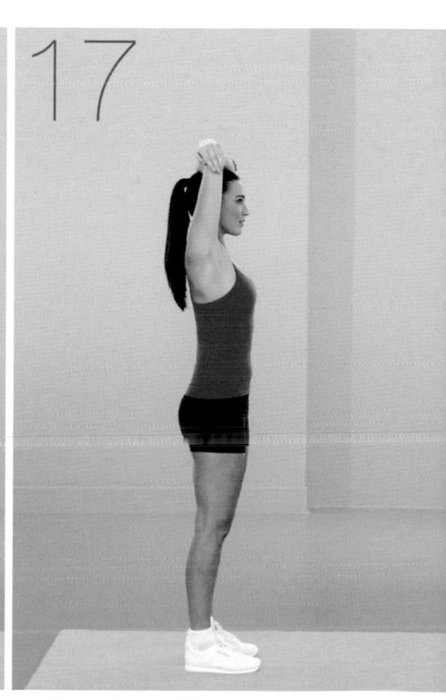

▲ **Cool down,** Triceps Stretch, page 54

>> **floor** plank/child's pose

22 **Plank** Walk forward and place your forearms on the mat, elbows directly under your shoulders, palms facing in, hands in loose fists. Tighten your abdominal and back muscles to keep your torso lifted in a straight line from head to toe. Tuck your toes under slightly: you will feel a stretch in your calves. Hold the position, breathing naturally.

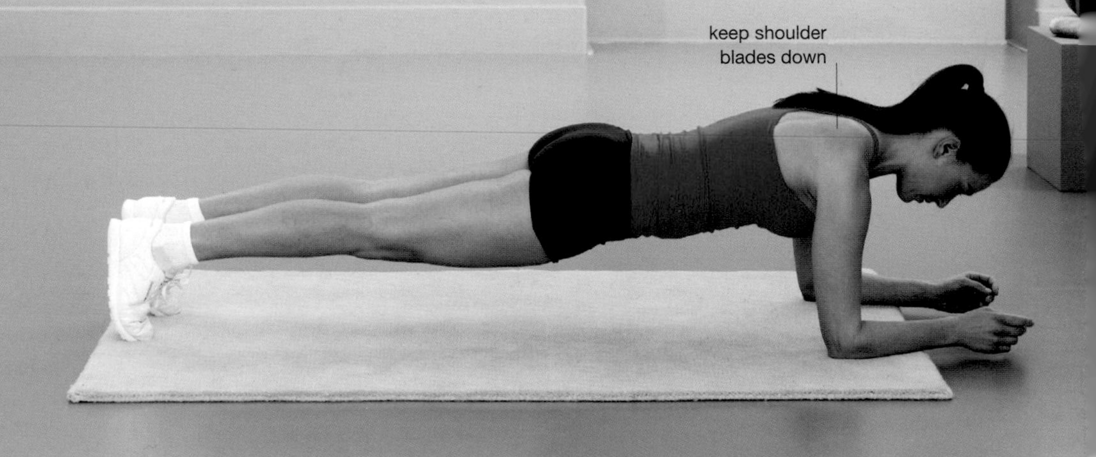

23 **Child's Pose** Bend your knees and reach back with your hips until your buttocks rest on your heels. At the same time round forward, curving the spine, forehead toward floor. Reach your arms to the front to stretch your lats, chest, and shoulders. With every exhale, sink deeper into the position; mind and body calm. Move back into the plank, bending your elbows and straightening your legs. Finally, repeat the Child's Pose.

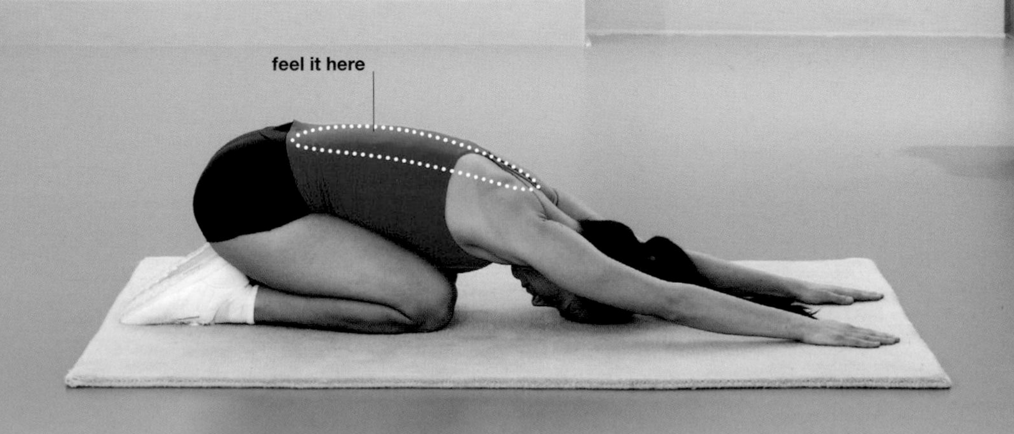

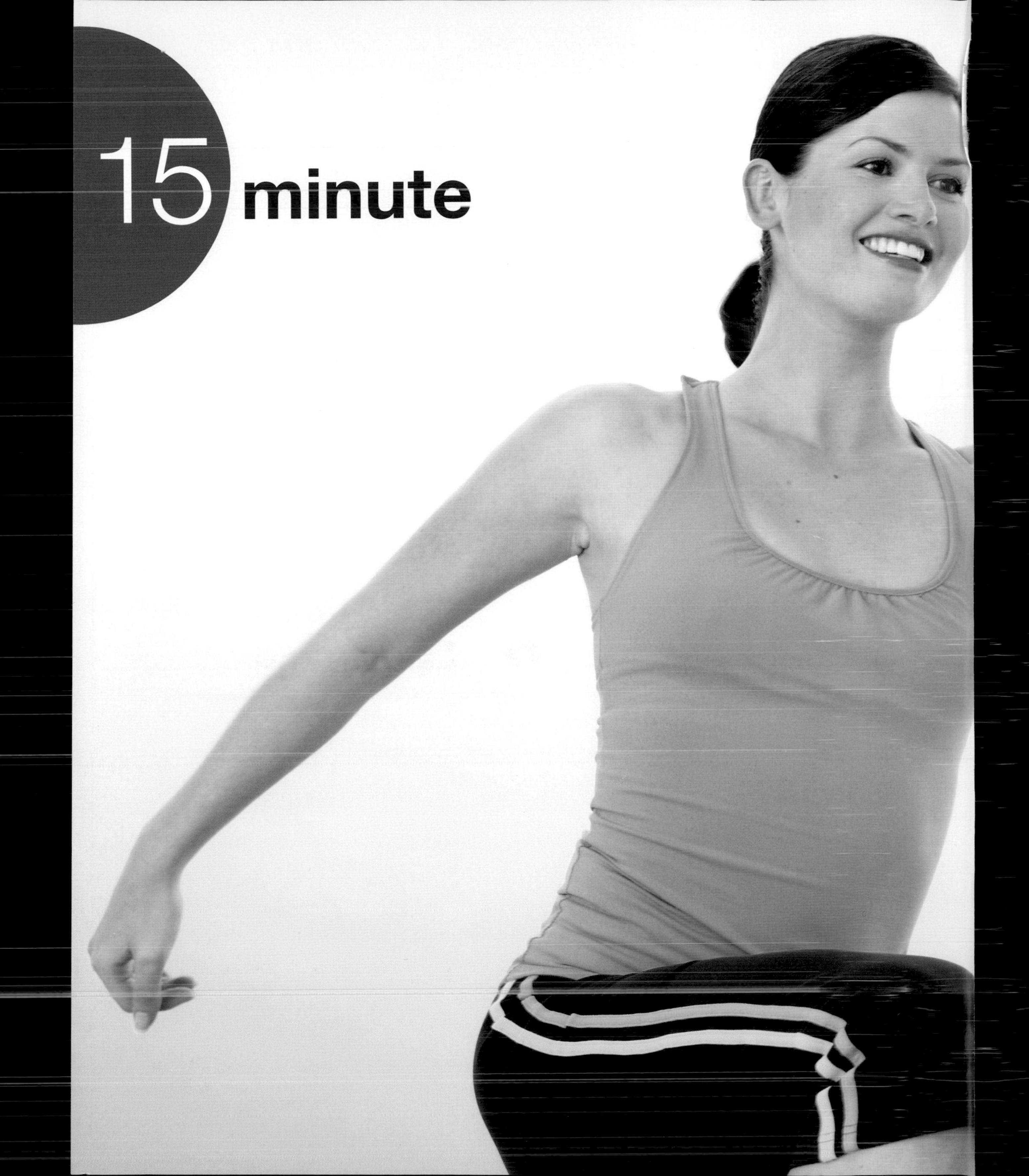

15 minute

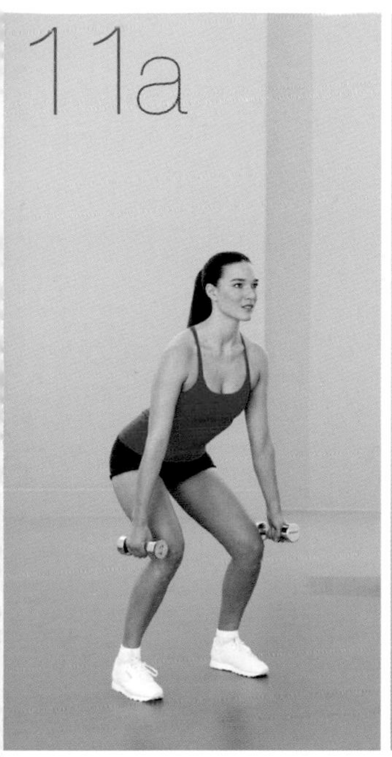

▲ **Resistance,** Squat with Knee Lift, page 50

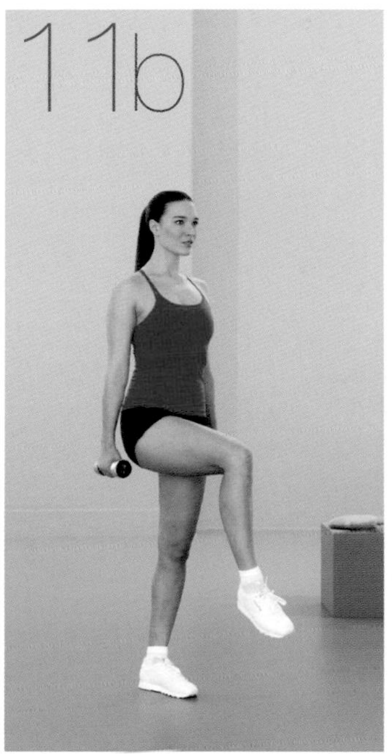

▲ **Resistance,** Squat with Knee Lift, page 50. Repeat Steps 8-10

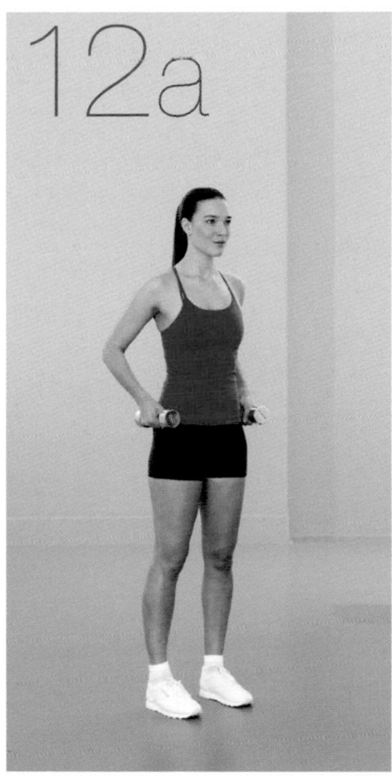

▲ **Resistance,** Lunge & Row, page 51

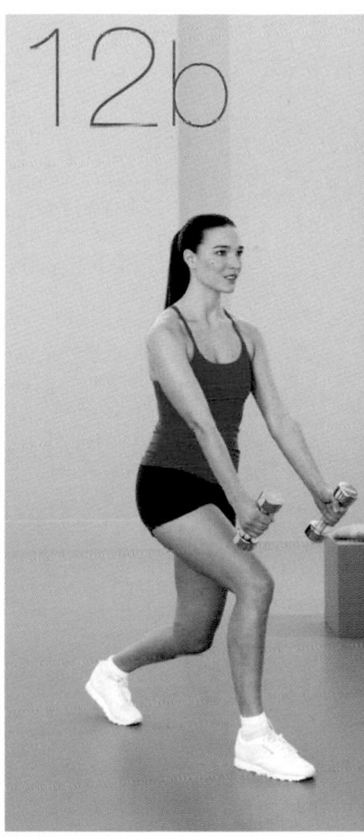

▲ **Resistance,** Lunge & Row, page 51. Repeat Steps 8–10

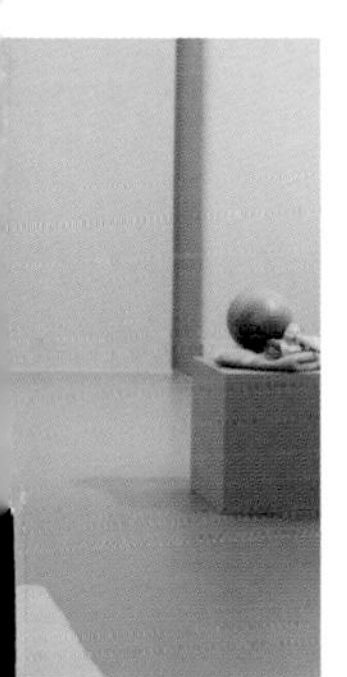

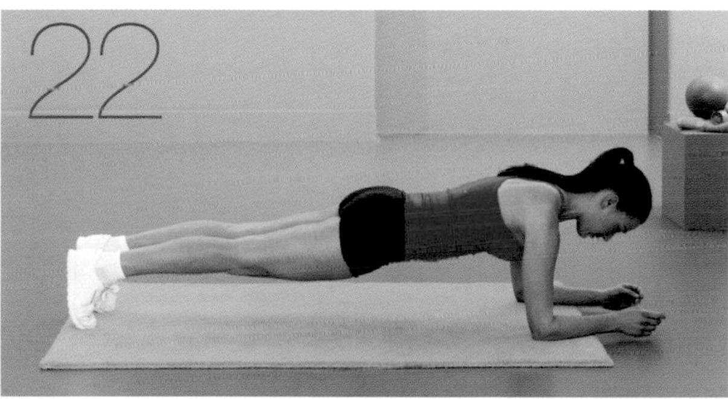

▲ **Cool down,** Plank, page 57

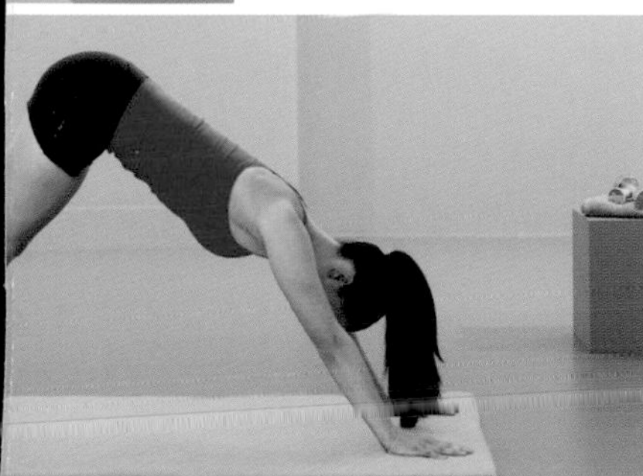

vnward Dog, page 56

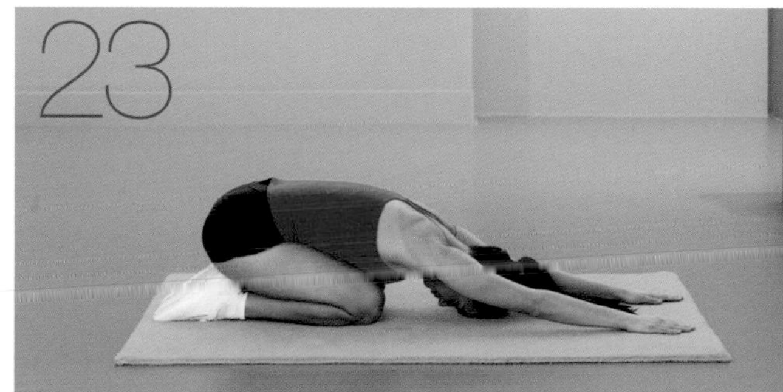

▲ **Cool down,** Child's Pose, page 57

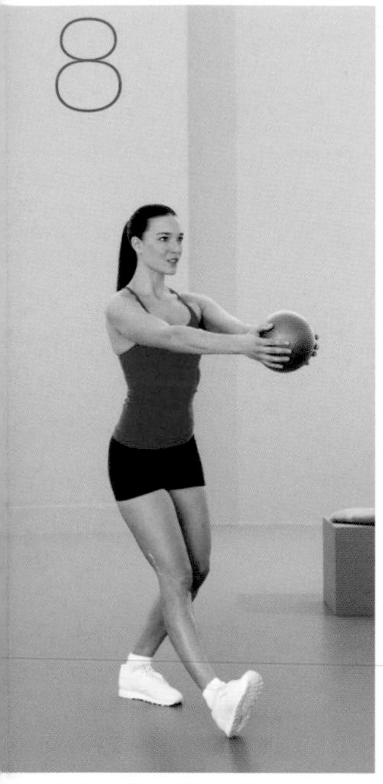

▲ **Cardio,** Step & Dig, page 48

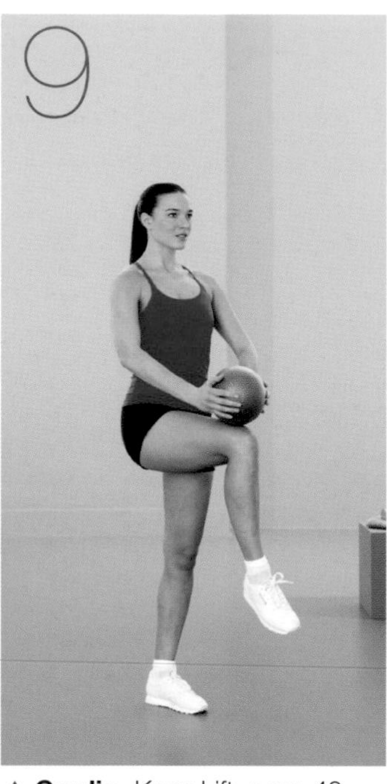

▲ **Cardio,** Knee Lift, page 48

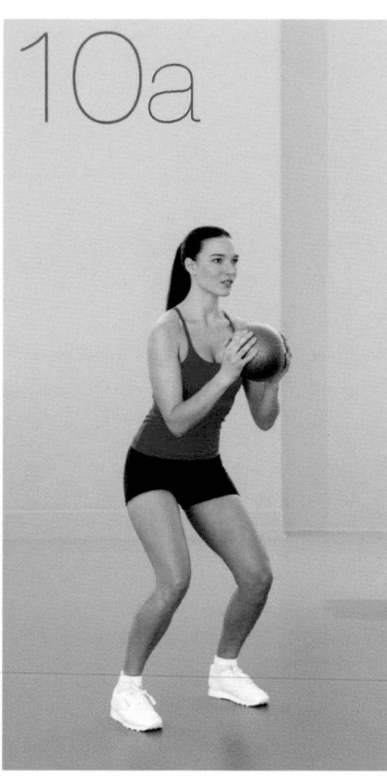

▲ **Cardio,** Squat Plus, page 49

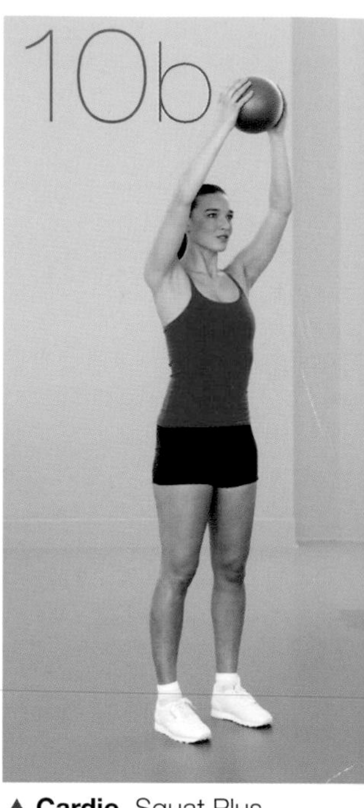

▲ **Cardio,** Squat Plus, page 49

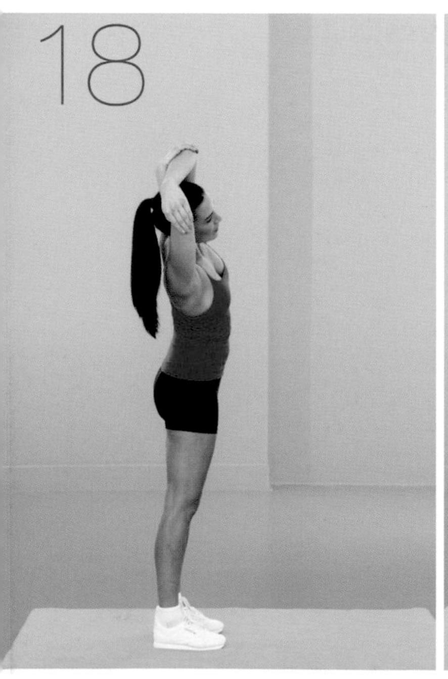

▲ **Cool down,** Side Bend, page 55

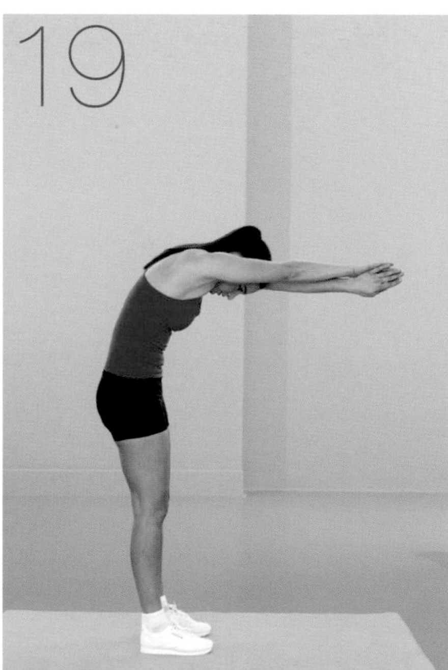

▲ **Cool down,** Forward Bend, page 55

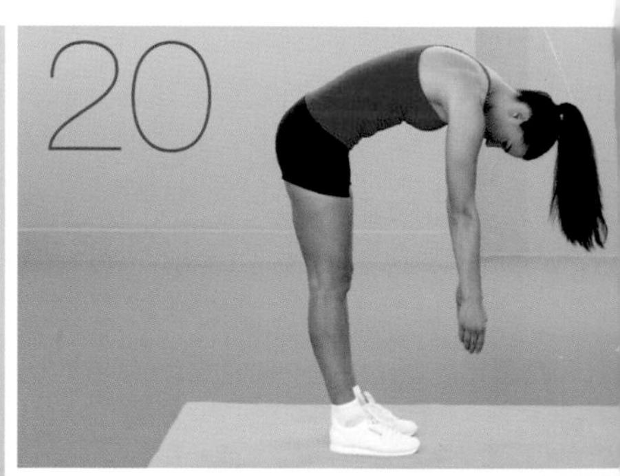

▲ **Cool down,** Spinal Roll-down, page 56

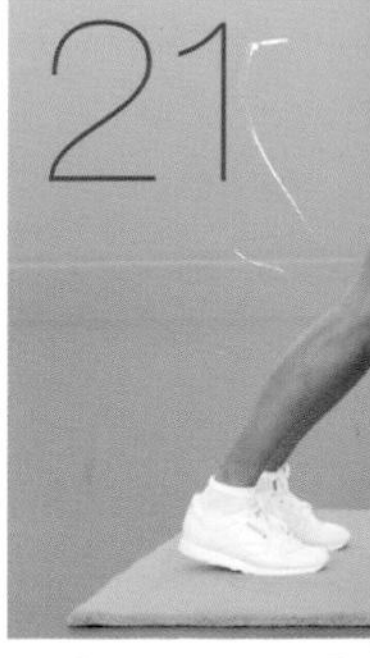

▲ **Cool down,** D

>> **frequently** asked questions

As you gradually work through the exercises, you may have questions about your progress and the effectiveness of your workout. This selection of questions focuses mainly on the issue of incorporating weights and how best to use them.

>> Aren't I too old, overweight, or out of shape to lift weights?

Whatever your age and current fitness level, you can train your cardiovascular system to develop more stamina and energy; build muscle to increase lean body mass and strength; and stretch out your muscles for greater ease of movement. If you are just starting out, begin with Step-Touch (see p18) and gradually progress. After four weeks, see if you can repeat it for a 30-minute workout. After eight weeks, advance to Beach Ball (see p42).

>> Will lifting weights make me look masculine?

The truth is that rather than causing women to build bigger muscles, weight training generally creates a "tighter" physique. You will have a flatter tummy, shapelier arms, firmer legs, and look great in a little black dress. The propensity to put on muscle is largely due to how much testosterone you secrete, and women produce only about one-tenth the amount that men produce.

>> How do I know the right starting level of weights for the different exercises?

You should be able to finish all repetitions while maintaining proper form. Your muscles need to adjust gradually to the new demands as tendons and ligaments need time to adapt. Gradual conditioning of connective tissue strengthens the joints and prevents injuries. Even if you are capable of lifting heavy weights, if you haven't previously trained with weights, you need to build up slowly.

>> I'm not sure I'm using the free weights properly. Please could you advise?

Your pacing and breathing are extremely important when you are using weights in your workouts. Lift the weights on a count of two, pause for a moment, and then lower on a count of four. Move through the full range of motion, maintaining tension when you lift the weight (or your body weight) against gravity, for example when you bend your elbow upward in a biceps curl or when you come up from a squatting position. See Squat with Knee Lift (p50) and Lunge & Row (p51) for examples of weights use.

>> I'm finding it easy to lift and lower the weights—am I working hard enough?

The goal in strength training is to work to muscular failure, always maintaining correct form. You should be working to the point of volitional fatigue ("I can't do any more") and your muscles should feel tired and weak as you finish your repetitions. Muscles build by a cycle of microdamage (lifting weights) and repair of the muscle fibers (your rest days); as the muscle repairs it gets stronger.

>> What are the benefits of working out with free weights, rather than using a weight machine?

Weight machines support your body in the correct position, and, generally, allow you to lift more weight than if you were using free weights. However, free weights highlight imbalances in the body, since you use them with individual limbs; they can be an effective tool for correcting these imbalances and for bringing the body into alignment. They make weight-lifting more like a sport.

>> Aren't aerobic activities the most efficient type of exercise to lose weight?

Aerobics plus weight training is the best formula for weight loss. Aerobic exercise burns calories and reduces fat stores from the whole body, while weight training develops leaner, toned muscles as you lose fat. Each pound of muscle that you gain raises your metabolic rate by about 50 calories per day, so you are burning more calories around the clock.

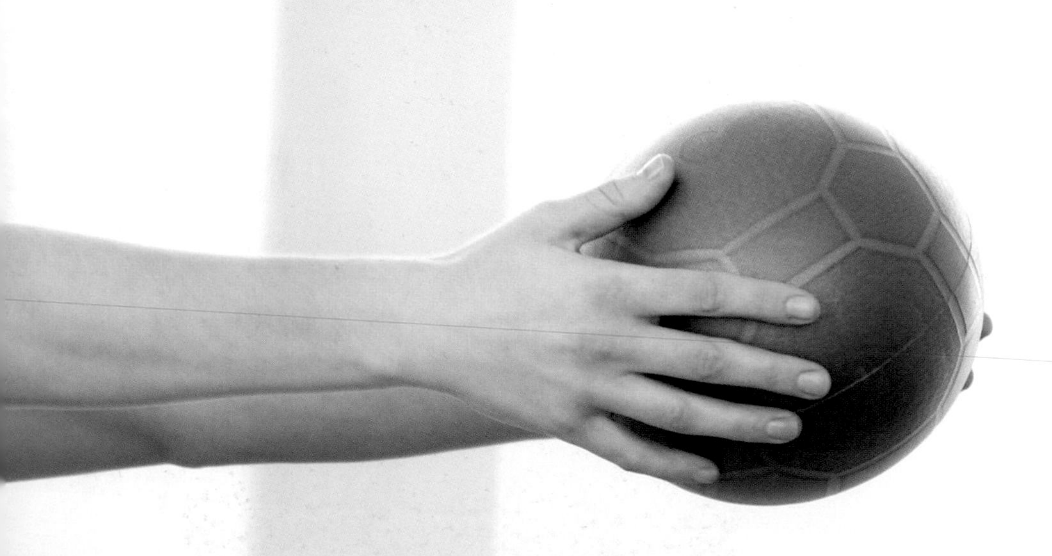

15 minute **summary**

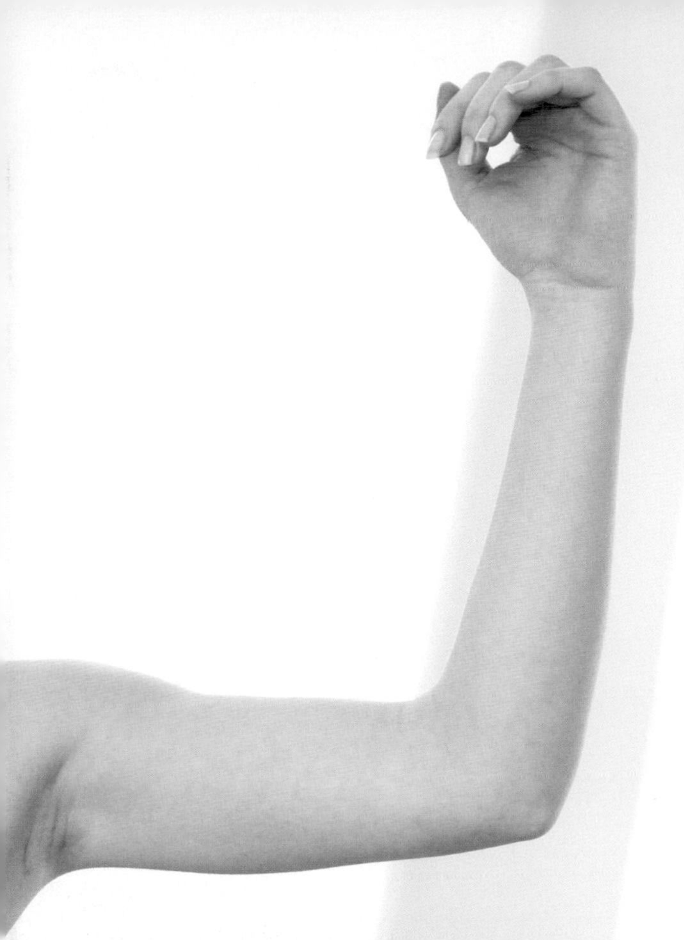

hop, jig, & jump workout >>

Experience the childlike joy of hopping and jumping as you release endorphins with this upbeat workout

>> **warm up** bend & raise/double arm swing

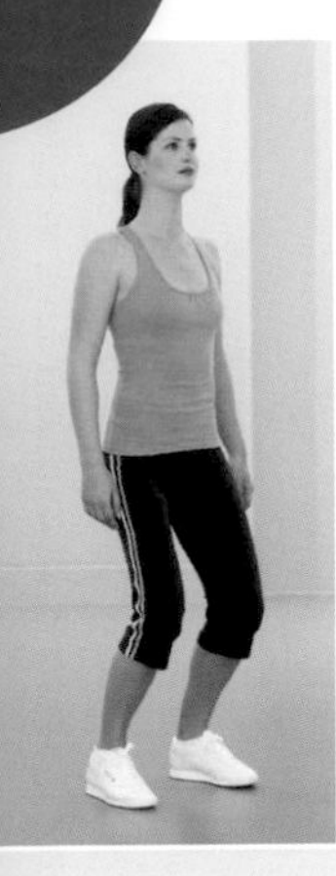

1 **Bend & Raise** Stand with your feet parallel, hip width apart, knees soft, arms by your sides. Tighten your abdominals and lift your chest. Bend your knees (see inset) then straighten your legs. Shift your weight to the balls of your feet and lift your heels, resisting the floor. Continue bending and then rising up, allowing your arms to swing naturally forward, for a total of 8 times.

2 **Double Arm Swing** Continue to bend your knees rhythmically as you swing your arms to back and front. From the starting position of bent knees (see inset), feet flat on the floor, straighten your legs and swing your arms behind. Bend your knees again as your arms pass through the center and then swing them in front as you straighten your legs. Repeat for a total of 8 swings, back to front.

look straight ahead
shift weight to balls of feet

swing arms forward as legs straighten
keep heels down

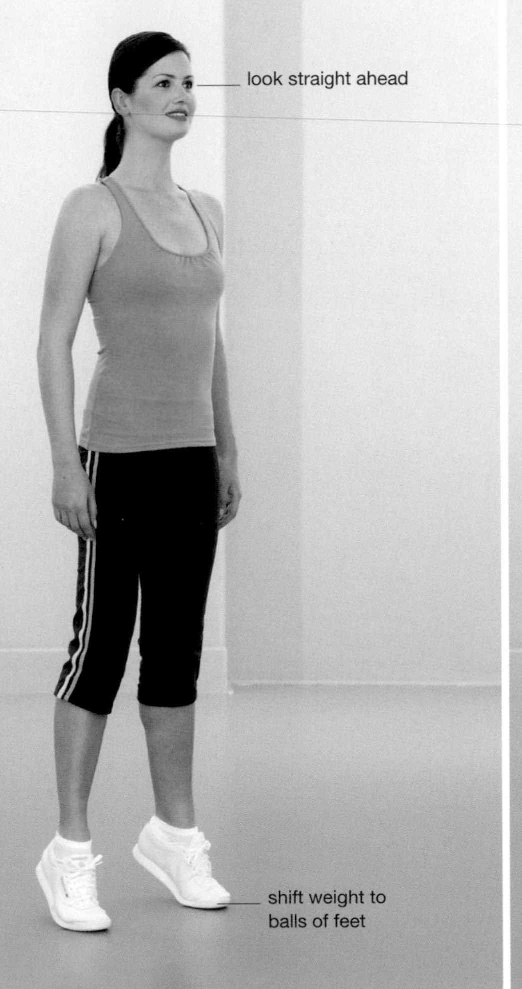

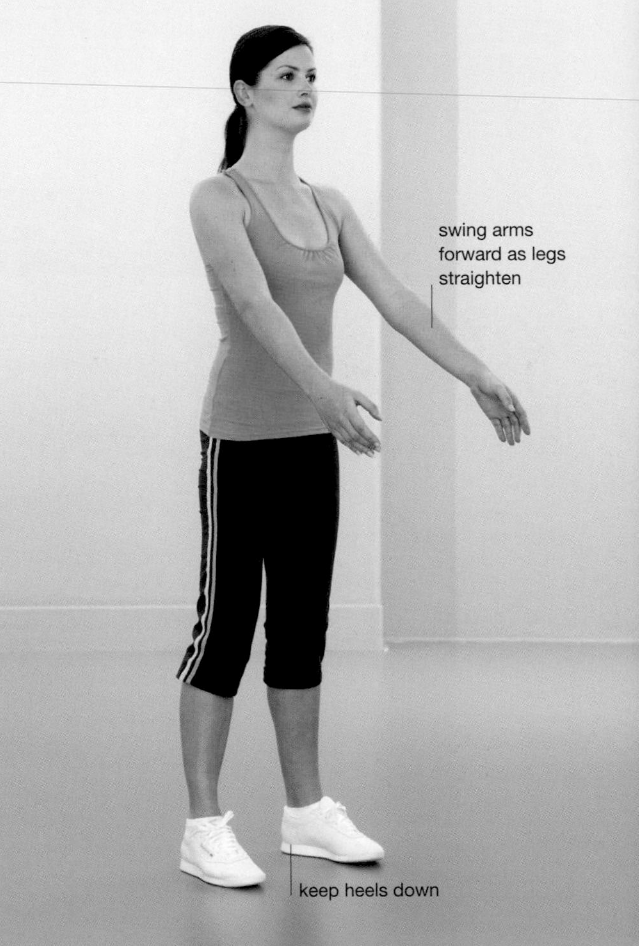

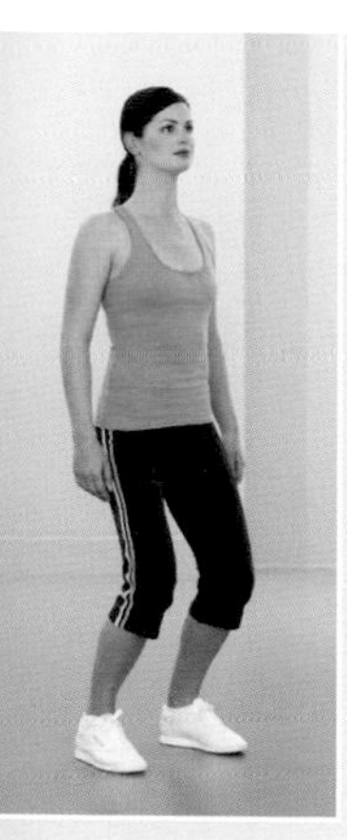

3 Single Arm Swing
Continue to bend your knees rhythmically, but change the arms, swinging one forward and the other back every time you straighten your legs. Keep your heels down, knees in line with toes. Keep your shoulder blades down as you swing your arms. Your chest stays lifted, chin level. Repeat, alternating arms, for a total of 8 reps (1 rep = both sides).

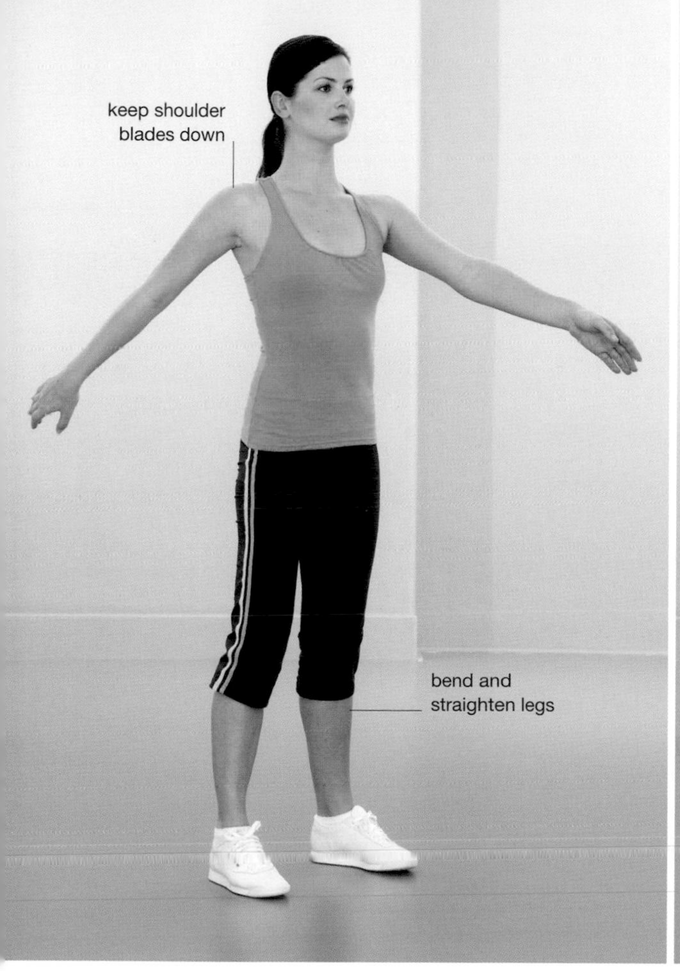

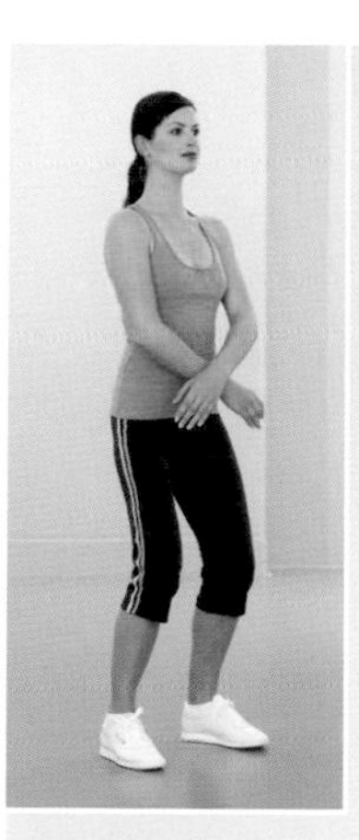

4 Cross & Open
Continuing with rhythmic knee bends, change your arms to cross in front as you bend your knees and then lift them out to the sides as you straighten your legs. Keep your shoulder blades down as you lift your arms to shoulder height, palms down. Bend and straighten, lifting your arms out to the sides, 16 times.

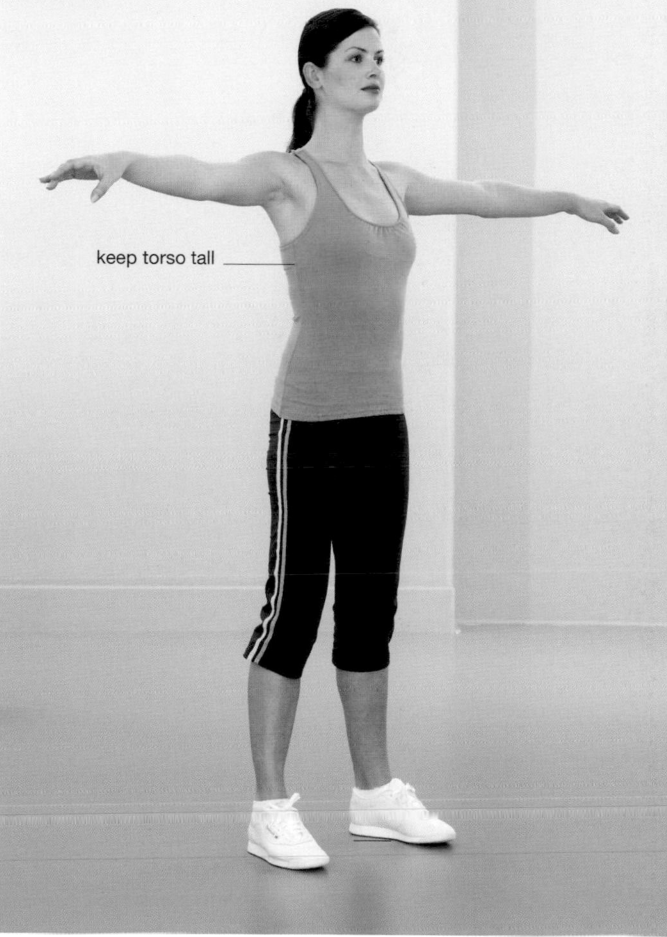

>> **warm up** lateral lift/jumping jack

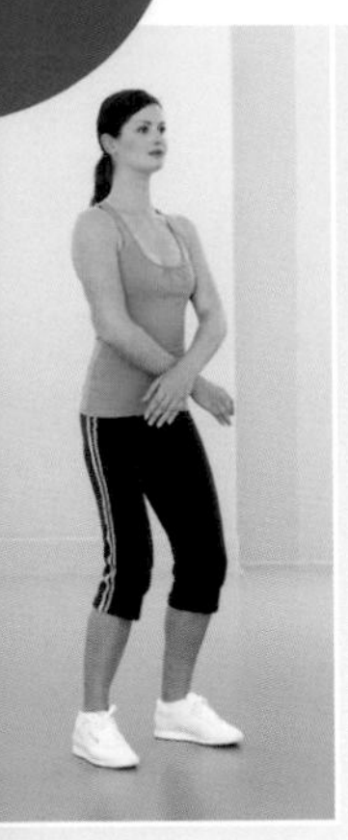

5 **Lateral Lift** Arms stay the same as you bend and straighten your knees, but you add a side leg lift. Bend your knees as you cross your arms in front, then straighten both legs and lift one to the side as you raise your arms. Keep your hips level, shoulders down. Repeat, alternating legs, for a total of 8 reps (1 rep = both sides).

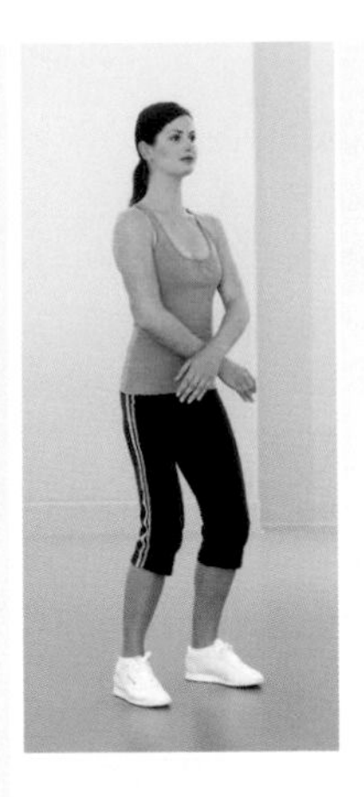

6 **Jumping Jack** Continue to raise and lower your arms, but change your legs. As you cross your arms in front, jump your feet together. As you raise your arms to shoulder height, tap one foot out to the side. Alternate sides for 8 reps (1 rep = both sides). **Repeat Steps 5–1 (in reverse) to complete your warm up.**

lift arms to shoulder height
lift leg to the side
bend and straighten legs

tap toe out to the side

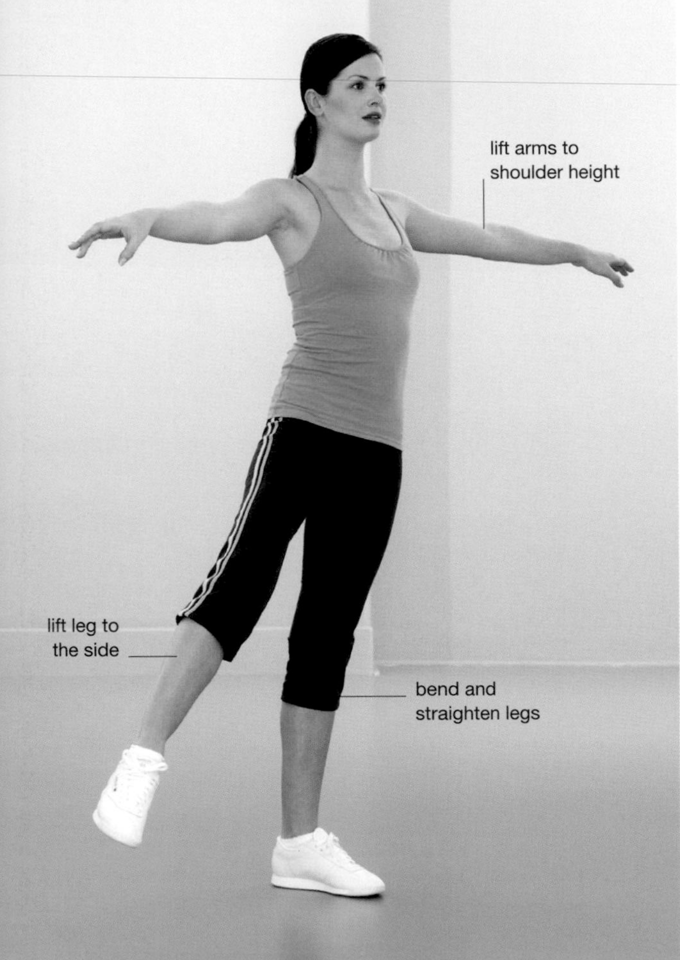

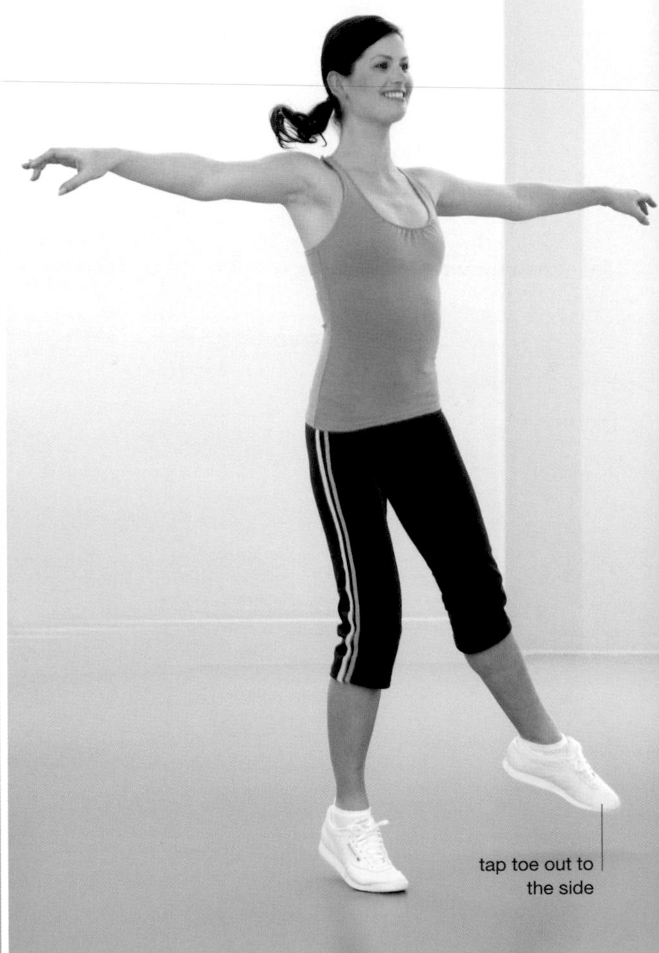

>> **resistance** hip hinge & reverse fly

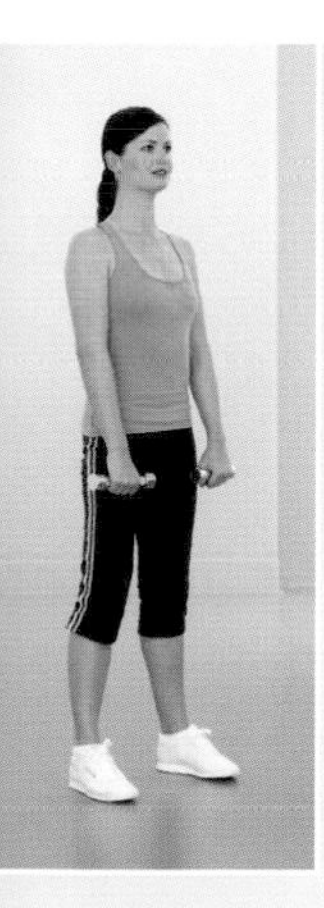

7a **Hip Hinge & Reverse Fly** Pick up two small weights for your first resistance exercise. Stand up straight, feet parallel, hip width apart, shoulders down. Hold a weight in each hand in front of your thighs, palms facing back. Bend your knees as you hinge forward from the hips, maintaining neutral spine alignment. The weights are now directly under your shoulders.

7b Inhale, then, as you exhale, raise your arms to the sides, in line with the shoulders, to shoulder height. Keep shoulder blades together as you lift your arms, elbows rounded, palms backward. Inhale and lower your arms, then exhale as you straighten your hips and knees to return to start position (see inset). Repeat combination for 8 reps.

keep spine straight, parallel to floor
hold weights directly under shoulders

squeeze shoulder blades together
feel it here

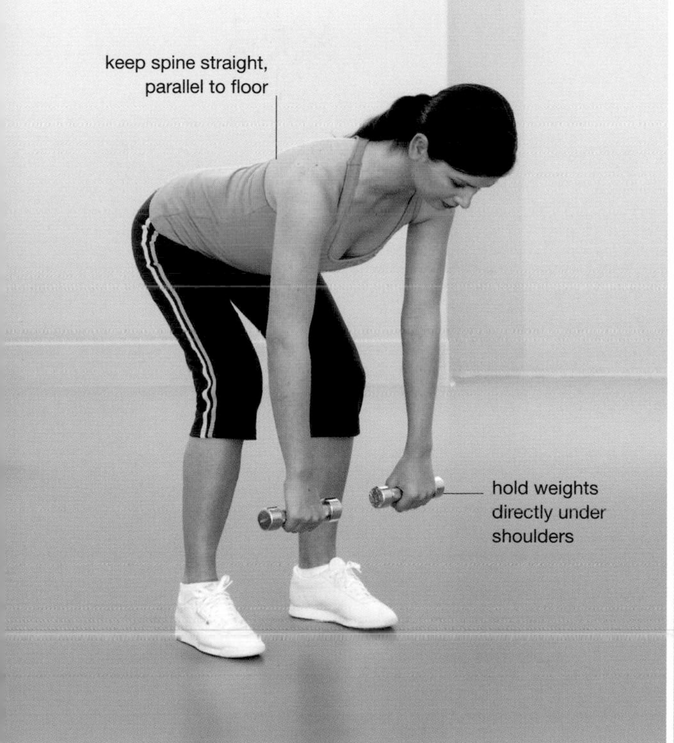

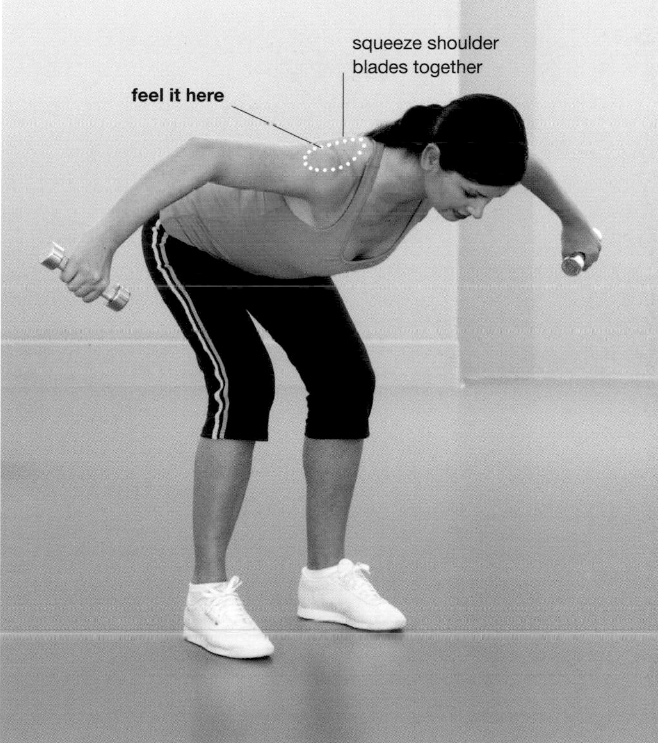

>> **cardio** step-hop/jig

8 **Step-Hop** Put down the weights for the first cardio interval. Stand with your feet parallel, hip width apart, arms by your sides. Step forward with one leg and hop on it, as your raise the other knee to hip height. The arm opposite the raised leg swings forward, elbow bent. Lower the leg and step back to the starting position. Alternate legs, swinging your arms in opposition, for a total of 6 reps (1 rep = both sides).

9 **Jig** To begin, jump in place, feet hip width apart, hands on your hips. Hop on one leg, extending the other leg on a diagonal, digging your heel into the floor, toe pointing toward the ceiling. Bring the exended leg back and repeat on the other side. Keep your upper body vertical, chest lifted, eyes looking straight ahead. Alternate legs for a total of 8 reps (1 rep = both sides).

keep arms close to your sides
step forward and hop

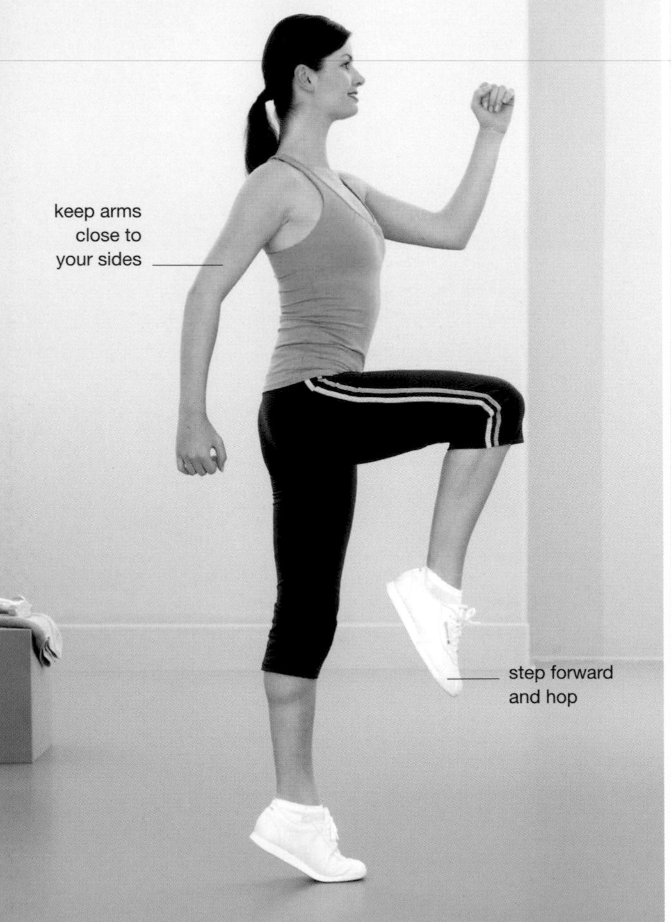

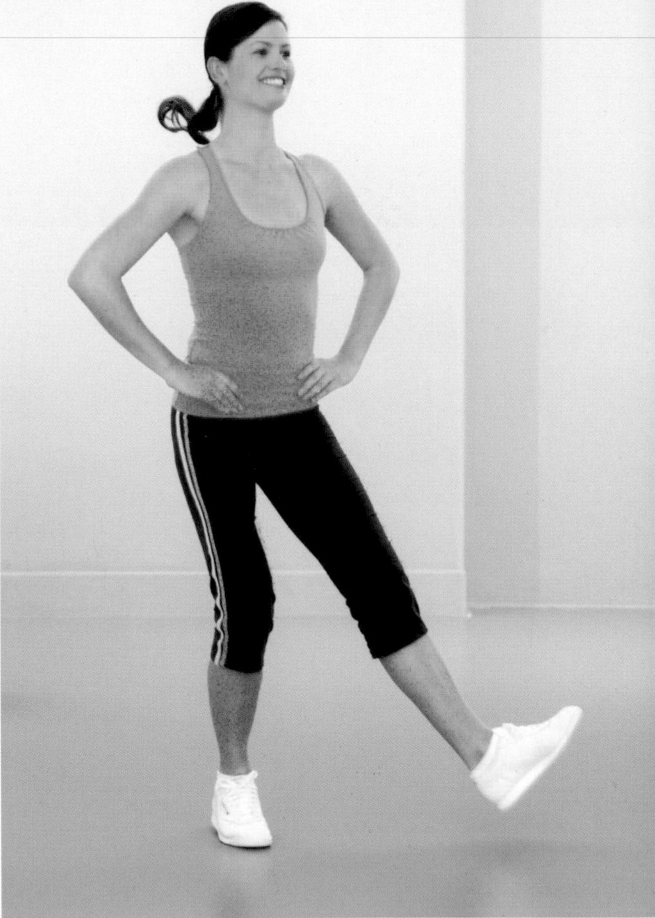

resistance lunge

10 **Jump & Twist** With your feet together, arms out to the sides, contract your abdominals and jump up, rotating your hips to one side. Turn your hips, knees, and feet as a unit. Land with your knees bent. Keep your torso upright, your shoulders facing forward. Alternate sides for a total of 8 reps (1 rep = both sides). **Steps 8–10 complete your cardio interval, which you will repeat after each resistance exercise.**

keep shoulders facing forward
land with knees bent

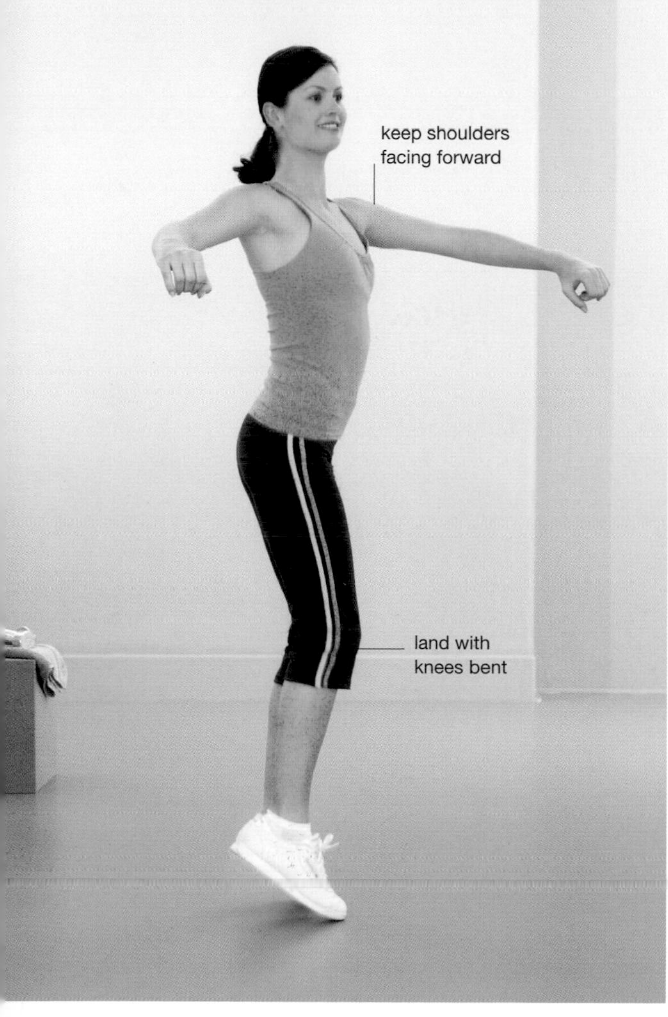

11a **Lunge & Twist** Pick up one large free weight. Step forward with one leg into a staggered lunge position. Hold the weight with both hands horizontally in front of your waist, elbows bent. Keep your weight centered between your legs, your back heel down and your feet parallel. Your shoulders should be square to the front, your eyes looking straight ahead.

heel down

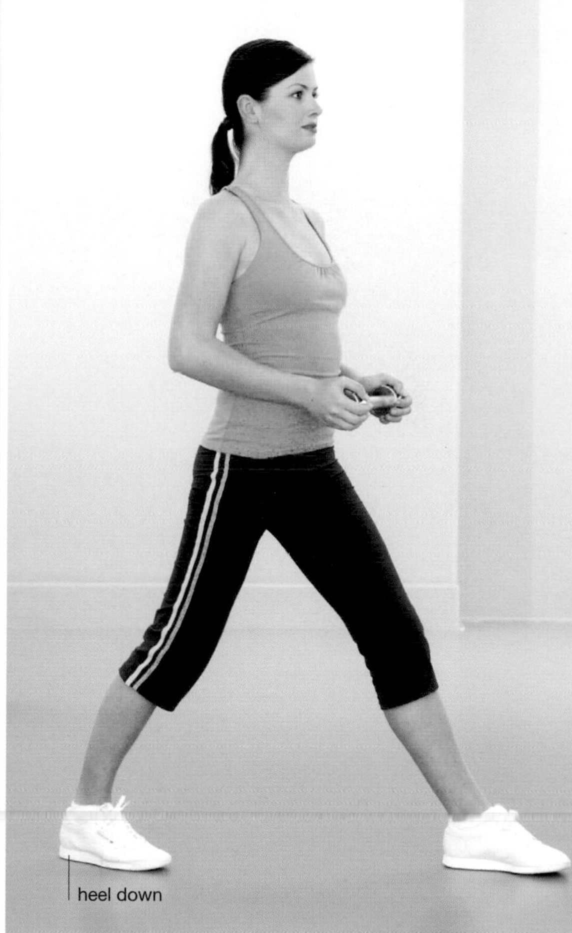

>> **resistance** lunge & twist

11b Inhale as you bend both knees into a low lunge. Bend your front knee at a right angle directly over the ankle, the thigh parallel to the floor; bend your back knee close to the floor with the back heel lifted. As you come into the lunge, twist through your torso, reaching the weight toward your little toe. Keep your shoulder blades drawn together and your head and neck aligned with your spine, being careful not to round the upper back.

11c Exhale as you return to the starting position and then lift the weight high on a diagonal above your opposite shoulder, elbows bent. Keep looking forward. Do 6 reps of the sequence, bending your knees into a lunge as you lower the weight before lifting it again. Switch sides for another 6 reps. **Then do your next cardio interval, Steps 8–10 (pp72–73).**

keep spine straight
lift heel up

twist through torso
feel it here

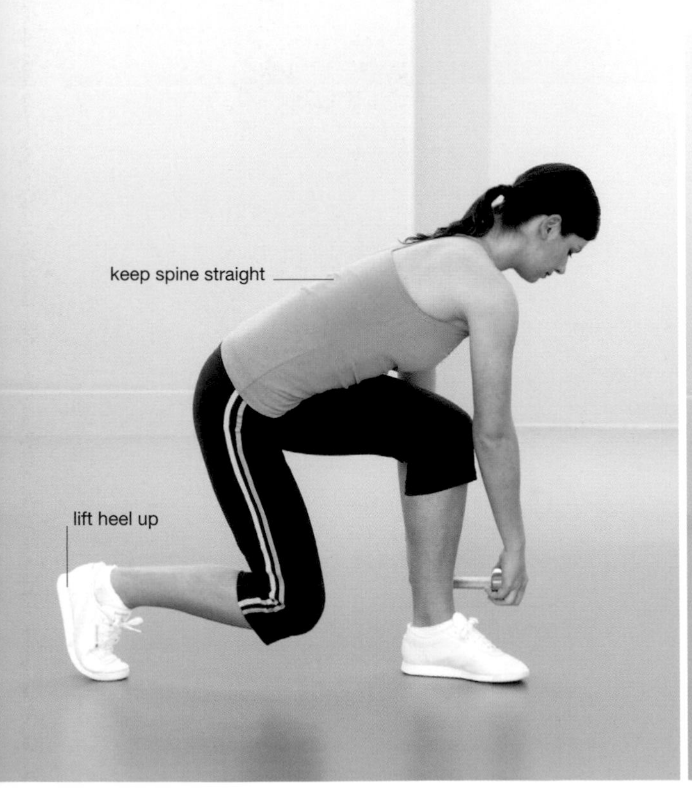

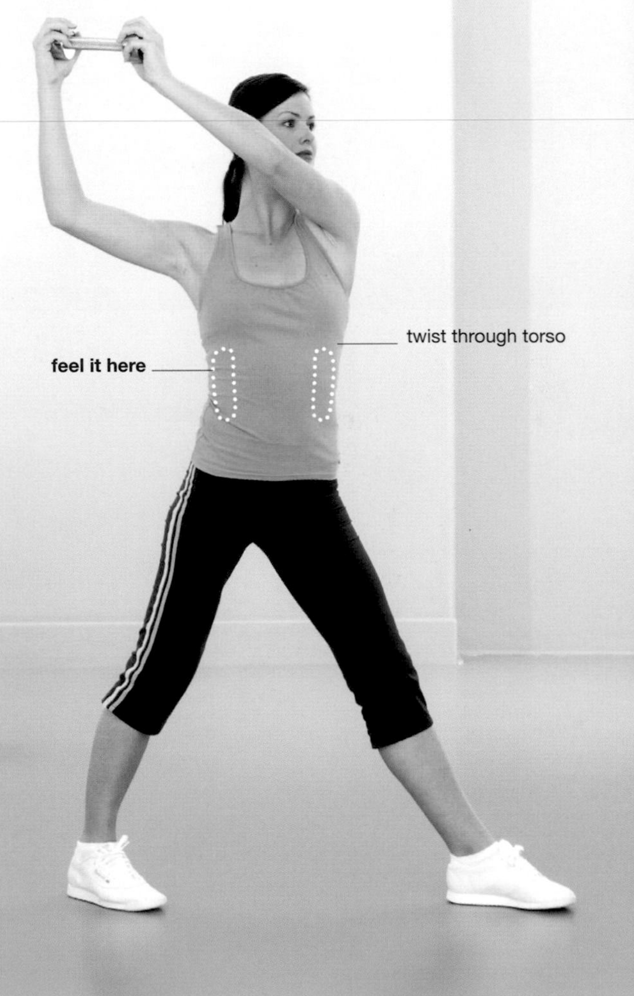

>> **resistance** side-squat, jump

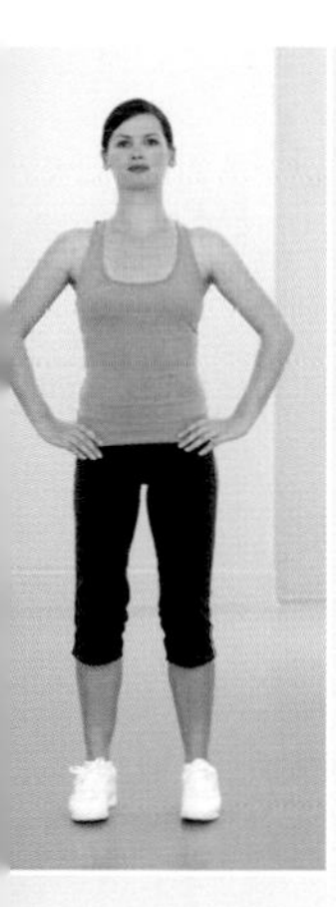

12a **Side-Squat, Jump** Stand with your feet parallel, hip width apart, knees soft, your hands on your hips. Step one leg to the side so that your feet are shoulder width apart. Shift your weight back onto your heels as you bend your knees into a squat. Reach back with your hips, keeping your chest lifted.

keep chest lifted
step to the side before squatting

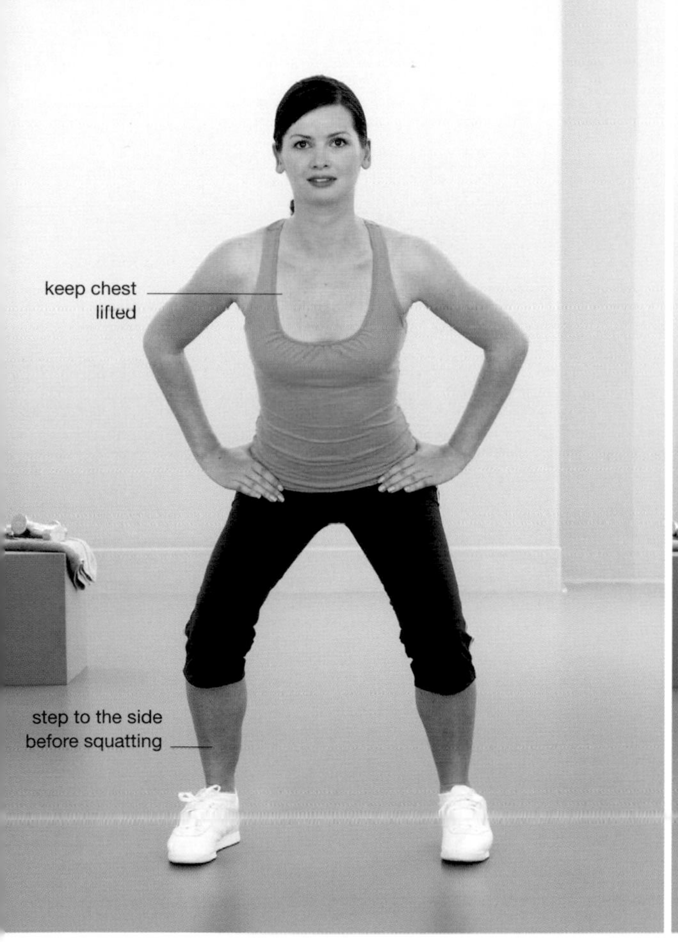

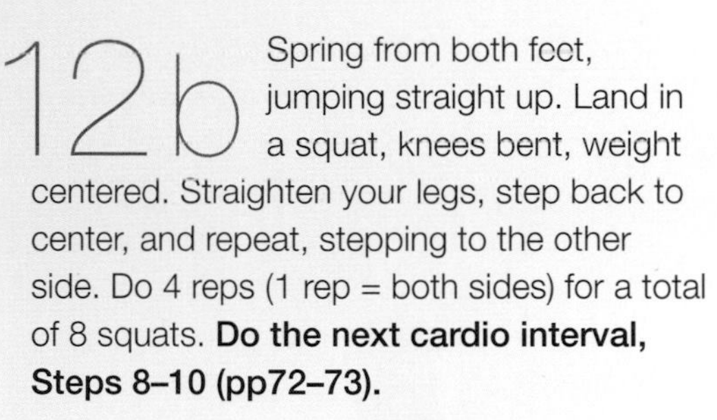

12b Spring from both feet, jumping straight up. Land in a squat, knees bent, weight centered. Straighten your legs, step back to center, and repeat, stepping to the other side. Do 4 reps (1 rep = both sides) for a total of 8 squats. **Do the next cardio interval, Steps 8–10 (pp72–73).**

jump several inches

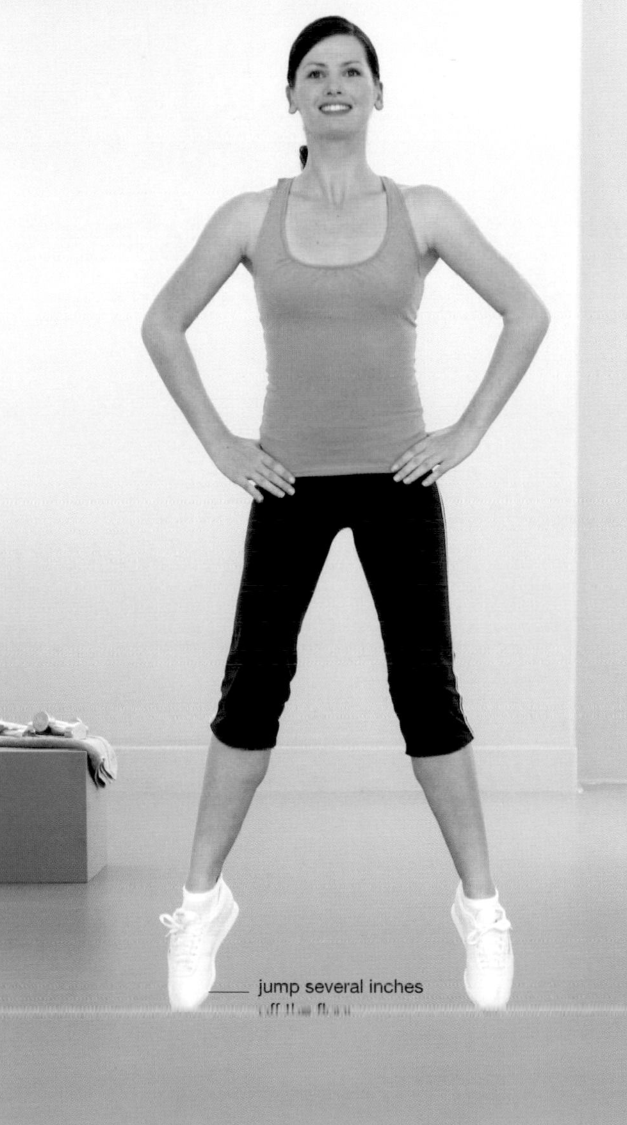

>> **resistance** balance & press/plié & curl

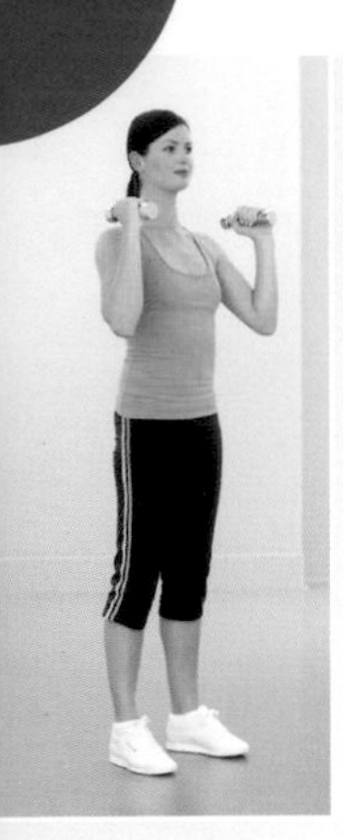

13 **Balance & Press** Stand with feet parallel, hip width apart. Hold two small weights at shoulder height. Exhale, extending one arm, lifting opposite knee. Balance, inhale and step in place, alternating sides for 8 reps (1 rep = both sides). **Do your next cardio interval, Steps 8–10 (pp72–73).**

keep palms facing in
lengthen through spine to maintain balance

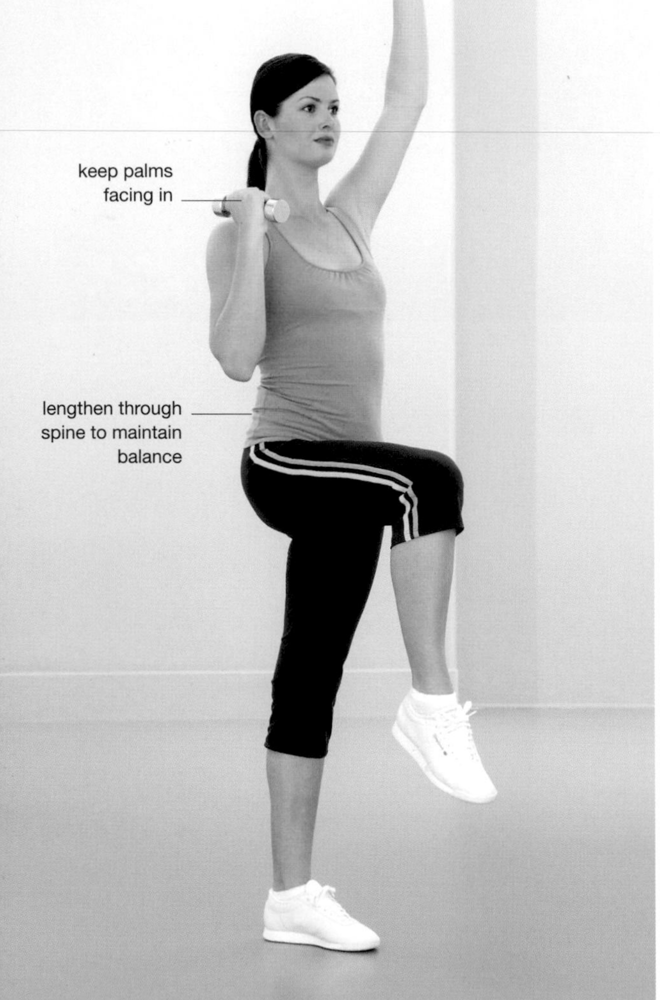

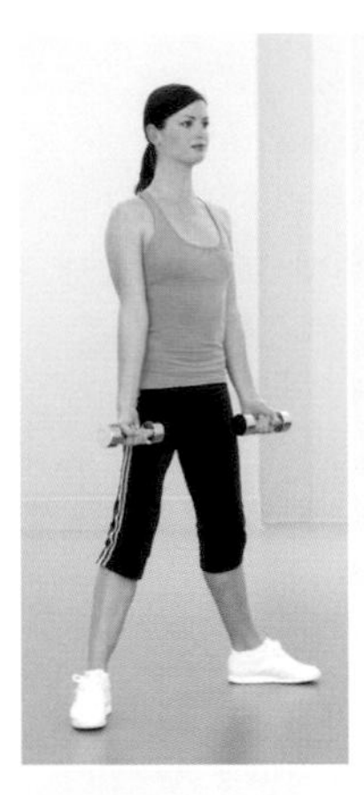

14 **Plié & Curl** Pick up two large weights, holding one in each hand. Stand in a wide stance, legs turned out to 45°. Keep your arms by your sides. Inhale and bend your knees and elbows at the same time, lifting the weights toward your shoulders. Exhale as you straighten your arms and legs. **Do your next cardio interval, Steps 8–10 (pp72–73).**

feel it here
hold elbows close to sides

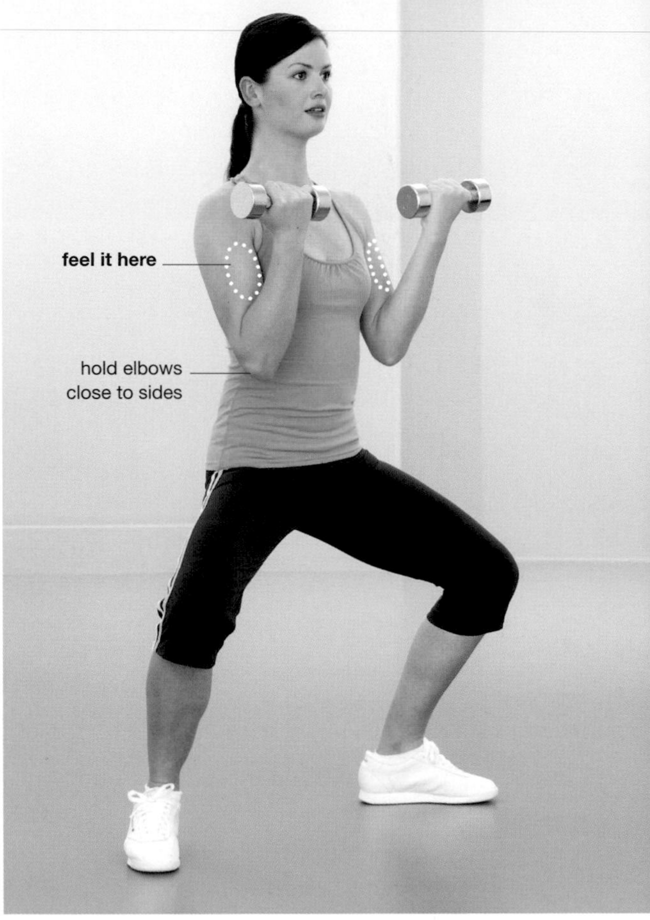

>> **resistance** lateral lift

15a **Lateral Lift** Pick up two small weights. Stand with your feet parallel, hip width apart, knees bent. Hold one weight in each hand, arms by your sides, palms facing inward. Make sure your torso is aligned and ready for action: stack your ribs over your hips, engage the abdominals, draw your shoulder blades down, and lift your chest.

15b Inhale, then exhale as you straighten your legs, lifting one to the side, as you raise both arms to shoulder height, palms down. Your arms should be straight but not stiff. Inhale, then return to the starting position, bending the knees and squaring the hips. Alternate legs, lifting both arms every time for 12 reps (1 rep = both sides).

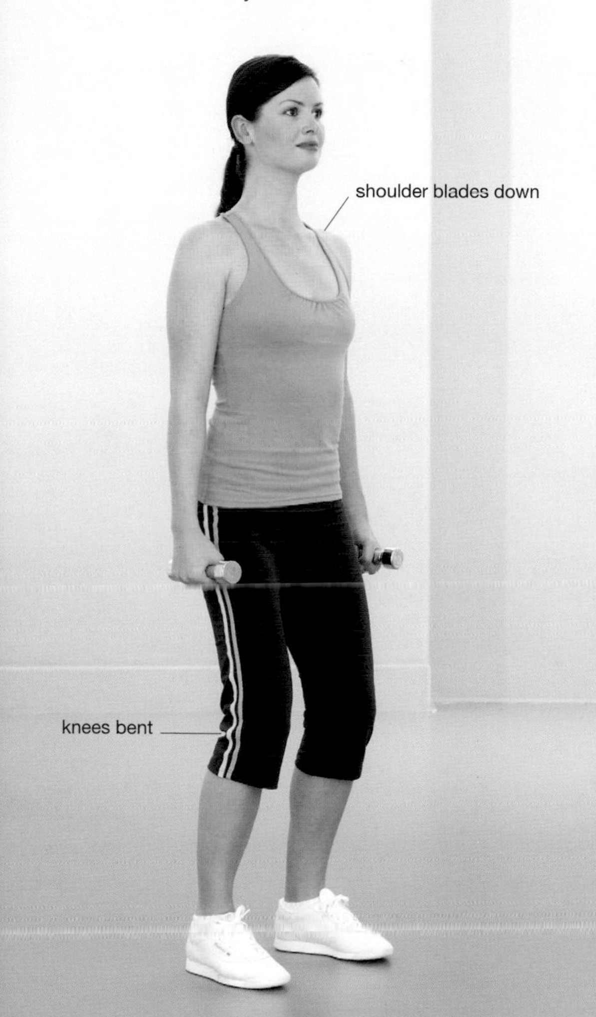

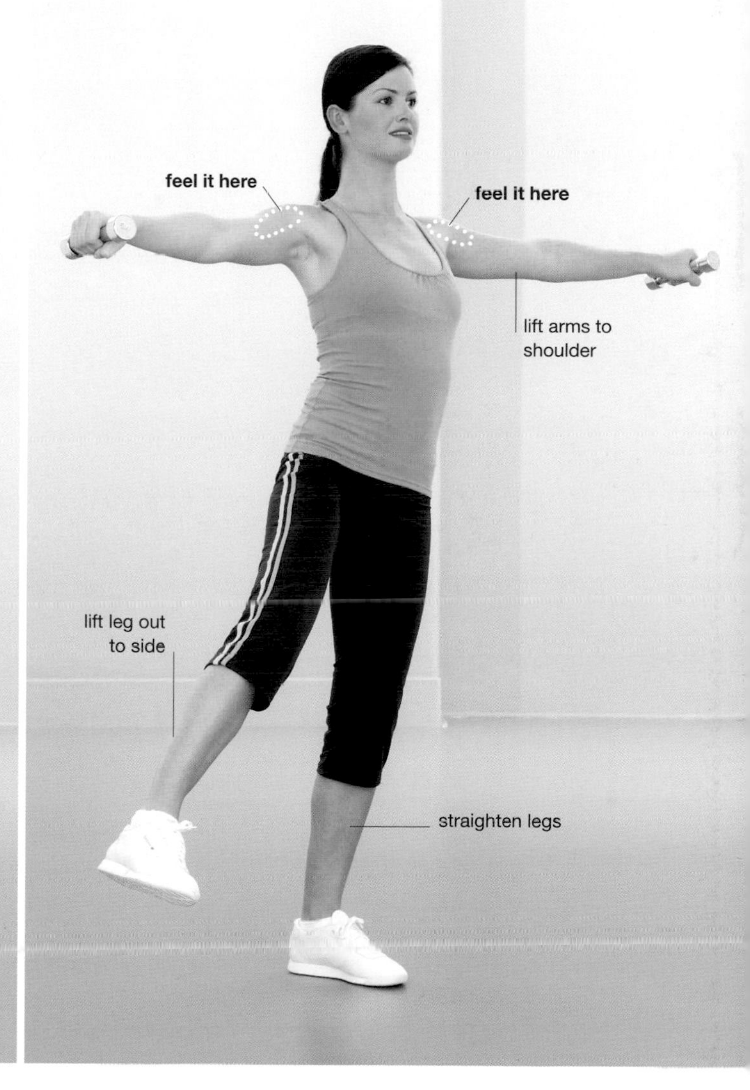

>> **cool down** flat back stretch/spinal twist

16 **Flat Back Stretch** Get your mat for the cool down, and stand with your legs hip width apart, hands on your hips. Lengthen through the spine, lifting the top of your head toward the ceiling. Draw your shoulder blades down and together. Bend forward from your hips until your back is parallel to the floor, still elongating the spine by reaching your head forward. Keep your knees straight, but not locked. Breathe deeply while you hold the stretch.

feel it here
keep legs straight
but not stiff

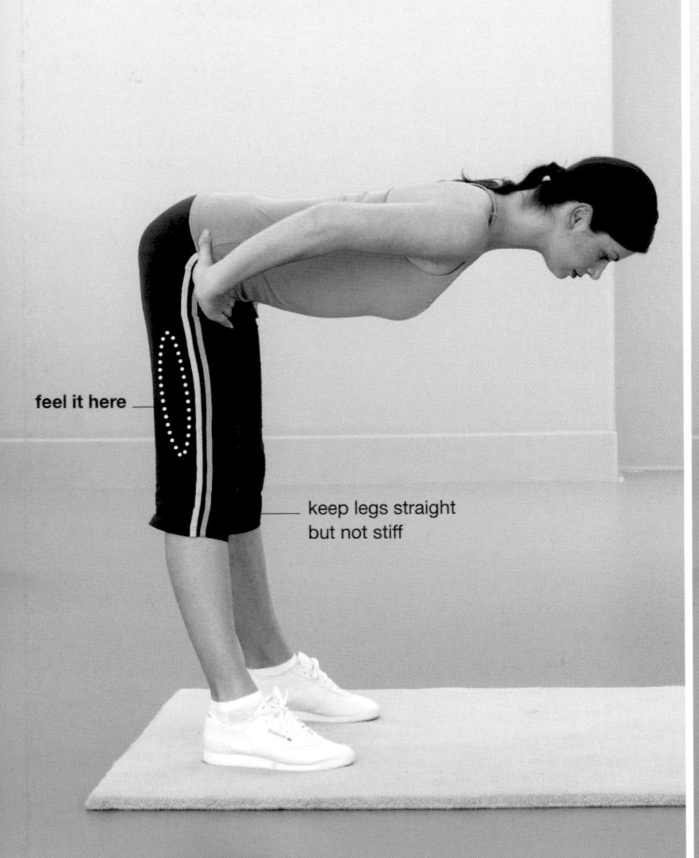

17 **Spinal Twist** From the flat back position, reach one hand across your body to the opposite foot, and lift the other arm straight up to the ceiling, palm forward. If you are able, press the heel of the supporting hand down on the mat. However, you may be more comfortable resting it on your ankle. Keep your knees straight and your hips level. Breathe naturally throughout, then switch sides and repeat.

keep hips level
feel it here

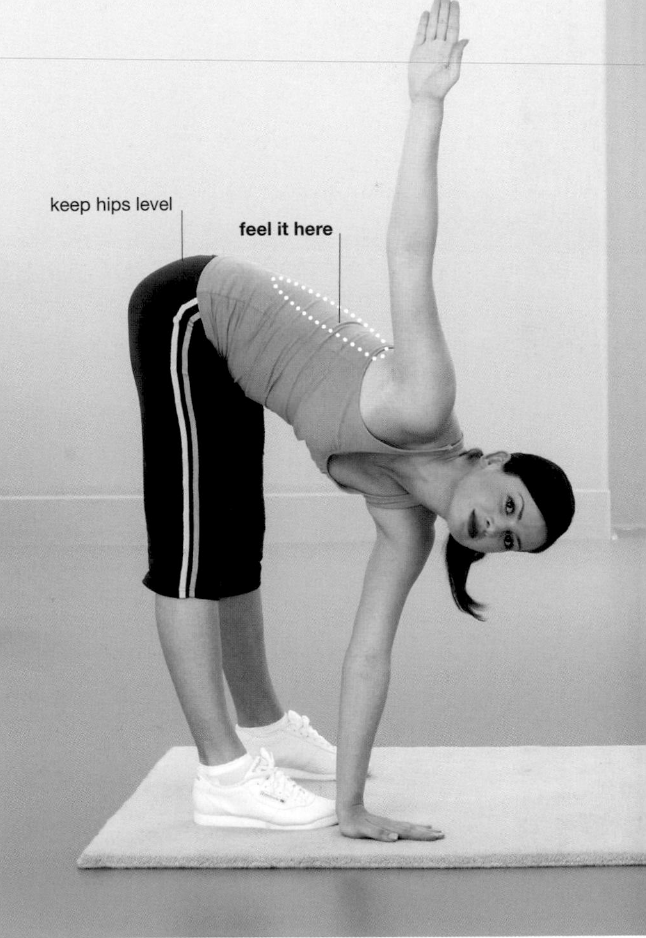

>> **cool down** glute stretch/arm & leg lift

head and neck
aligned with spine
place feet parallel,
hip width apart

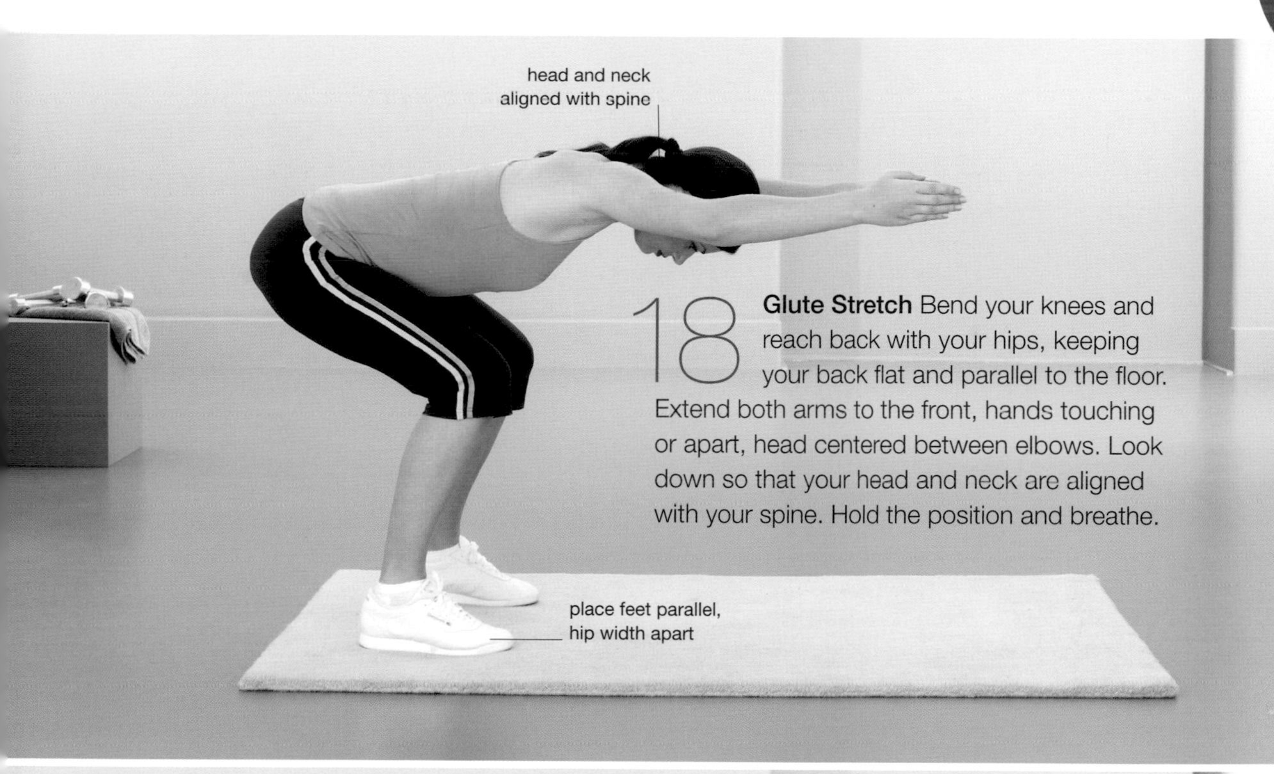

18 **Glute Stretch** Bend your knees and reach back with your hips, keeping your back flat and parallel to the floor. Extend both arms to the front, hands touching or apart, head centered between elbows. Look down so that your head and neck are aligned with your spine. Hold the position and breathe.

19 **Arm and Leg Lift** Kneel on all fours, wrists beneath shoulders, knees under hips. Lift one leg to the back, keeping the knee straight, then reach forward with the opposite hand. Use deep breathing to increase the stretch, reaching further on every exhale.

hold leg at
hip height

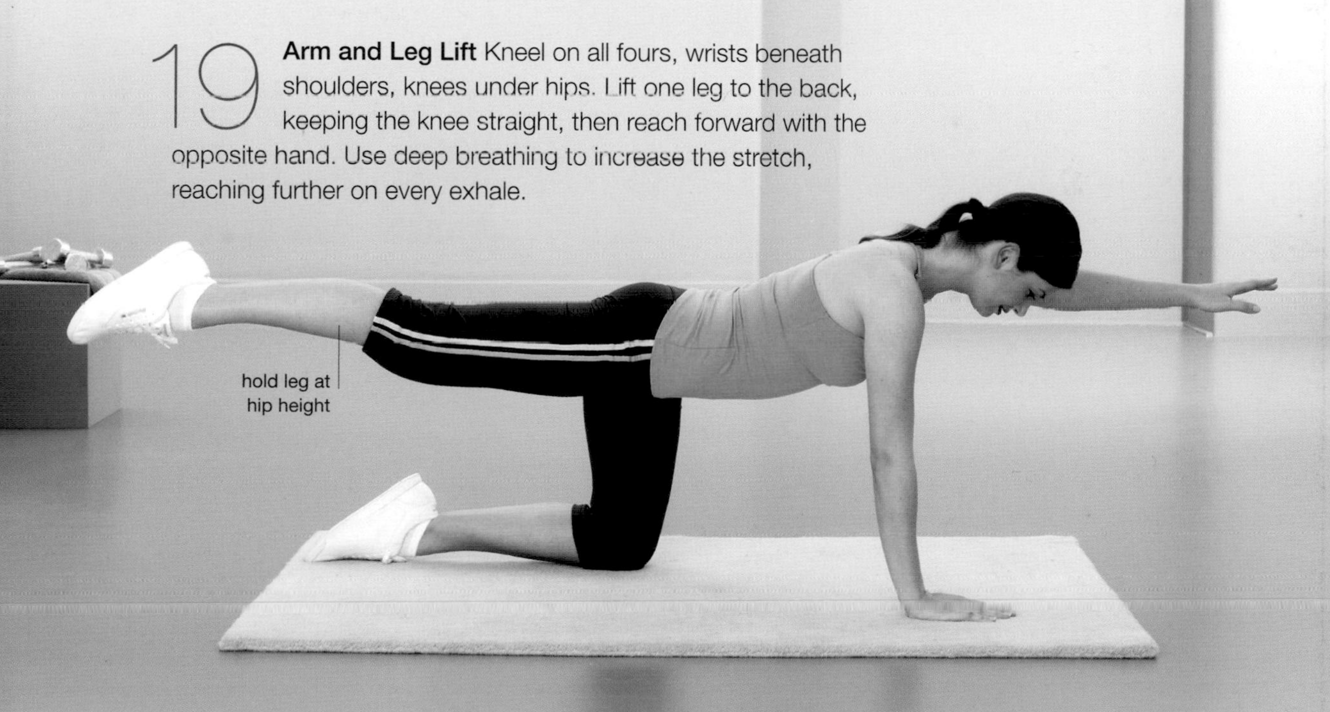

>> **cool down** calf stretch/spinal curve

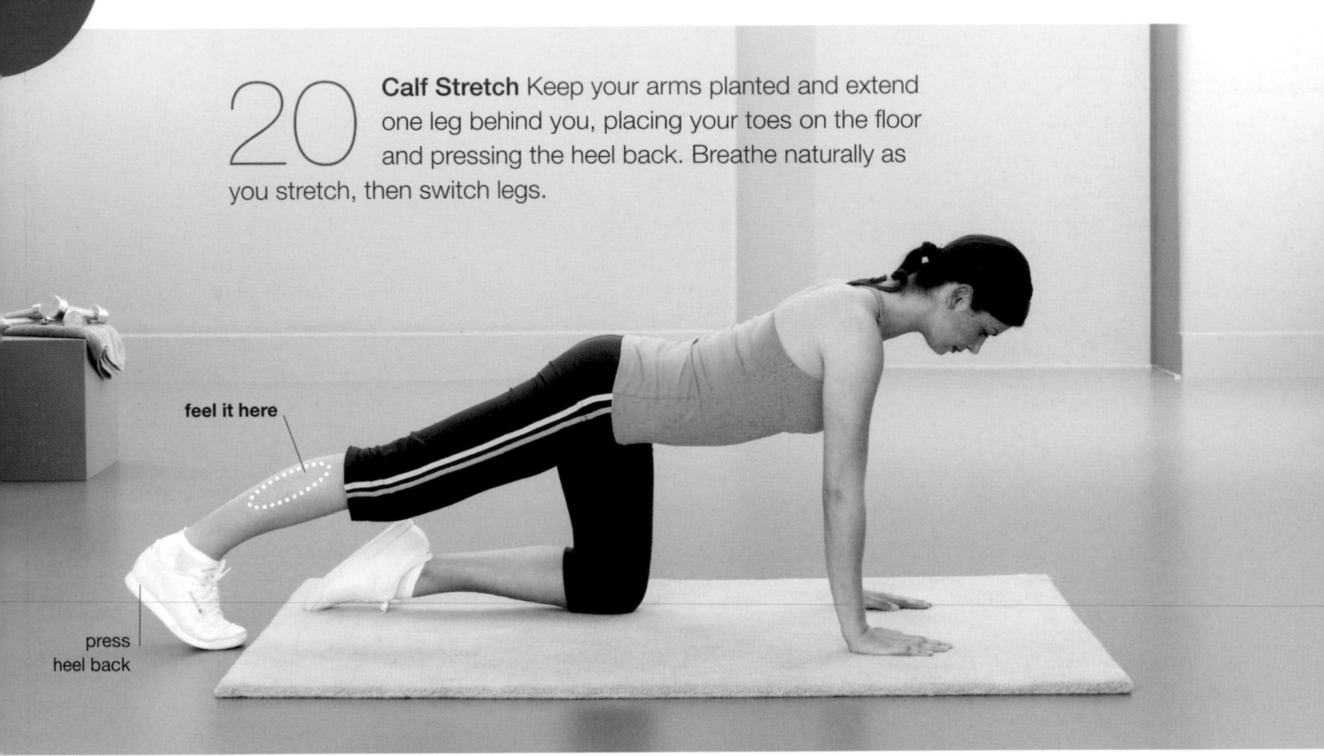

20 **Calf Stretch** Keep your arms planted and extend one leg behind you, placing your toes on the floor and pressing the heel back. Breathe naturally as you stretch, then switch legs.

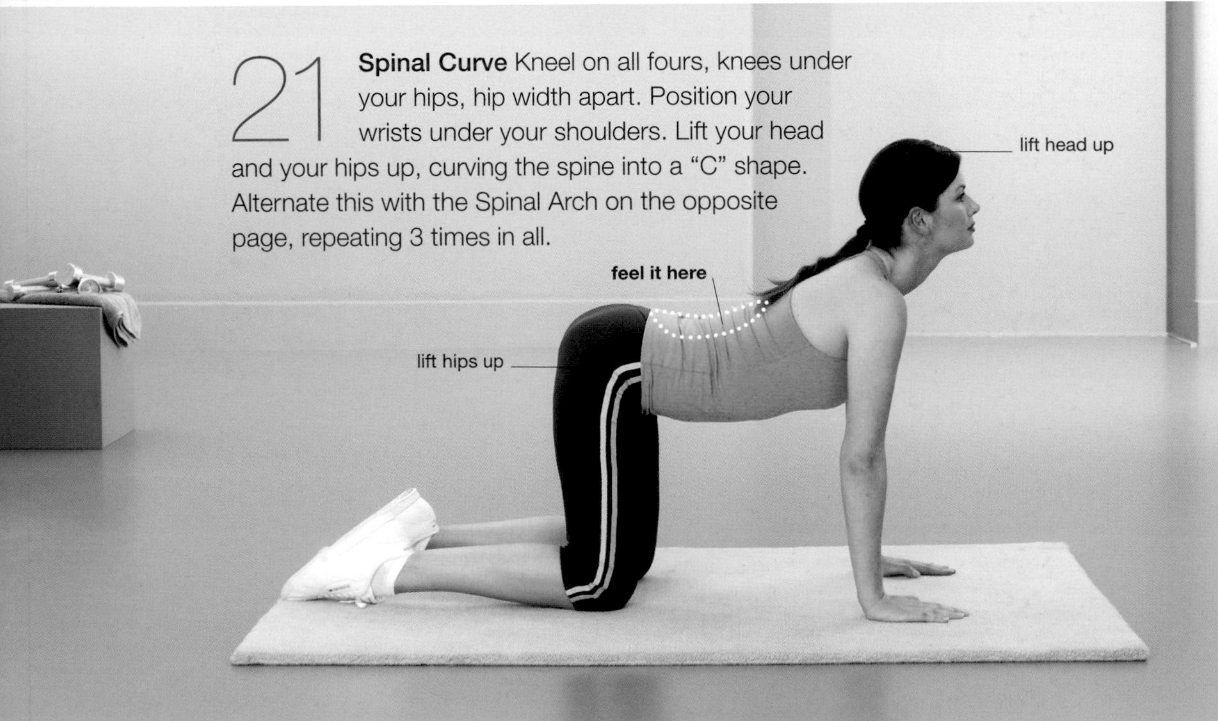

21 **Spinal Curve** Kneel on all fours, knees under your hips, hip width apart. Position your wrists under your shoulders. Lift your head and your hips up, curving the spine into a "C" shape. Alternate this with the Spinal Arch on the opposite page, repeating 3 times in all.

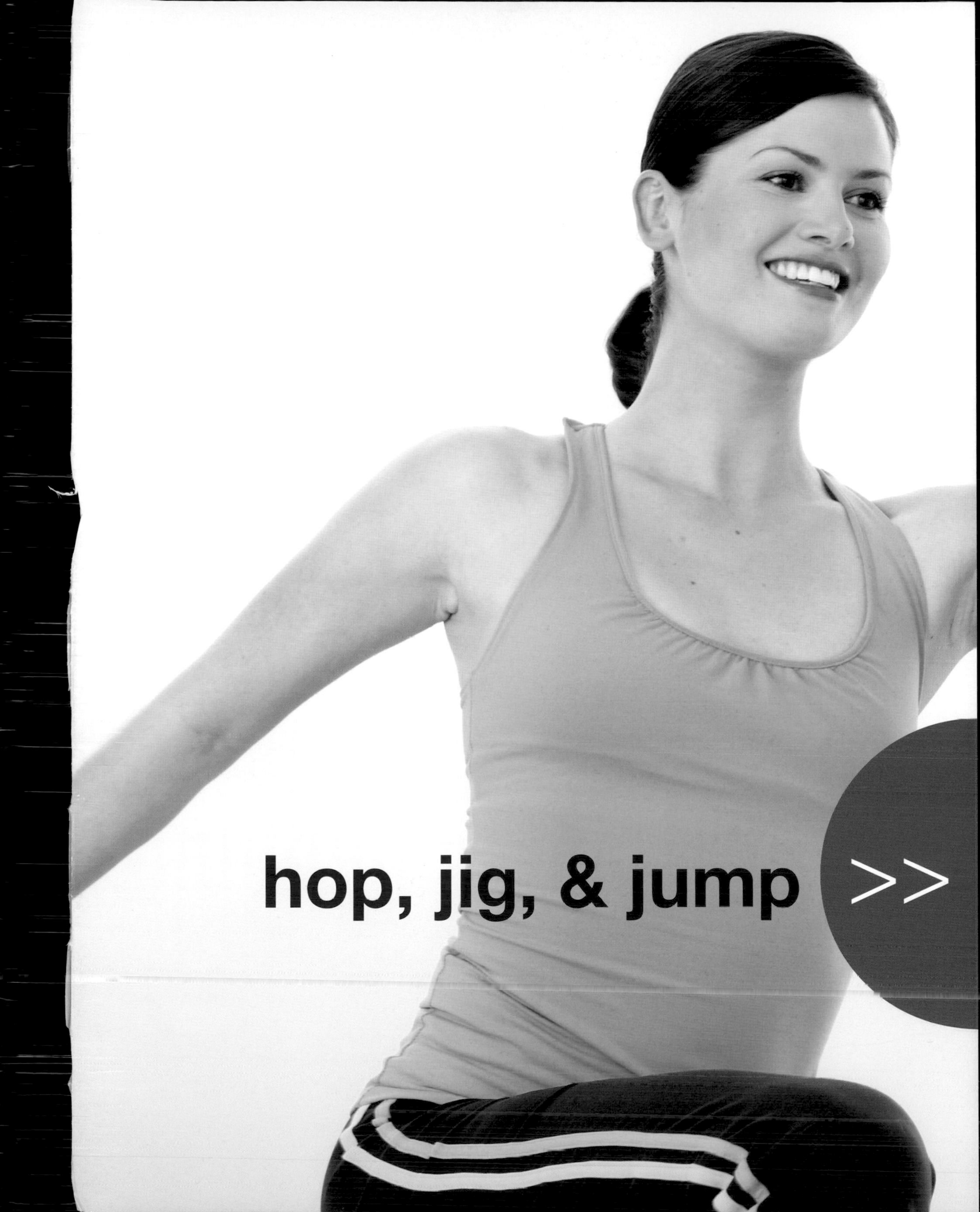

hop, jig, & jump >>

hop, jig, & jump at a glance

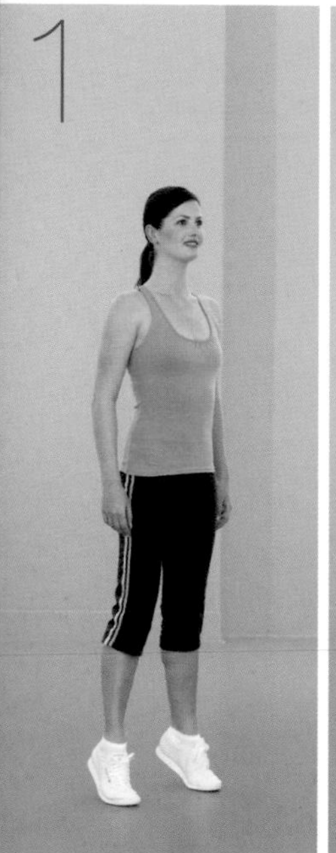

▲ **Warm up,** Bend & Raise, page 68

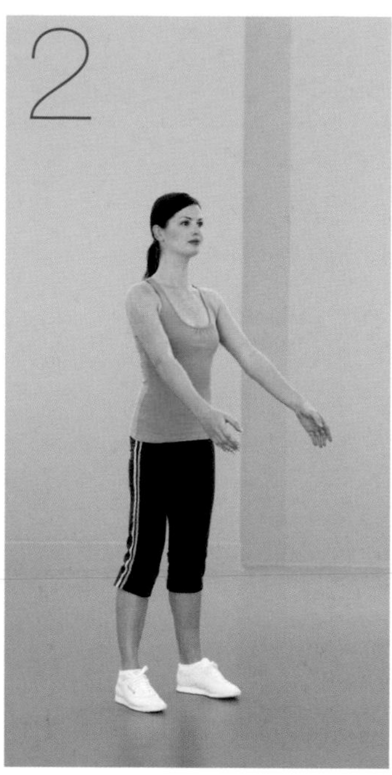

▲ **Warm up,** Double Arm Swing, page 68

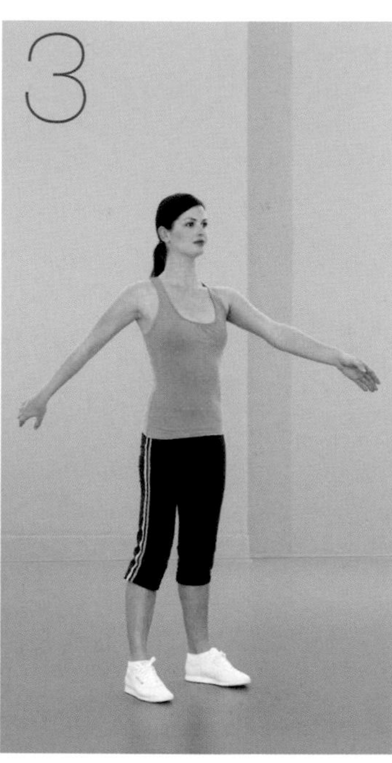

▲ **Warm up,** Single Arm Swing, page 69

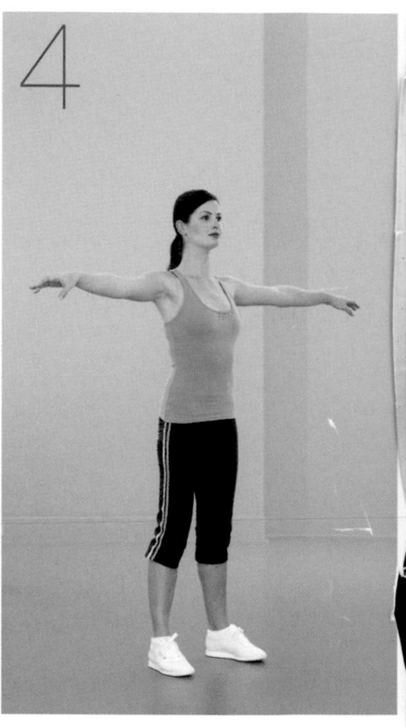

▲ **Warm up,** Cross & Open, page 69

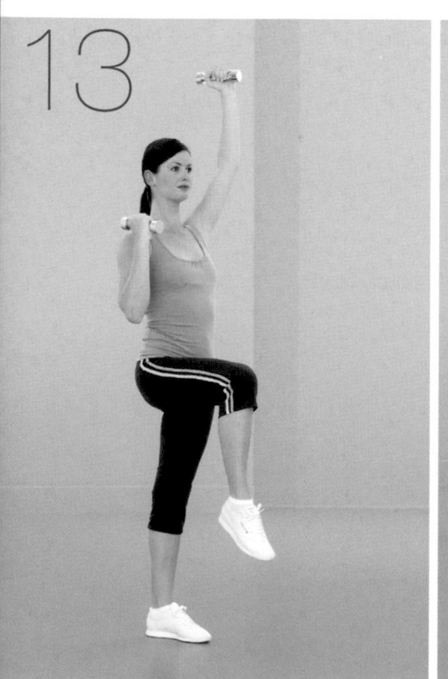

▲ **Resistance,** Balance & Press, page 76. Repeat Steps 8–10

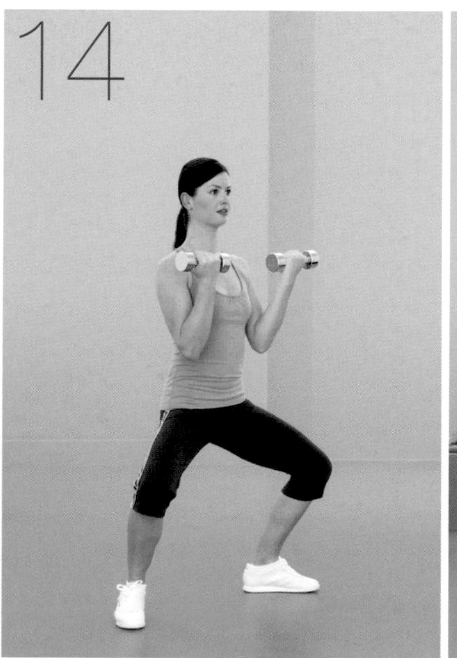

▲ **Resistance,** Plié & Curl, page 76. Repeat Steps 8–10

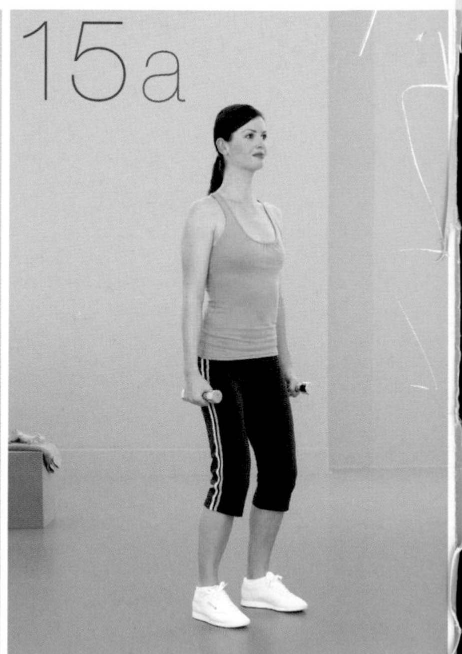

▲ **Resistance,** Lateral Lift, page 77.

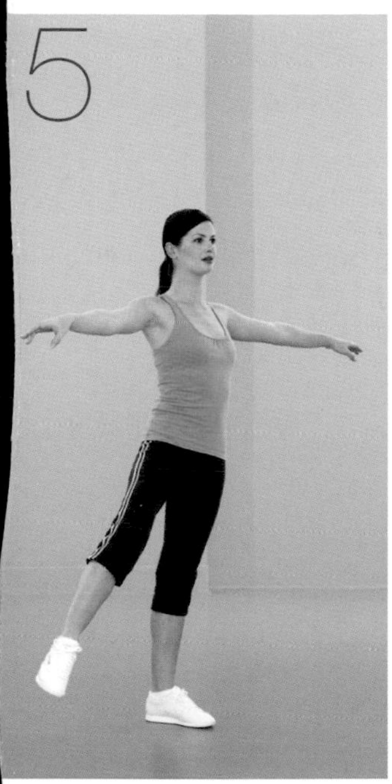

▲ **Warm up,** Lateral Lift, page 70

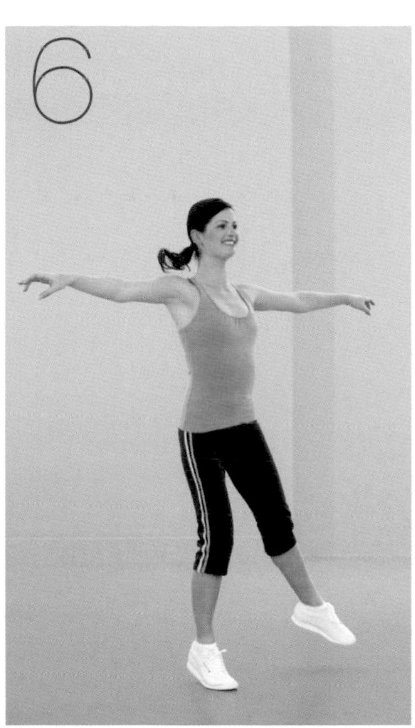

▲ **Warm up,** Jumping Jack, page 70. Repeat Steps 5–1

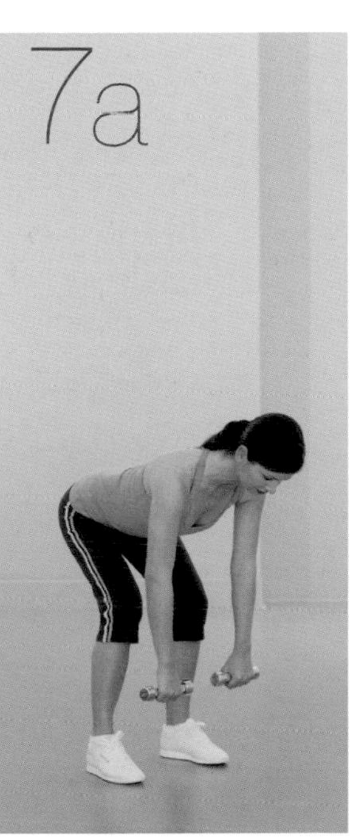

▲ **Resistance,** Hip Hinge & Reverse Fly, page 71

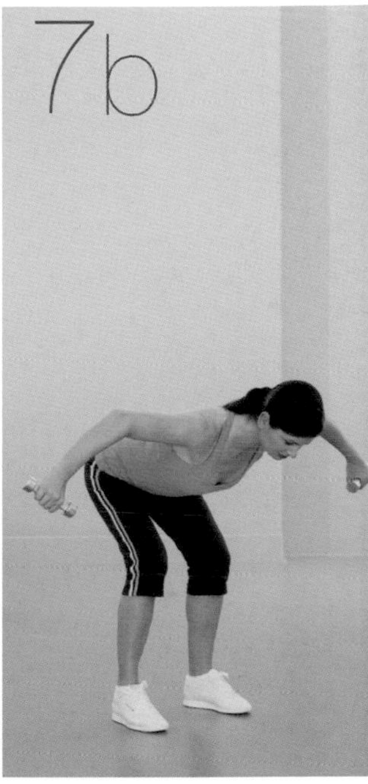

▲ **Resistance,** Hip Hinge & Reverse Fly, page 71

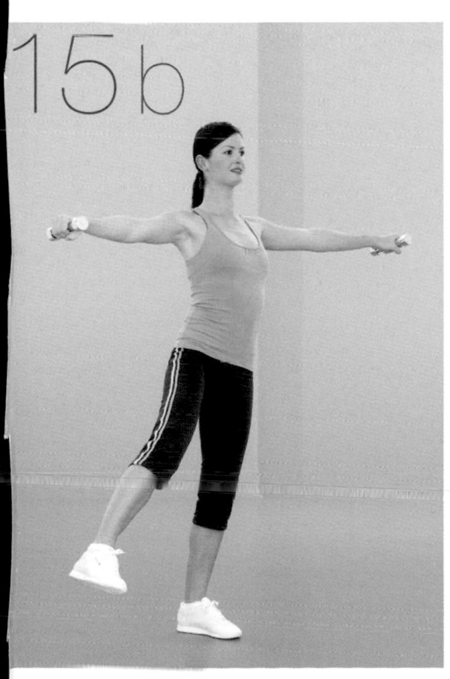

▲ **Resistance,** Lateral Lift, page 77.

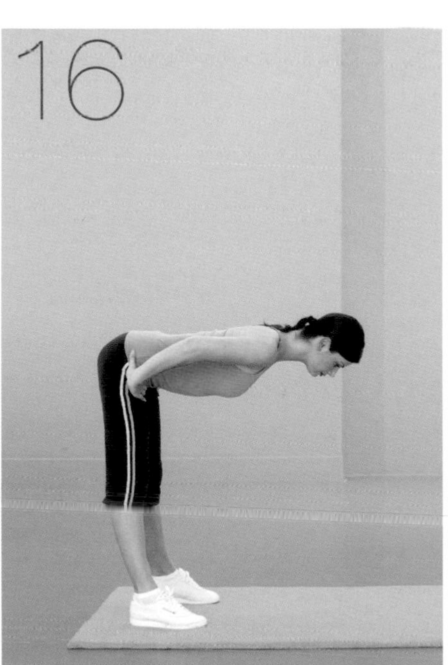

▲ **Cool down,** Flat Back Stretch, page 78

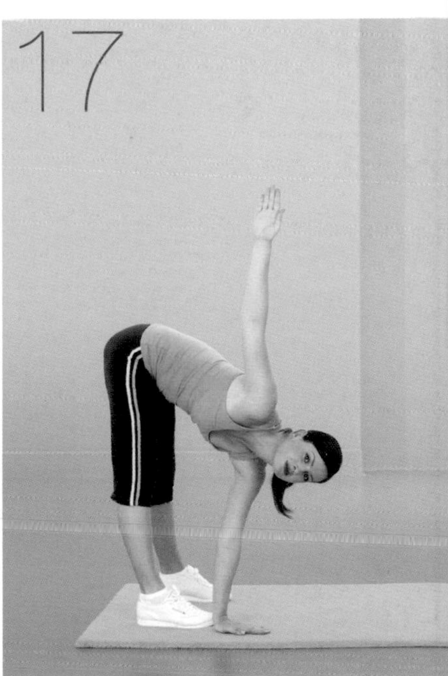

▲ **Cool down,** Spinal Twist, page 78

>> cool down spinal arch/child's pose

22 **Spinal Arch** Start from a kneeling positon, knees under hips, wrists under shoulders, your back neutral. Then arch your spine, rounding it up to the ceiling by tucking your hips under and dropping your head between your arms. Alternate this with Spinal Curve (opposite page), repeating 3 times in all.

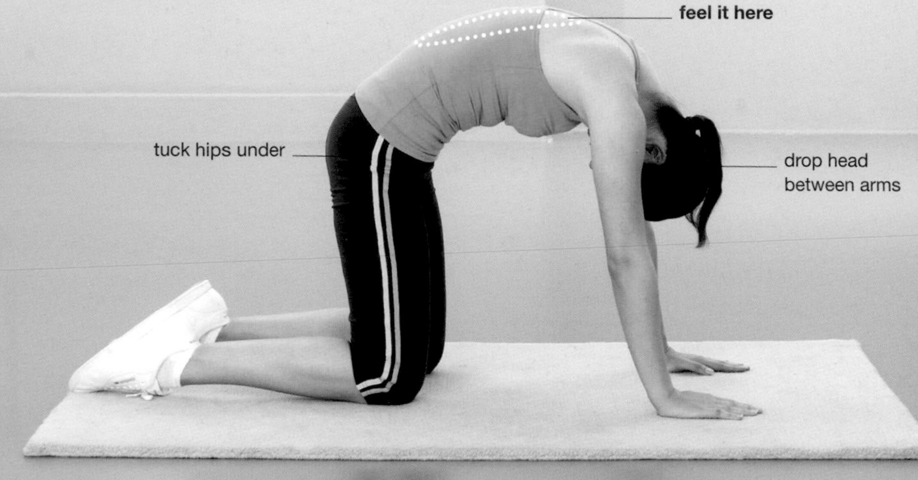

23 **Child's Pose** Sit back, reaching your hips toward your heels, at the same time rounding forward and extending your arms in front of you until your head rests on the mat. Keep your elbows off the mat to get the best stretch. Sink down into the position, holding for 3 deep breathing cycles, and sinking deeper into the position with each exhalation.

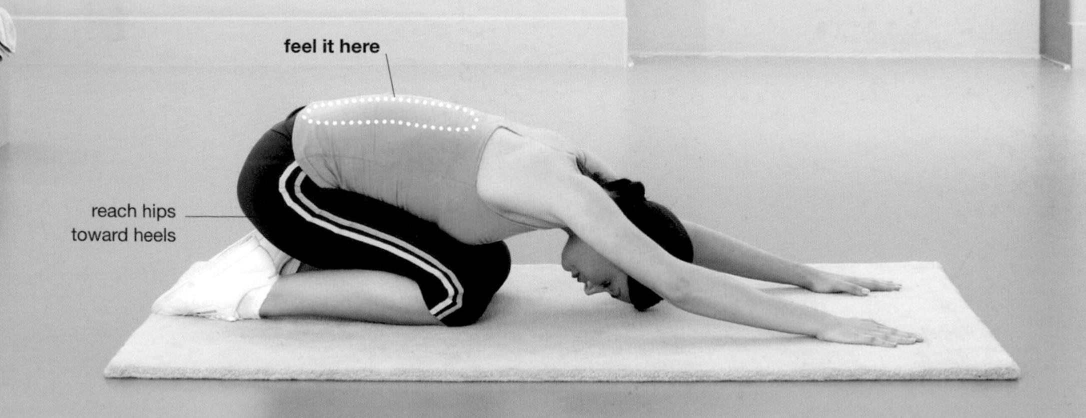

>> **frequently** asked questions

Even when you have the best intentions, it can be difficult to maintain the motivation required to get the most from your workouts. There are common reasons why this happens, so if you find that you are feeling unmotivated, follow this advice to get back on track.

>> I'm finding it hard to establish a regular exercise routine. How can I start the habit?

With a basic workout taking just 15 minutes, it is more likely that you can't find the "right time" to exercise, rather than not having the time at all. Try to align your program with your personal preferences, and stick to a regular time—if you find you have more energy in the morning, plan to exercise then. A little advance planning in terms of your goals and expectations can go a long way to keeping you on track. And remember to stay positive and focused on what you *can* achieve, rather than what you can't.

>> I'm finding the workout rather easy—am I working hard enough?

The routines cover a range of intensities, so explore them all to find the ones that challenge you appropriately. Step-Touch (see p18) is the most gentle; if it is too easy, you might use it as a warm up for one of the other more vigorous routines. Lunge Around the Clock (see p90) is the most advanced in terms of the movements. In any workout, you can raise the intensity by increasing the range of motion: lift your legs higher, lengthen your reach, bend your knees deeper, jump higher or add a kick or a leg lift where it fits.

>> I'm finding the workout exhausting—what should I do?

If the weights are too heavy to complete the sequence in good form, use lighter weights. If the cardio intervals leave you breathless, you can modify the intensity by making the leg movements smaller or by leaving out the arm movements. If you are feeling very tired, march on the spot—it's important to keep moving to pump blood to the heart and brain, or else you may feel dizzy.

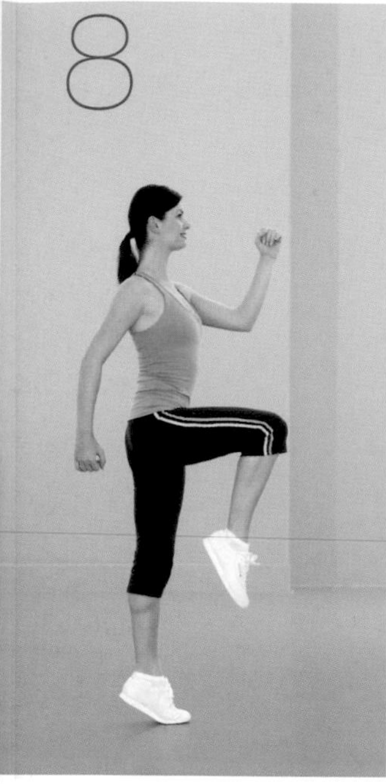

▲ **Cardio,** Step-Hop, page 72

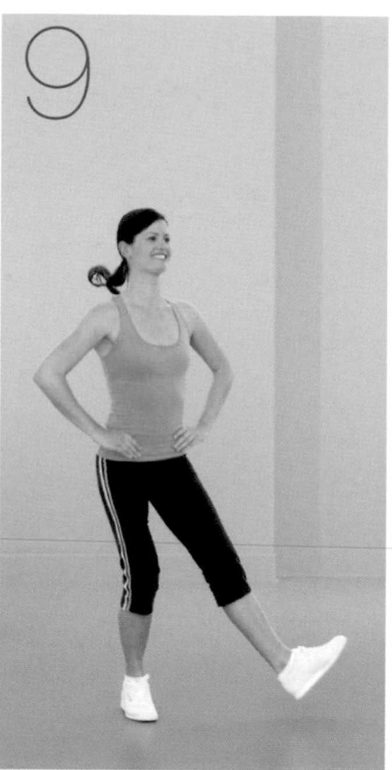

▲ **Cardio,** Jig, page 72

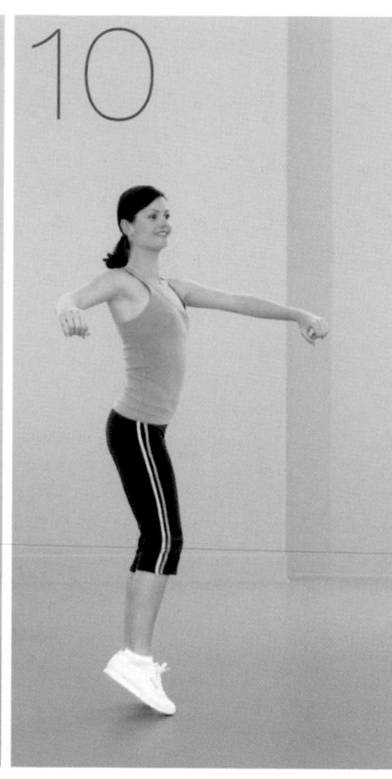

▲ **Cardio,** Jump & Twist, page 73

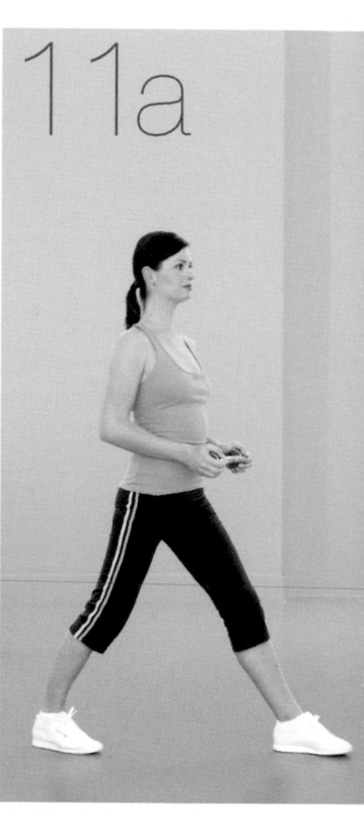

▲ **Resistance,** Lunge & Twist, page 73

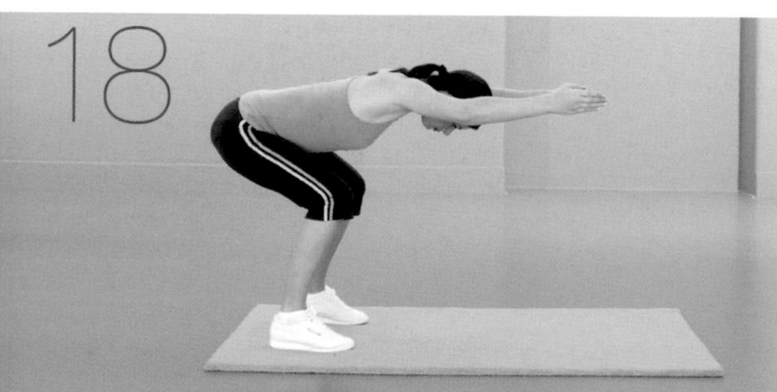

▲ **Cool down,** Glute Stretch, page 79

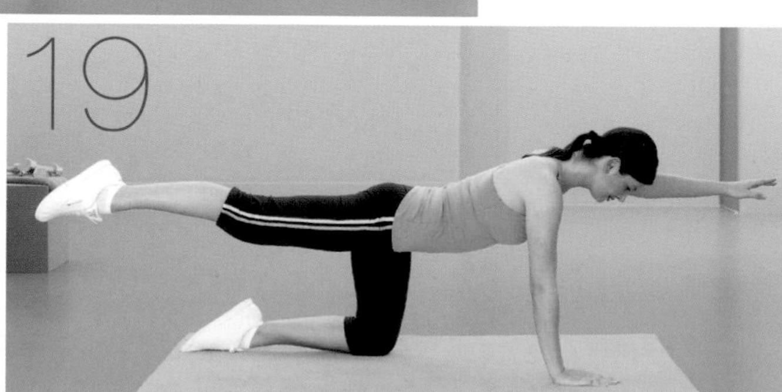

▲ **Cool-down,** Arm & Leg Lift, page 79

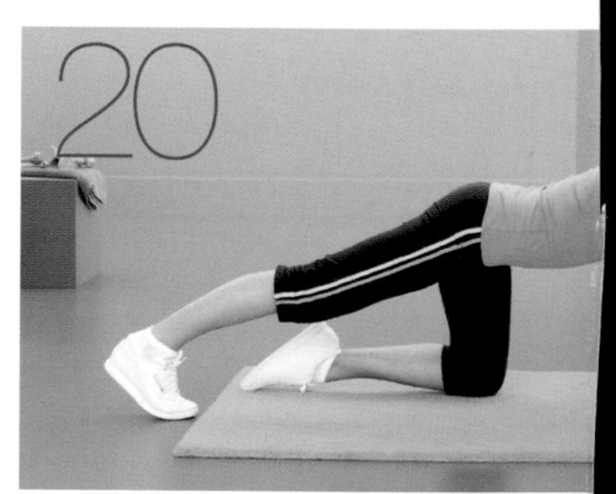

▲ **Cool down,** Calf Stretch, page 80

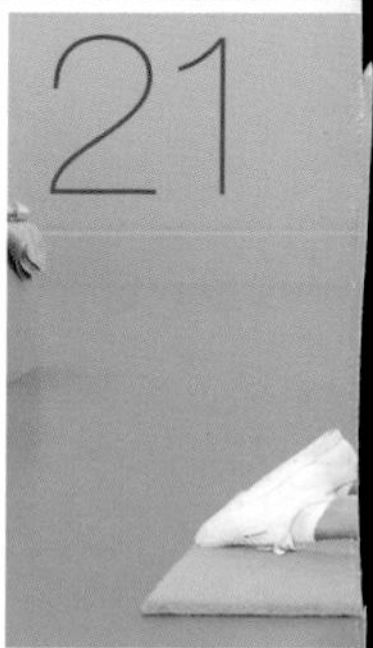

▲ **Cool down,** Sp

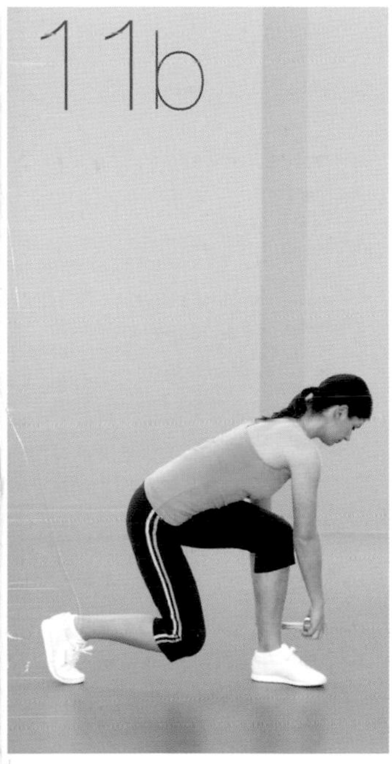

▲ **Resistance,** Lunge & Twist, page 74

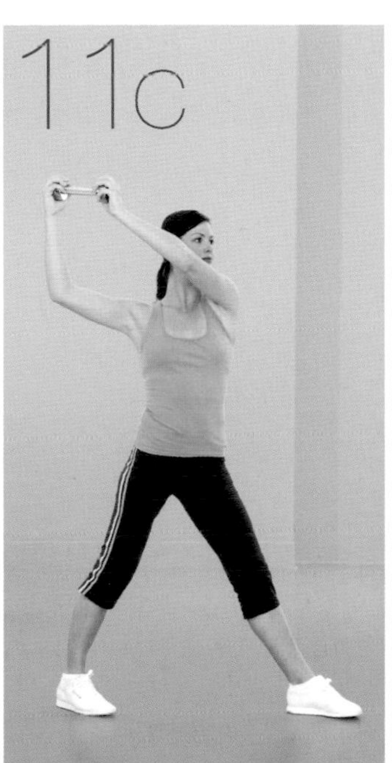

▲ **Resistance,** Lunge & Twist, page 74. Repeat Steps 8–10

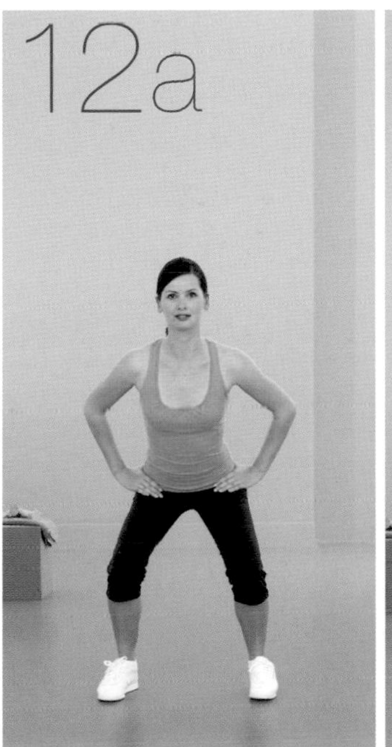

12b

▲ **Resistance,** Side-Squat, Jump page 75. Repeat Steps 8–10

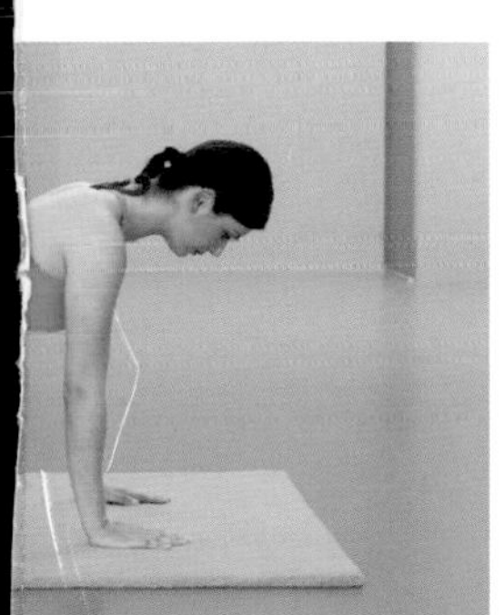

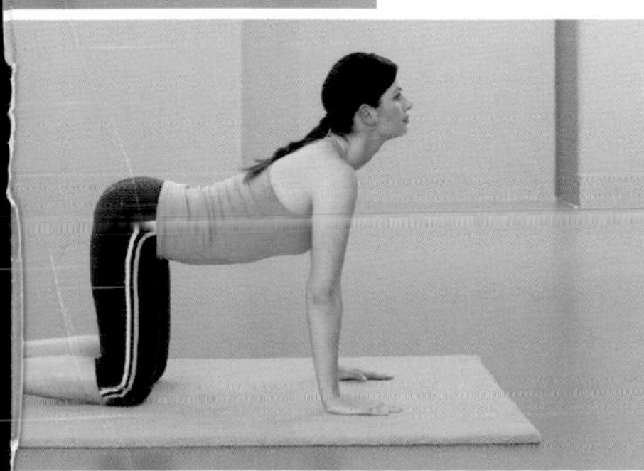

inal Curve, page 80

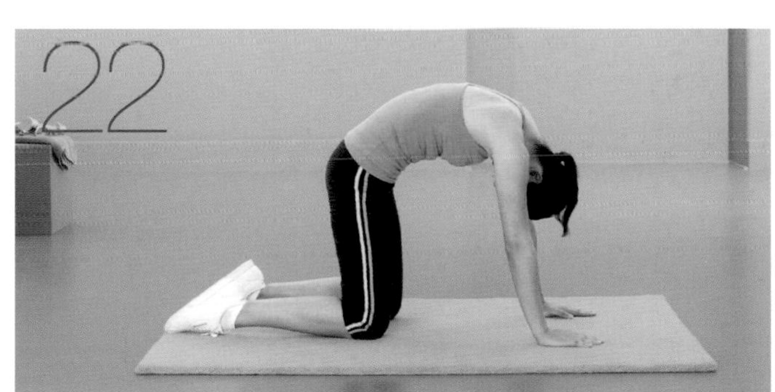

▲ **Cool down,** Spinal Arch, page 81

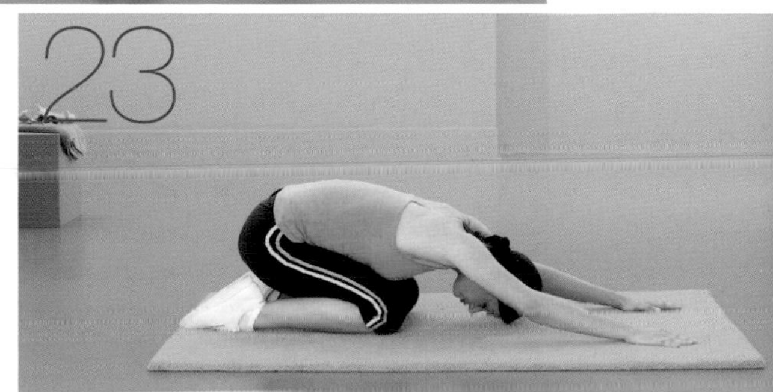

▲ **Cool down,** Child's Pose, page 81

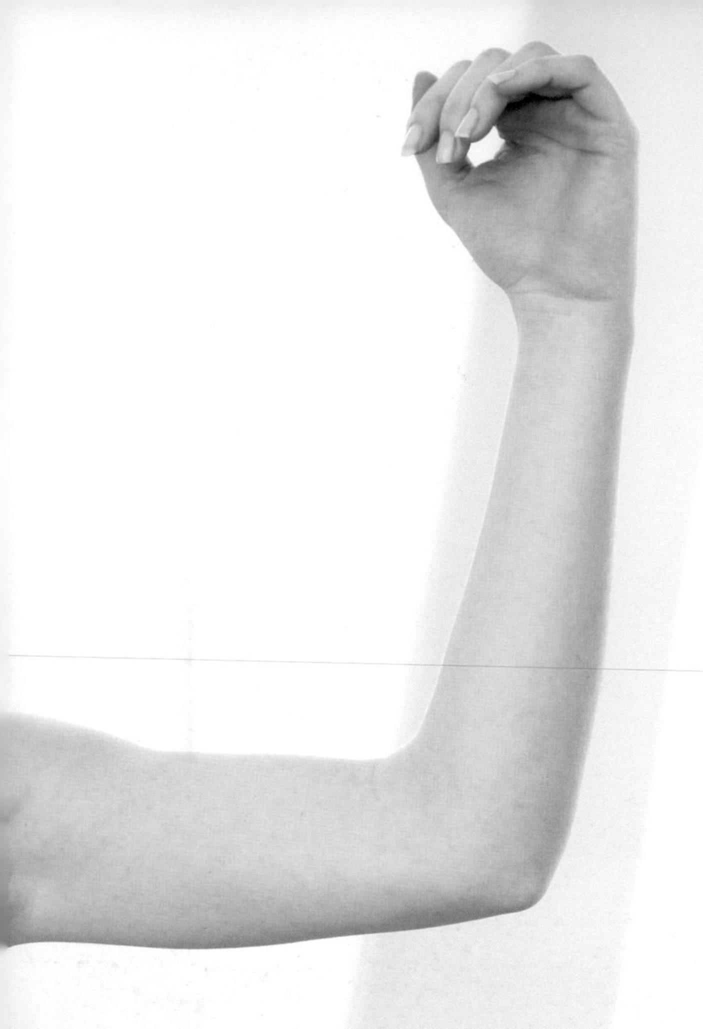

15 minute **summary**

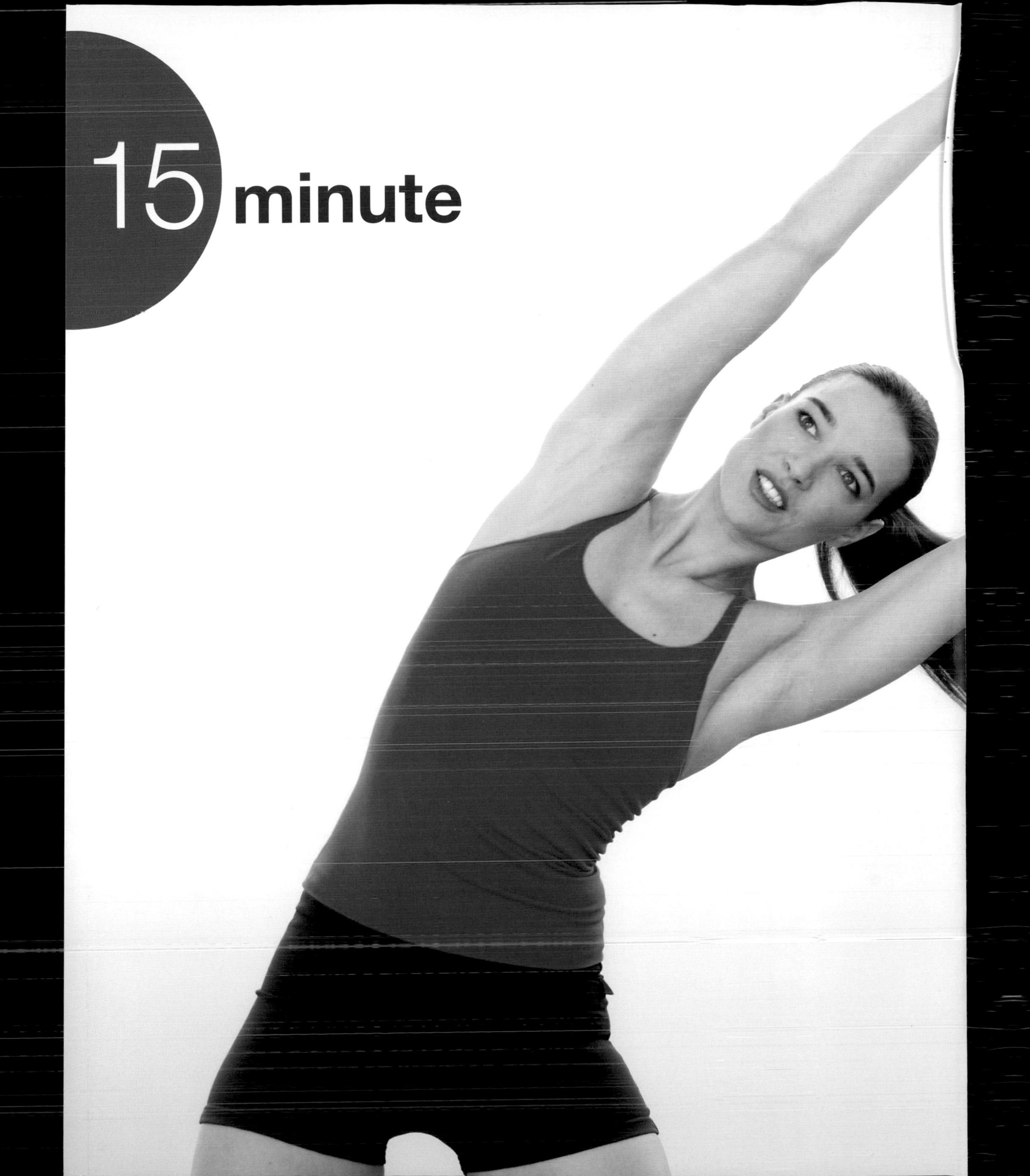
15 minute

>> How do I know which goals are realistic for me to achieve?

Devise a plan to make your intentions clear and focus your efforts. Establish control of the situation by ensuring that your goals are realistic and attainable. Begin and proceed at your own pace and be consistent. Define obstacles and find solutions ("I need to find time in my schedule"; "How can I make this convenient?"). Create a supportive environment and ask for the support of others (a friend or partner). Reward yourself healthfully—pamper yourself with a bubble bath or a massage (see SMART tips on goal setting, p10).

>> How do I know if I'm working at a safe level?

Your heart rate training range determines how hard you should work for light, moderate, and high-intensity levels. The traditional, easy-to-use formula of "220 minus your age" gives an estimate of your maximum heart rate (EMHR). Take 65–95 percent of your EMHR to develop a training range with a continuum of low to high intensity. Use the "talk test" as a simple measure of cardiovascular intensity: if you can't talk, the intensity is too hard; if you can sing, it's too easy.

>> My enthusiasm about exercising is starting to lag. How can I jump-start my motivation?

Goal setting is key to staying motivated. Create a goal that's out of your current reach, but still attainable. Pick a goal that is specific to your training, such as fitting into your skinny jeans. Remember that it's normal to have fluctuations in energy levels, but that doesn't mean you are backsliding. Keep your long-term goals in mind and do something every day to advance toward them. When you meet challenges, it's very satisfying and provides even more incentive.

>> I'm not sure the exercise is working. What should I feel the next day?

You may feel "awareness" of the muscles you worked. Starting gradually will minimize any muscle soreness: if you are just beginning an exercise program, or returning after a long absence, start with the Step-Touch program (see p18) three times a week. When that feels easy, progress by either doing it twice in a row for a 30-minute workout, or moving on the Beach Ball workout (see p42).

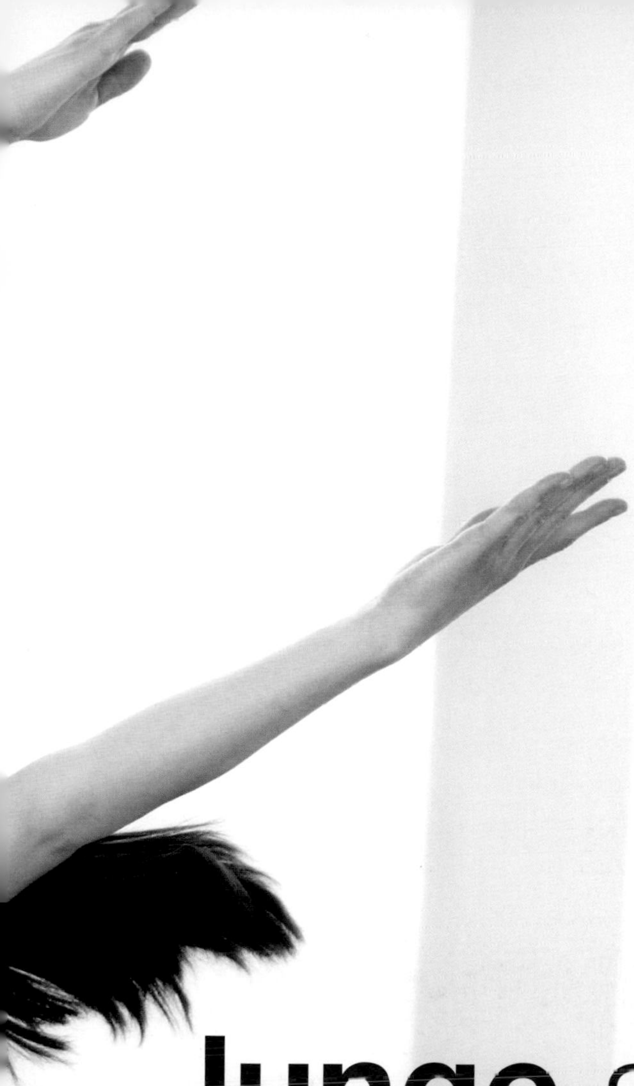

lunge around the clock >>

Challenge yourself with more complex moves to advance your skills and fitness levels

>> **warm up** front lunge/opposite arm raise

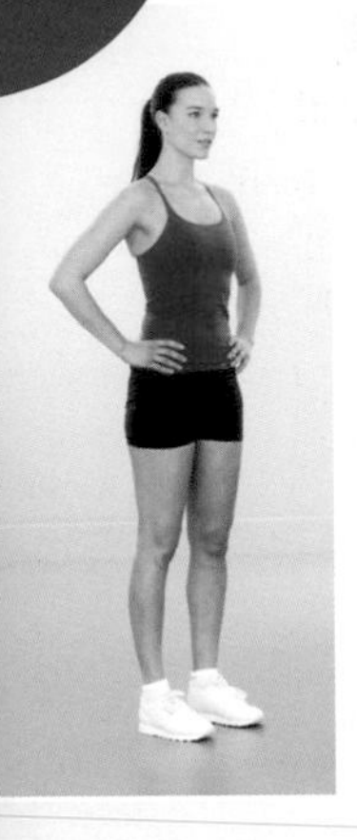

1 **Front Lunge** Stand with feet parallel, hip width apart, knees soft, hands on hips. Inhale as you step forward, bending knees slightly. Then exhale and push off with your front leg to spring back to the center. Alternate sides for 8 reps (1 rep = both sides).

2 **Opposite Arm Raise** Continue to lunge, alternating legs, and add your arms. From the starting position, feet parallel, hip width apart, step forward, bending your knees a little deeper, lifting your back heel and always keeping your knee over the ankle. At the same time, raise your hands to shoulder height, palms in, the opposite arm to the front and the other one behind. Keep your torso upright, chest lifted, chin level. Alternate legs and arms for 8 reps (1 rep = both sides).

bend knees
slightly

raise arms to
shoulder height
bend knees
a little deeper

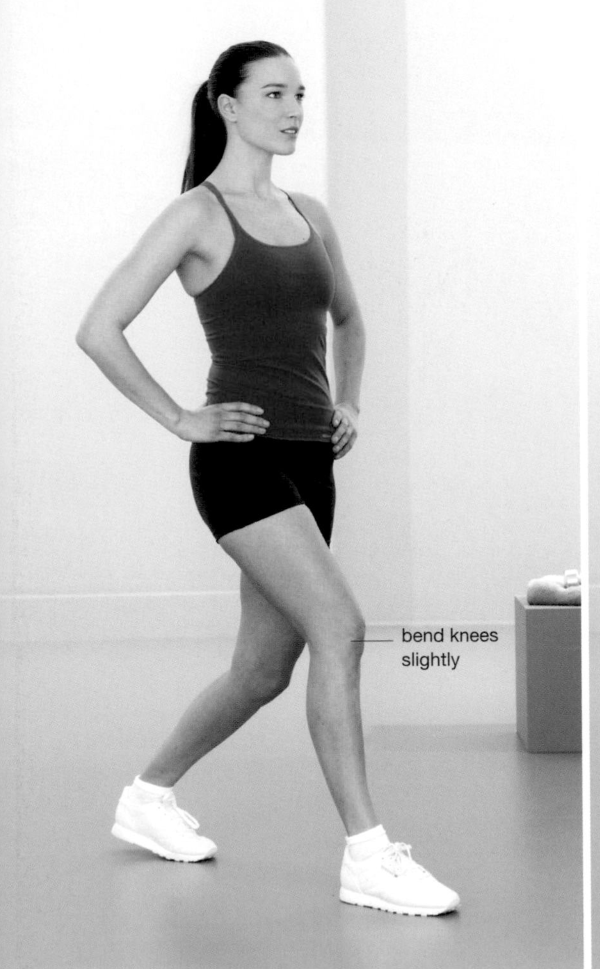

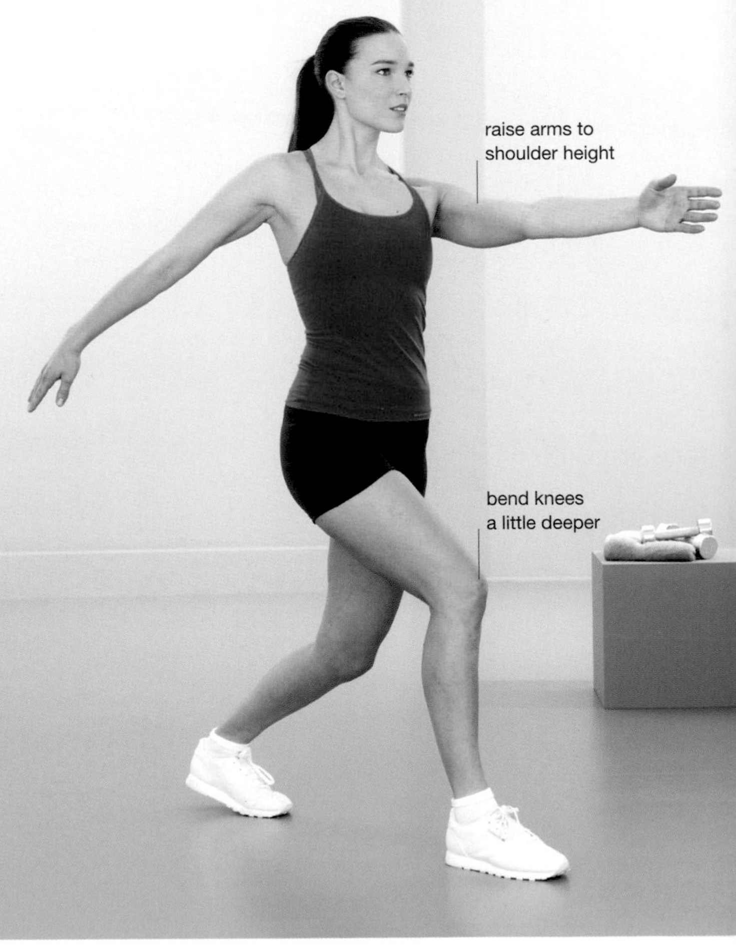

>> **warm up** arm reach/diagonal lunge

3 **Arm Reach** Continue to lunge, but now raise both arms to the front, lifting as you lunge, and increasing the bend in your knees. Pull your shoulder blades down and together to stabilize them as you extend your arms forward. Lower your arms to your sides as you return to center. Continue, alternating legs, for 8 reps (1 rep = both sides).

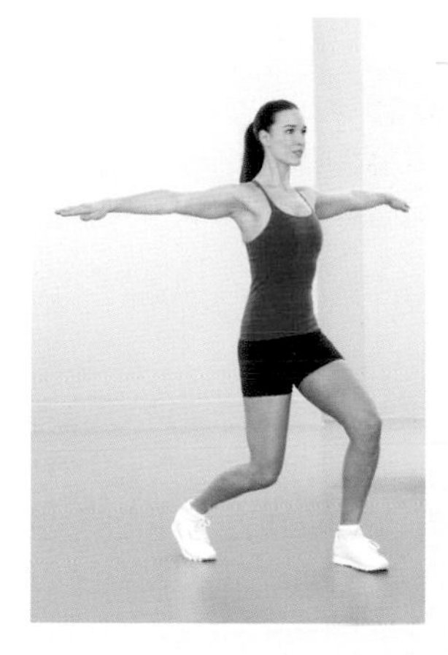

4 **Diagonal Lunge** From the center, pivot on the back foot and step out to 11 o'clock, lifting your arms to the sides. Spring back to center, lowering your arms, then lunge out on the opposite diagonal to 1 o'clock. Repeat for 8 reps.

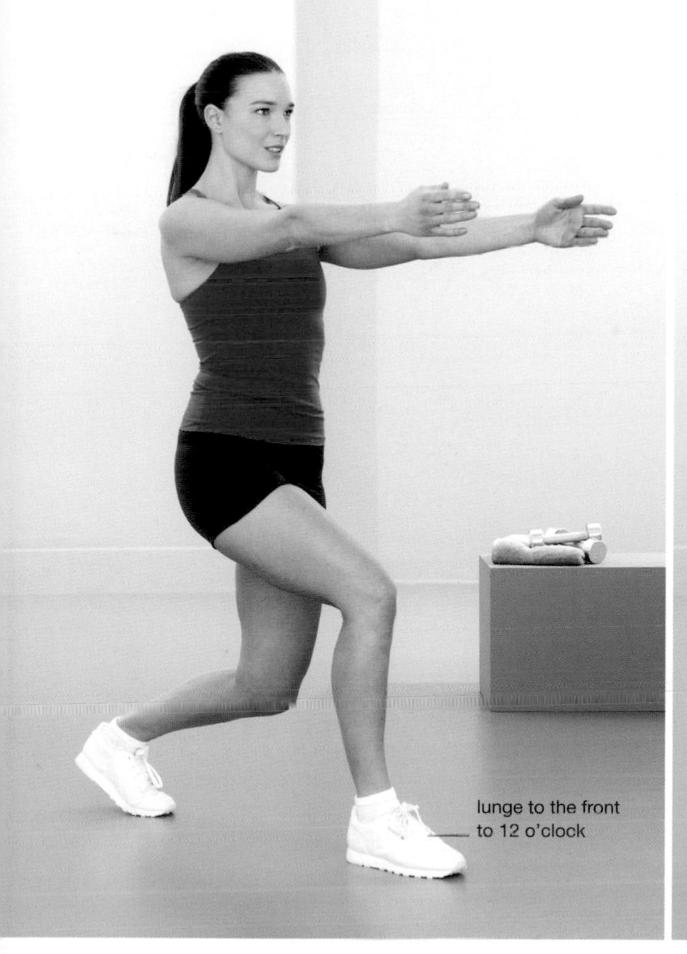

lunge to the front to 12 o'clock

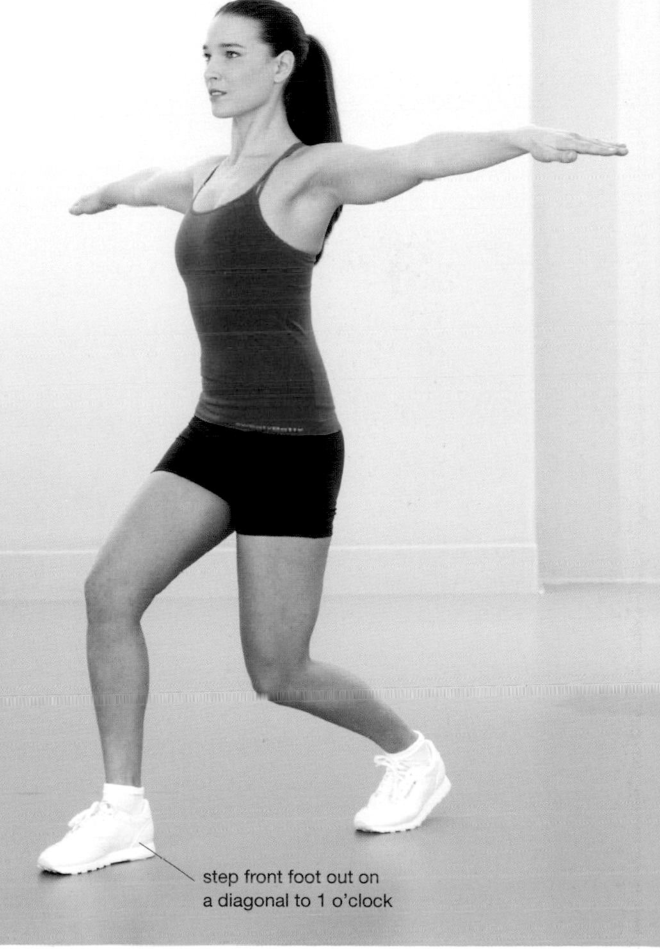

step front foot out on a diagonal to 1 o'clock

>> **warm up** side lunge

5a **Side Lunge** Stand with your feet parallel, hip width apart. Raise your arms to the sides at shoulder height, palms down. Keep your abdominals tight, hips square to the front, chest lifted. Draw your shoulder blades down and together as you prepare to lunge.

5b Inhale and step your left leg out to the side (9 o'clock), bending your knee. At the same time reach your arms high, turning the palms in, and flex your torso toward the center, bending sideways at the waist. Exhale and spring back to center, rotating the palms down as you lower your arms to shoulder height. Alternate sides (lunge to 3 o'clock) for 8 reps (1 rep = both sides).

keep leg straight
lunge to the side to 9 o'clock

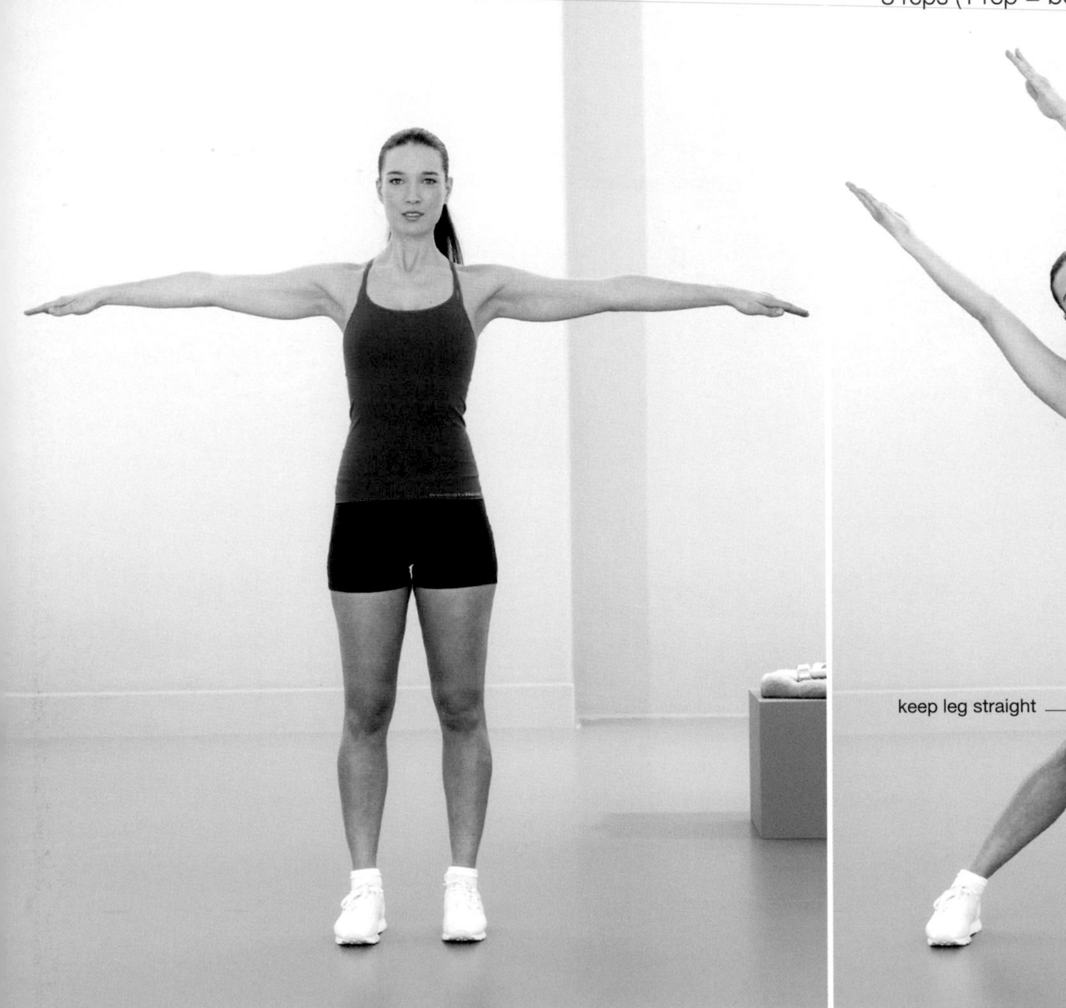

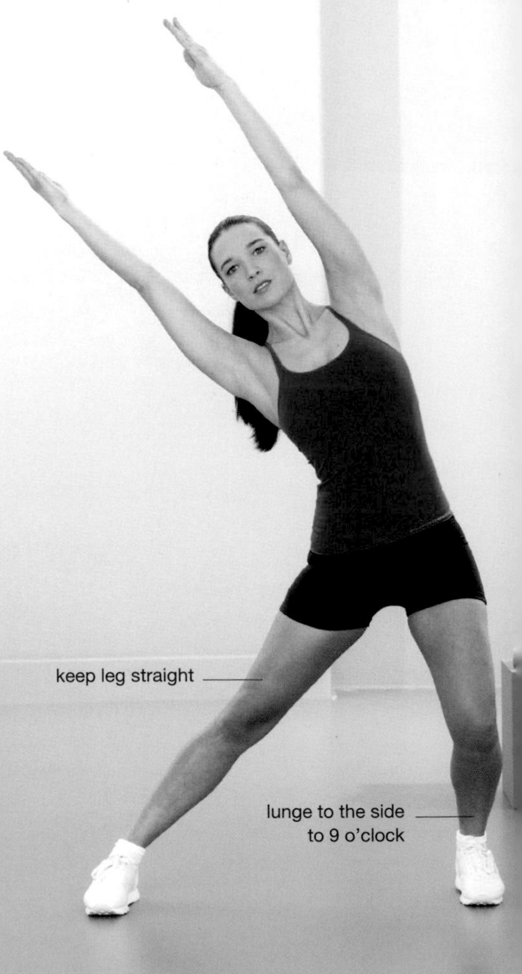

resistance squat

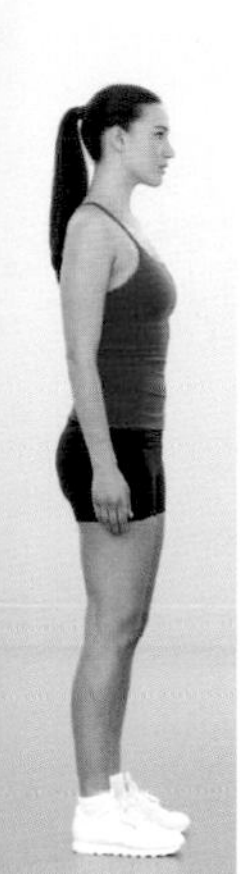

6 **Reverse Lunge** Start in the center position, feet parallel, arms by your sides. Inhale as you lunge to the back (6 o'clock), landing on the ball of your foot, and bending both knees. At the same time, reach both arms high in front, palms in. Exhale and return to center, arms by your sides. Repeat for 8 reps (1 rep = both sides). **Repeat Steps 5–1 (in reverse order) to complete your warm up.**

lunge back
to 6 o'clock

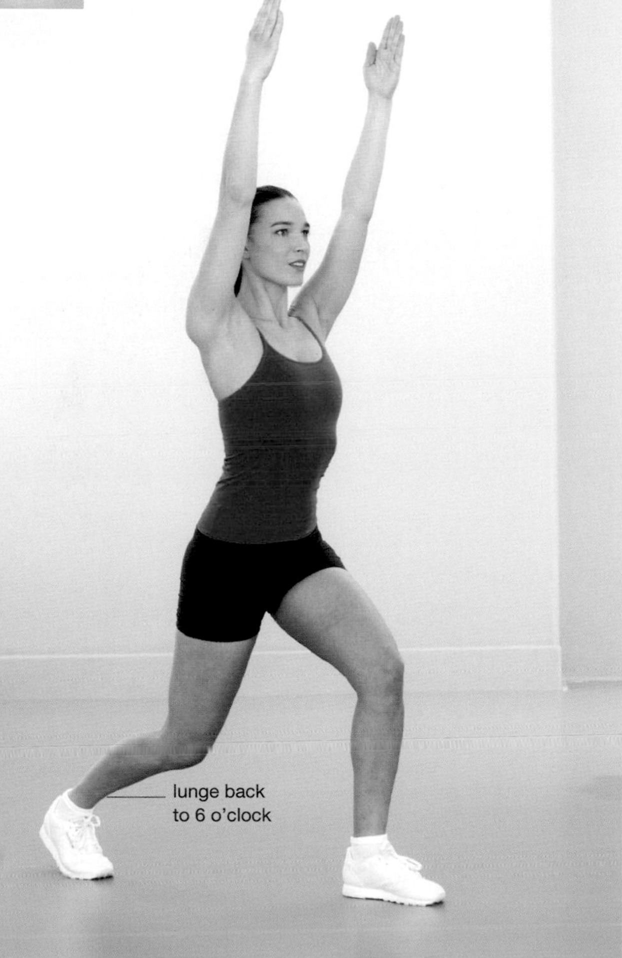

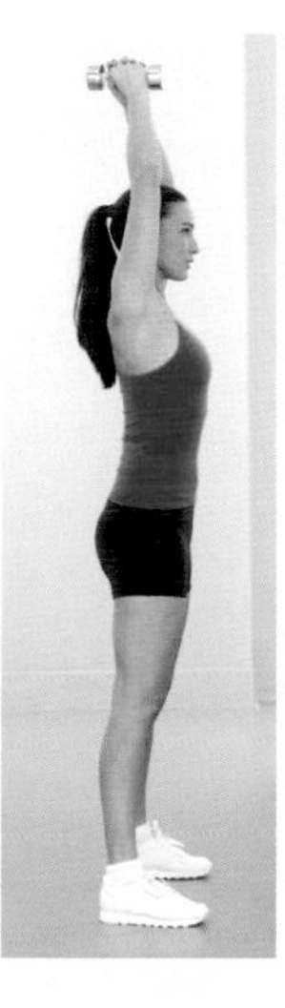

7 **Wood-Chop Squat** Pick up one large weight. Standing with your feet parallel, shoulder width apart, hold the weight overhead. Inhale as you squat, lowering the weight to your knees as if you are chopping wood. Exhale as you return to the starting position and repeat for 12 reps.

keep chest lifted
feel it here
keep knees

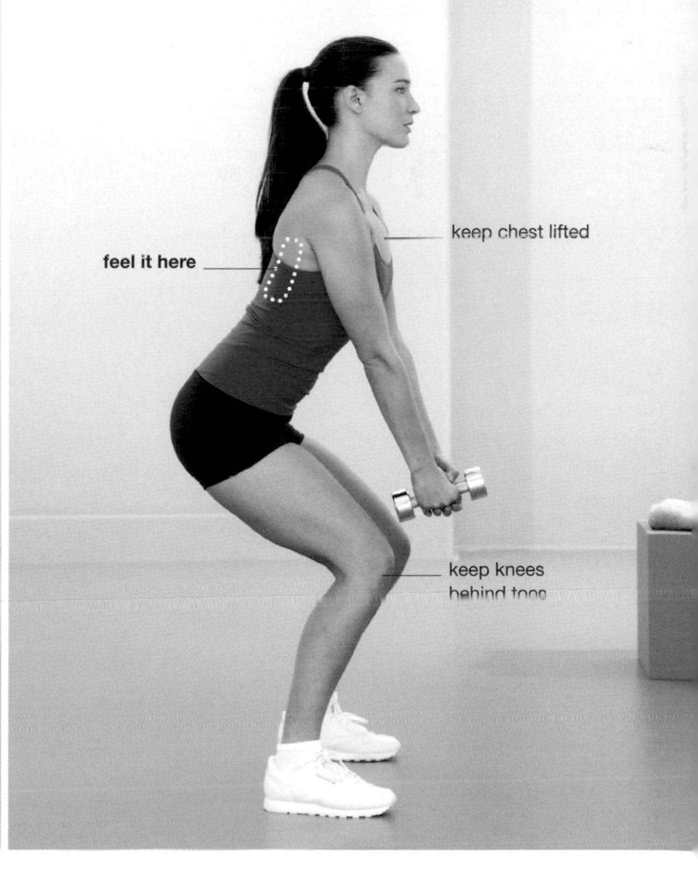

>> **cardio** curtsy lunge

8a **Curtsy Lunge** Put down the weight for your first cardio interval. Stand with your feet parallel, hip width apart, knees soft. Raise your arms out to the sides at shoulder height, palms down. Keep your elbows slightly rounded. Stand tall, lengthening through your spine by lifting the top of your head toward the ceiling and engaging the abdominals.

8b Step back on a diagonal, landing on the ball of your foot, heel lifted. Bend both knees and squeeze your shoulder blades together every time you curtsy. Keep your arms at shoulder height. Breathe naturally throughout. Repeat for 8 reps, alternating legs (1 rep = both sides).

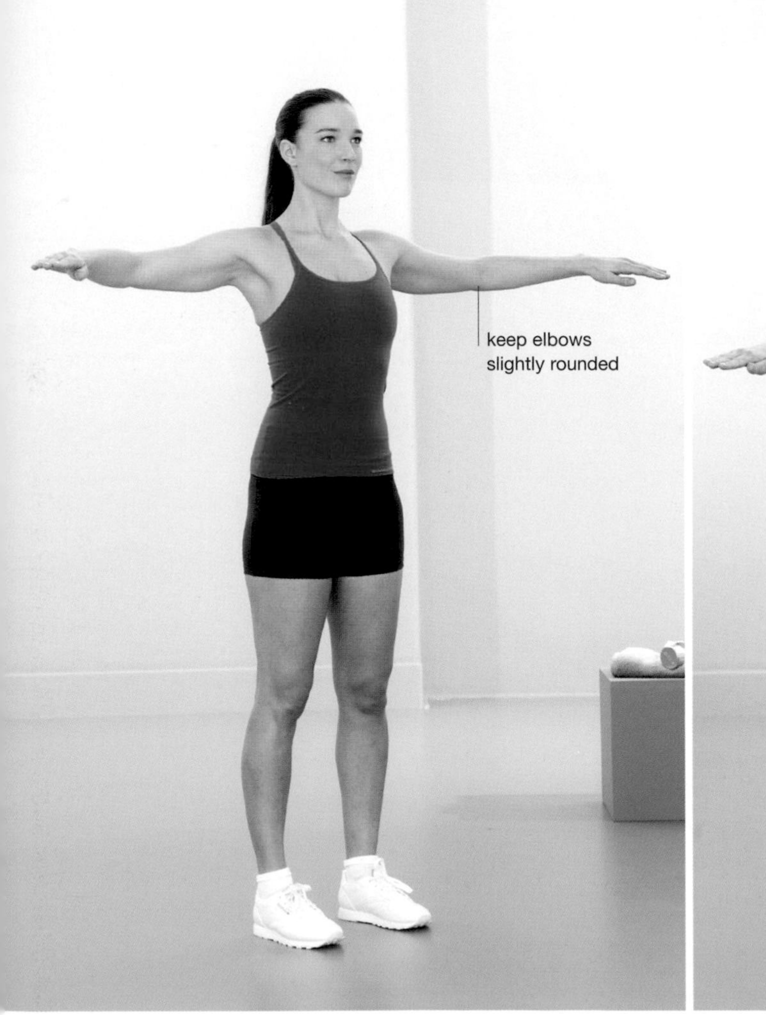

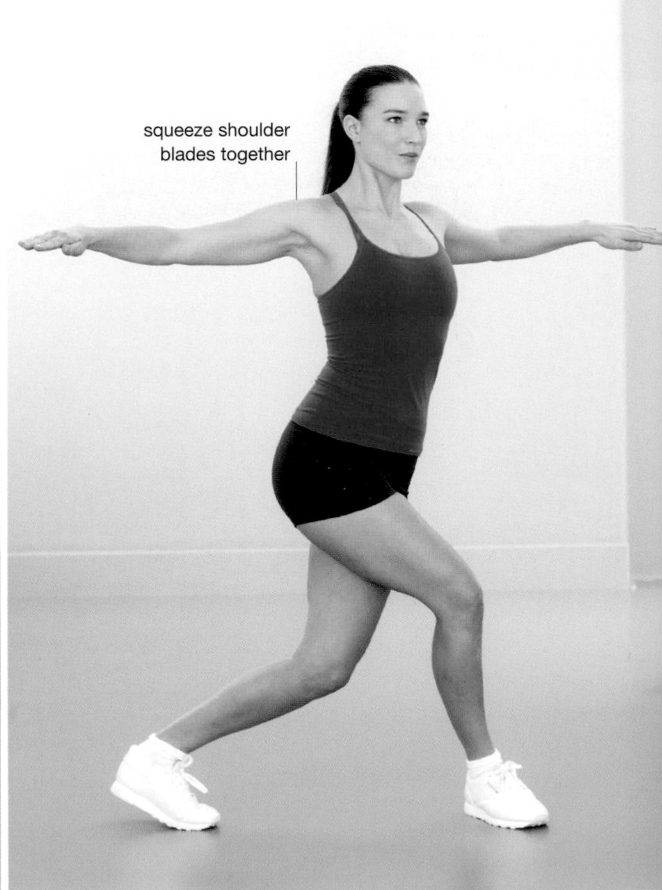

>> **cardio** charleston lunge

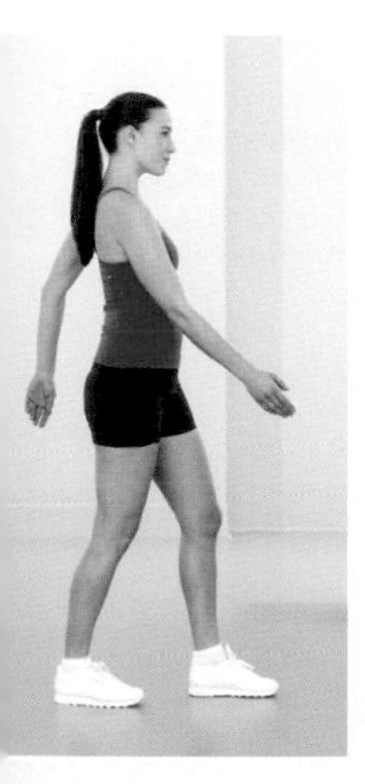

9a **Charleston Lunge** Step forward with the lead leg and kick the other leg in front of you, knee to hip height. Then swing the leg back and step in place. Swing your arms in opposition to your legs. Continue the movement with the Reverse Lunge (see 9b).

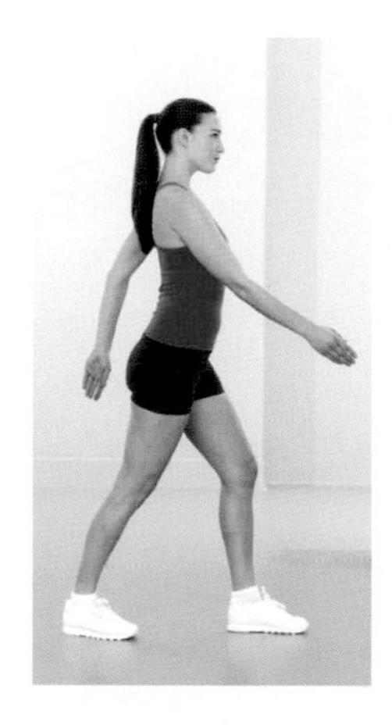

9b Reverse lunge with the lead leg. Continue a series of step, kick front (see 9a), step, lunge back. Switch arms with every leg change. Repeat 6 times. Change legs by substituting the last lunge with a step in place. Repeat the sequence 6 times on the other side.

swing arms in opposition to legs
lunge back with lead leg

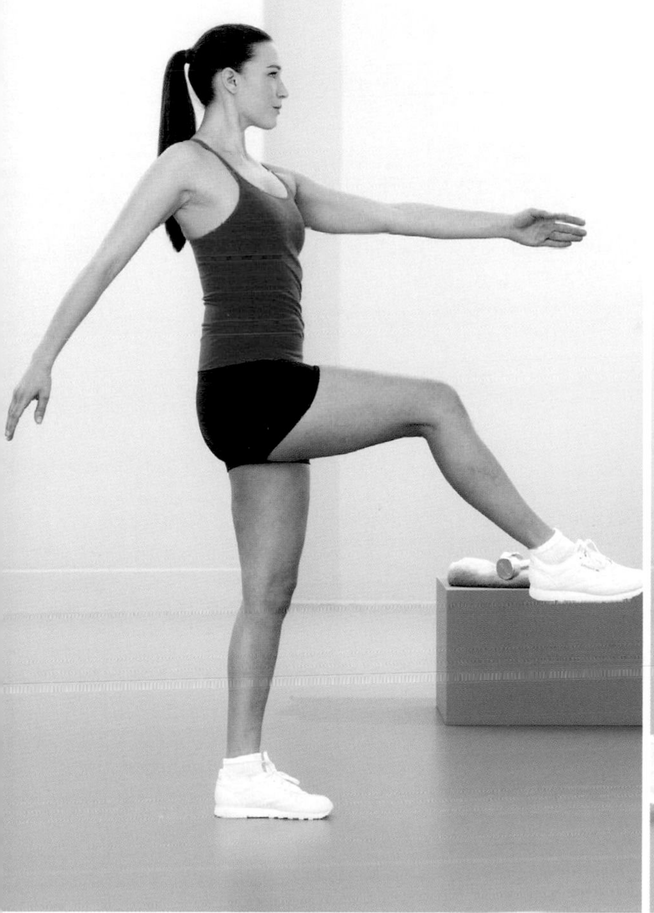

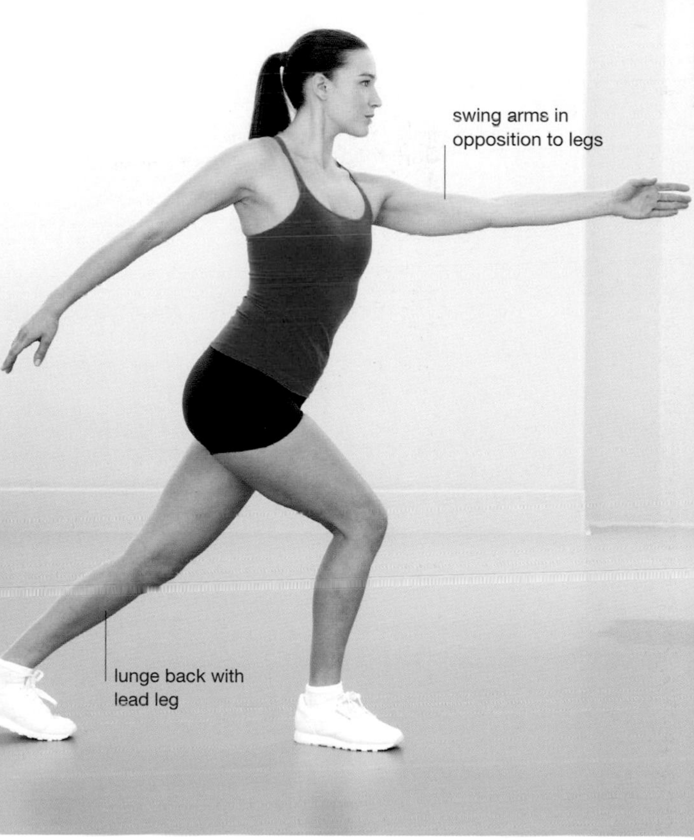

>> **cardio** push-off lunge

10a **Push-off Lunge** Start from a staggered lunge position, your front knee over the ankle. Your back heel should lift easily. Reach your arms overhead on a diagonal, palms in. Center your weight between your legs, torso square to the front, eyes looking forward. Prepare to push off with your back foot.

10b Push off with your back foot, shifting your weight to your front leg, and pump your knee to hip height. At the same time, bend your arms, pulling your elbows to your sides, hands to hip level. Balance for a moment on the supporting leg before lunging again. Repeat a total of 8 times, then change to the other side. Breathe naturally throughout. **You have now completed the cardio interval, which you will repeat after each resistance exercise.**

reach arms up on a diagonal
keep knee directly over ankle
prepare to push off

keep elbows bent close to sides
lift knee to hip height

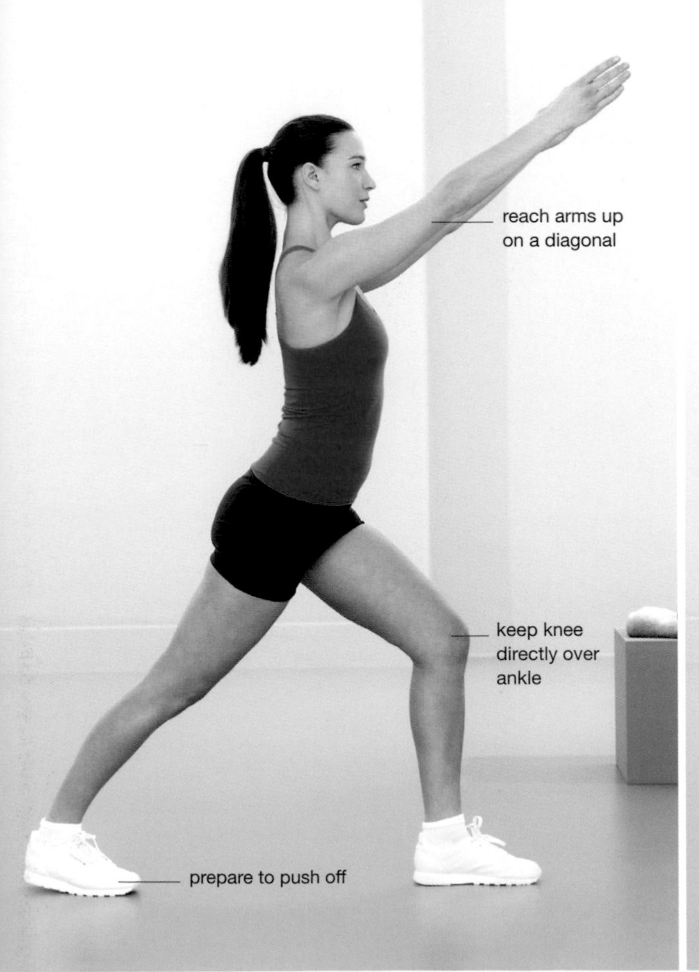

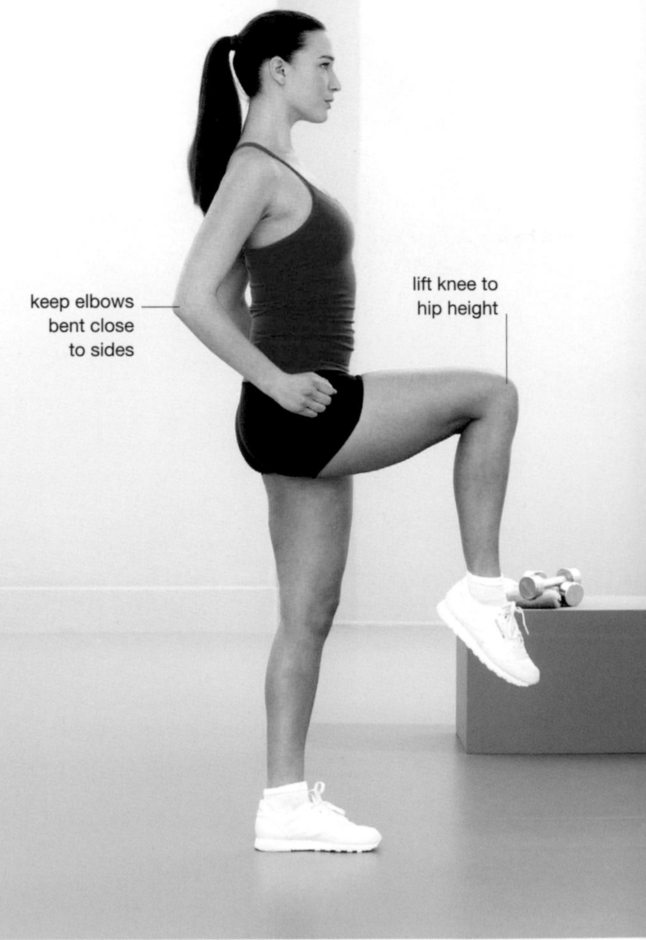

resistance plié & row/balance squat

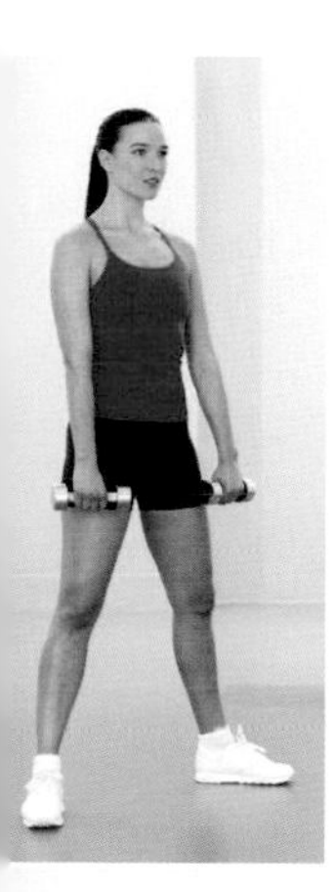

11 **Plié & Row** Pick up two small weights. Stand with your legs turned out, slightly wider than shoulder width apart. Hold a weight in each hand, arms straight down, palms facing back. Inhale as you bend your knees over your toes and pull the weights to your chest, elbows bending out to the sides. Exhale and straighten up, lowering the weights. Move up and down 12 times. **Do your next cardio interval, Steps 8–10 (pp96–98).**

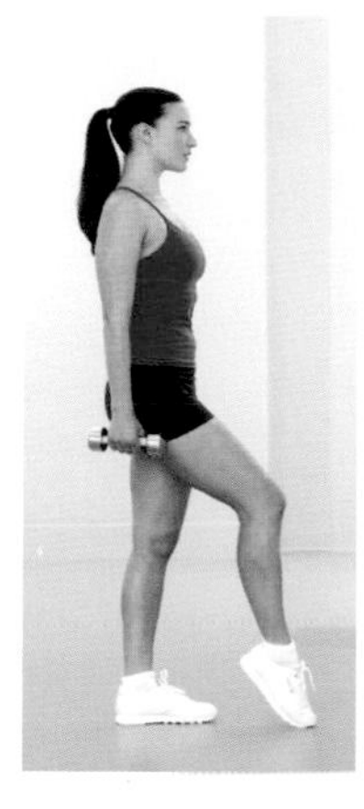

12 **Balance Squat** Stand with all your weight on one leg, the other leg resting lightly to the front. Inhale, reach back with your hips and squat on the working leg. Exhale up. Repeat 12 times, then change sides. **Do your next cardio interval, Steps 8–10 (pp96–98).**

feel it here
feel it here
keep elbows below shoulder level
turn legs out at the hips
place feet at 45° angles

keep torso upright or leaning slightly forward
rest front leg lightly for balance

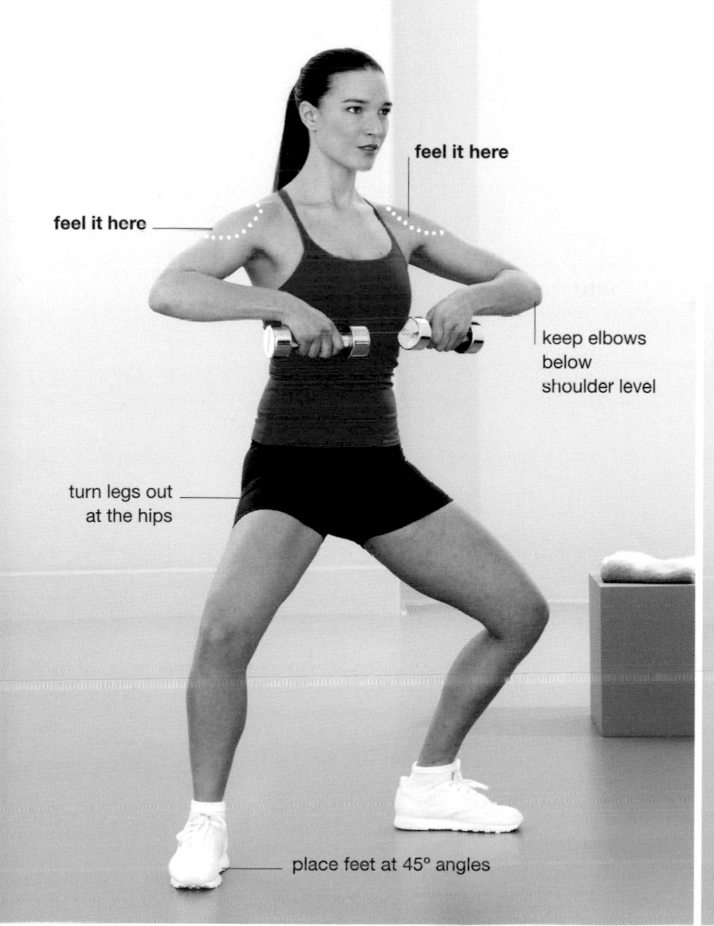

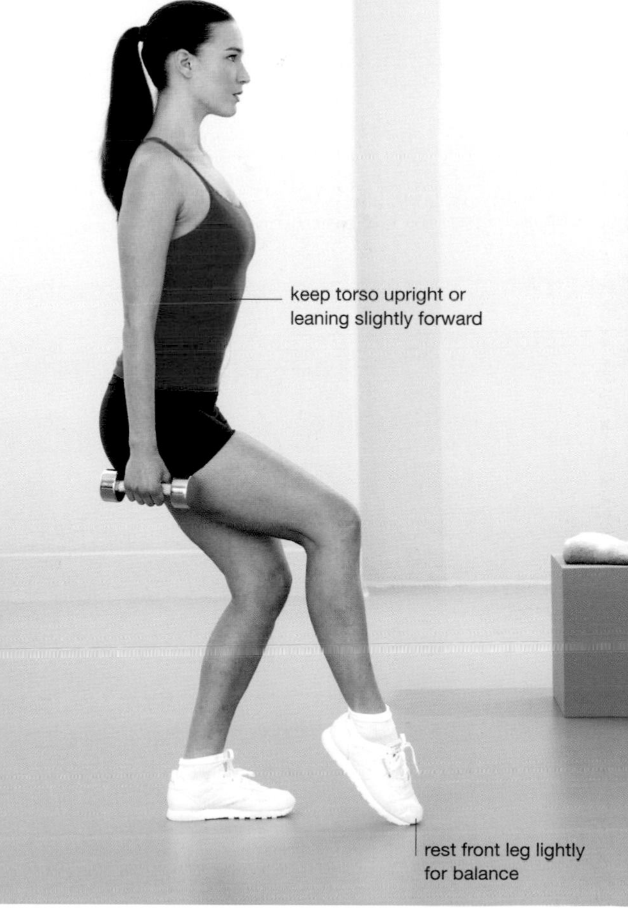

>> **resistance** bent-over row

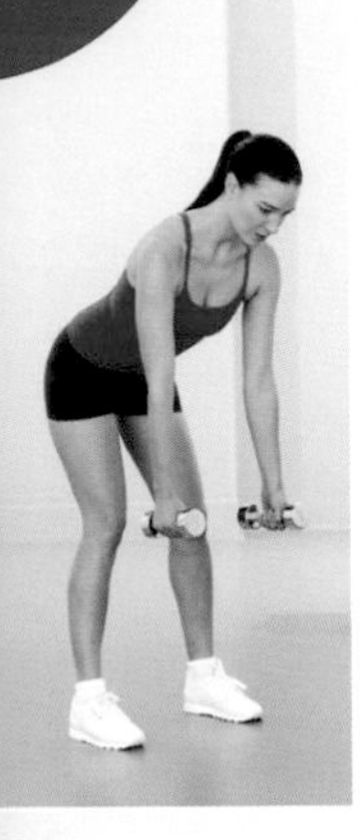

13a **Bent-Over Row** Pick up two weights. Stand with your feet parallel, shoulder width apart, holding a weight in each hand, arms by your sides, palms in. Bend your knees and hinge forward from the hips, keeping your spine in neutral alignment. Draw your shoulder blades together and exhale as you lift the weights, bending your elbows until the upper arms are parallel to the floor.

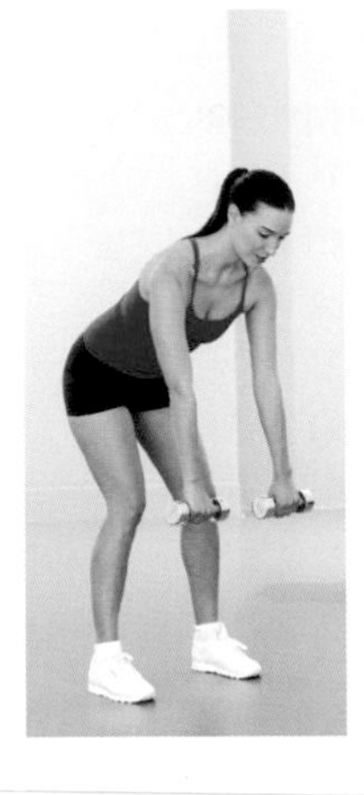

13b Lower the weights to the starting position and rotate your arms so that your palms face back. Pull your shoulder blades together and exhale as you bend your elbows out to the sides until your upper arms are parallel to the floor. Do 8 reps, alternating the position of the arms. **Do your next cardio interval, Steps 8–10 (pp96–98).**

keep elbows close to sides
feel it here
palms facing in

bend elbows out to sides
palms facing back
keep knees bent

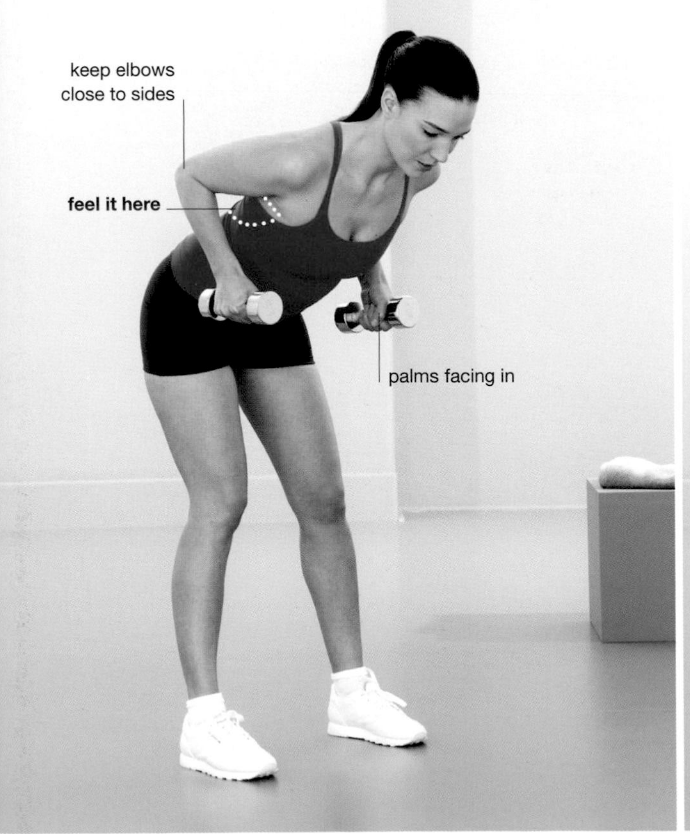

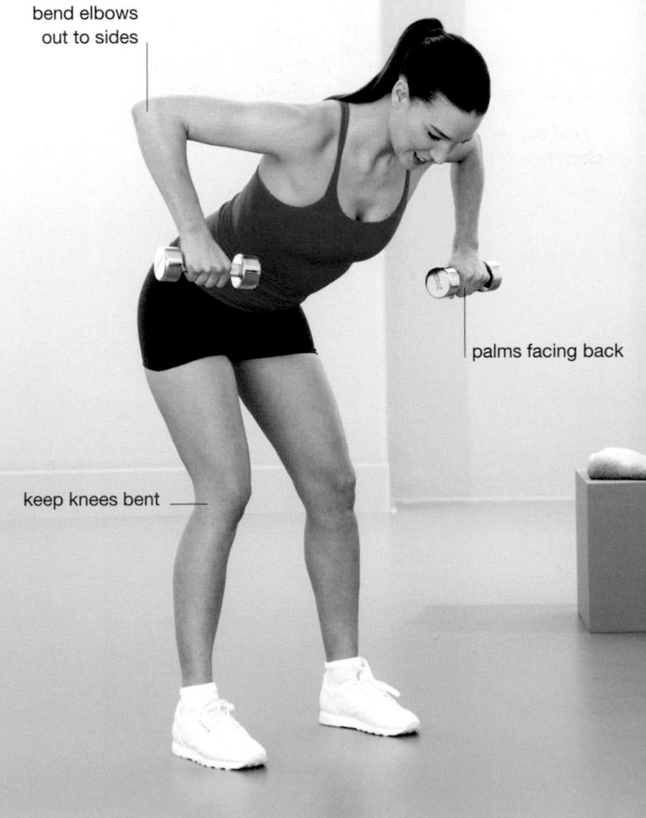

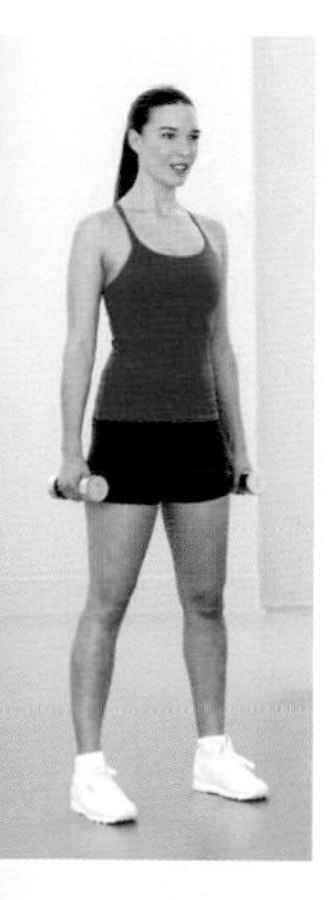

14a **Lift & Squat** Pick up two small weights. Stand feet parallel, shoulder width apart. Hold a weight in each hand, arms by your sides. Shift your weight to the balls of your feet and lift the heels high; at the same time, bend your elbows, lifting the weights toward your shoulders. Balance, then return to the starting position.

14b Plant your heels on the floor, shift your weight back, and bend your knees into a squat. At the same time, raise your arms behind you, elbows straight. Straighten up, then repeat the combination of rising onto the balls of the feet followed by squatting for 8 reps. Breathe naturally throughout. **Do your next cardio interval, Steps 8–10 (pp96–98).**

hold elbows close to sides
lift heels high
shift weight to balls of feet

feel it here
keep elbows straight, close to sides
shift weight onto heels

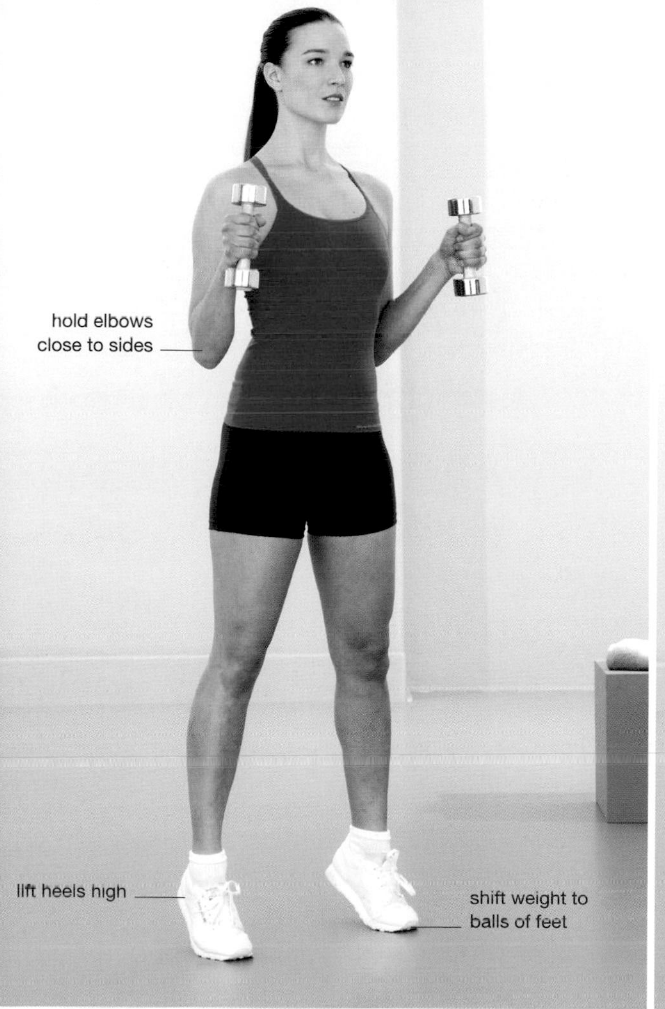

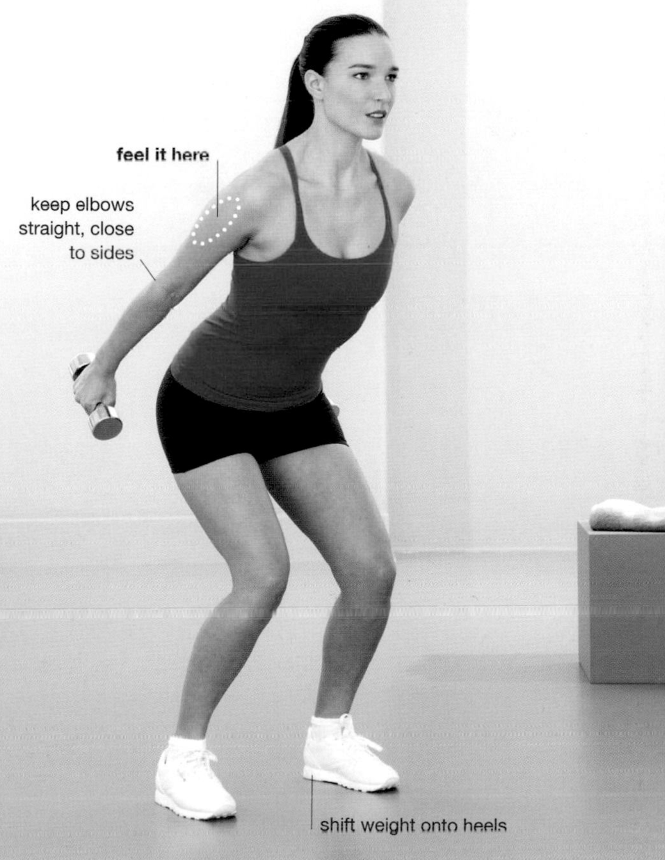

>> **cool down** upper body stretch/down dog

feel it here
keep shoulder blades down
breathe deeply throughout

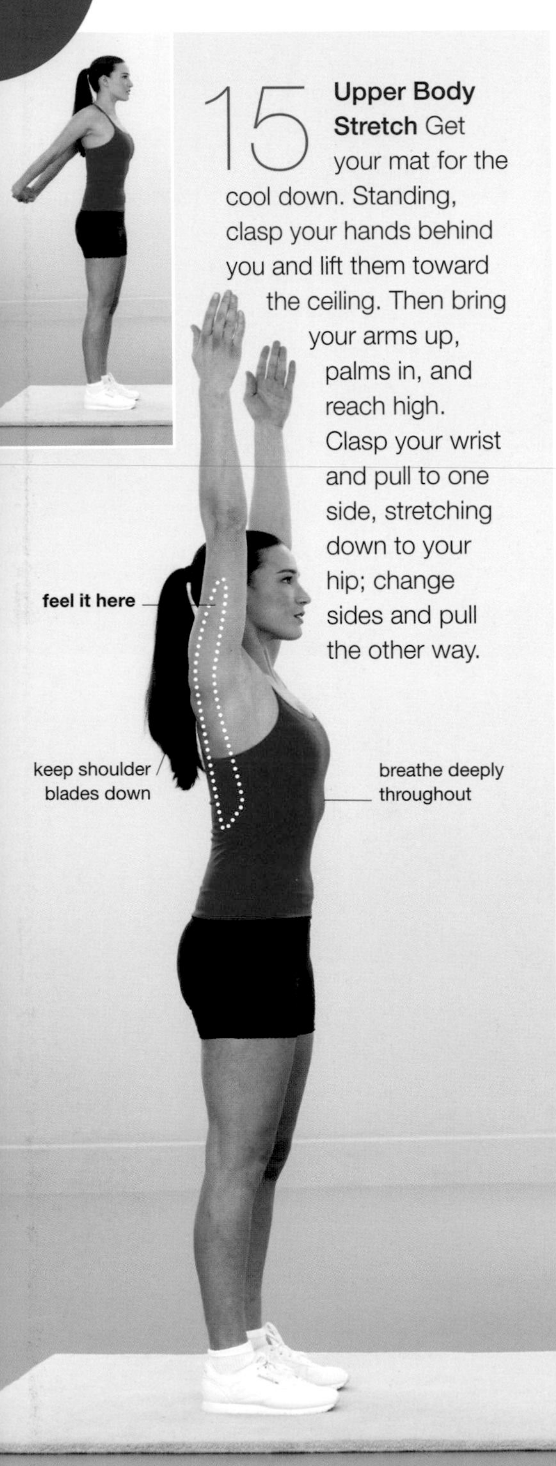

15

Upper Body Stretch Get your mat for the cool down. Standing, clasp your hands behind you and lift them toward the ceiling. Then bring your arms up, palms in, and reach high. Clasp your wrist and pull to one side, stretching down to your hip; change sides and pull the other way.

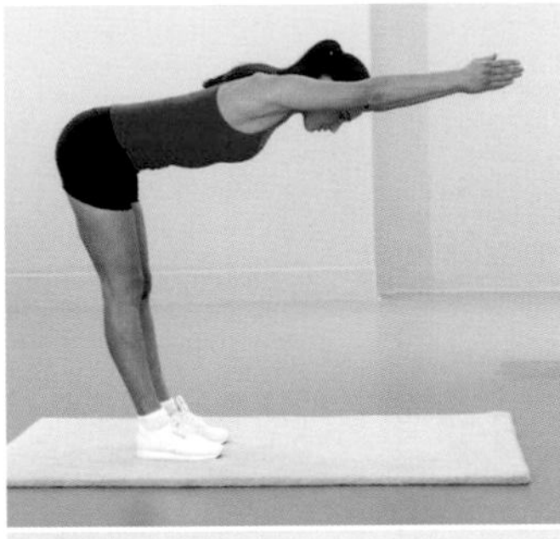

16

Upper Body Stretch/Down Dog Return to center and hinge forward from the hip; knees and back straight. Reach back with the hips as you extend the arms forward, lengthening the spine. Hold the stretch and breathe. Bend down, place your palms on the mat, and walk your hands forward into Down Dog, reaching your hips toward the ceiling and pressing your heels toward the mat. If necessary, bend your knees to release the hips and heels. Keep the breath flowing.

reach hips toward ceiling
lengthen through spine
align head and neck with spine
press heels toward mat

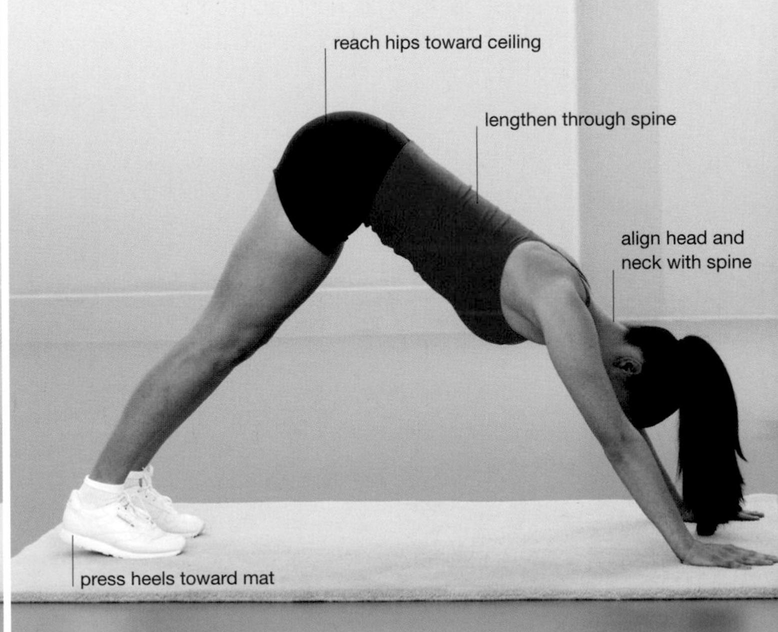

>> **cool down** half push-up & side plank

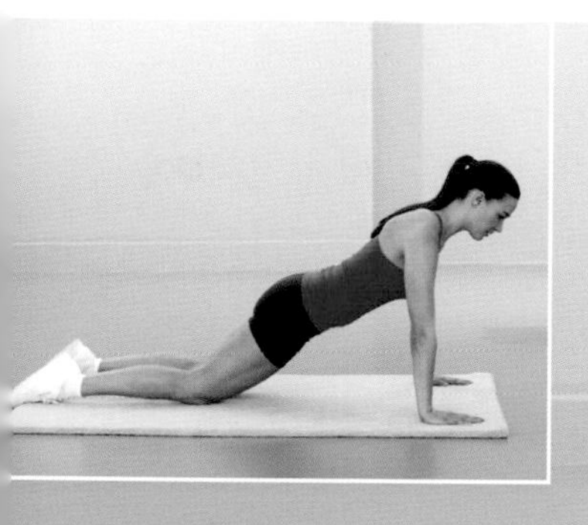

17a **Half Push-up & Side Plank** Kneel with your wrists under your shoulders, 3–4 in (7.5–10 cm) wider than shoulder width apart. Drop your hips and shift your weight forward so there is no direct pressure on the kneecaps. Inhale, bend your elbows out to the sides and lower your chest toward the mat. Exhale and push up.

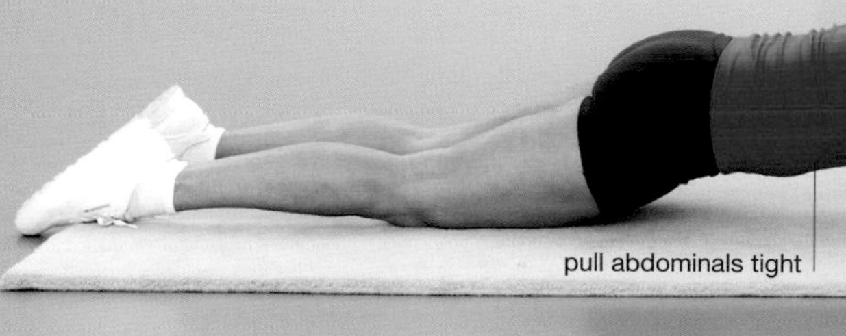

17b Turn onto your side, knees and lower legs stacked, hips and ribs lifted, a straight line from shoulder to knees. The supporting arm is straight, wrist directly under the shoulder. Reach your top arm to the ceiling, palm forward. Repeat the Half Push-up (see 17a) and then do a Side Plank to the other side, alternating for 3 sets (1 set = Push-up, Side Plank, Push-up, Side Plank).

reach top arm to ceiling

place supporting arm under shoulder

stack knees and lower legs

>> **cool down** child's pose/kneeling lunge

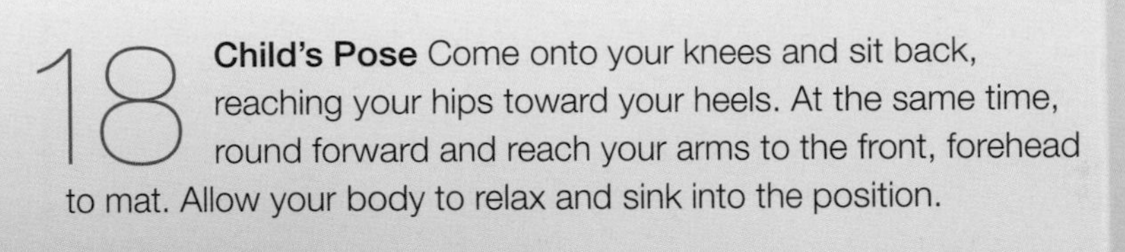

18 **Child's Pose** Come onto your knees and sit back, reaching your hips toward your heels. At the same time, round forward and reach your arms to the front, forehead to mat. Allow your body to relax and sink into the position.

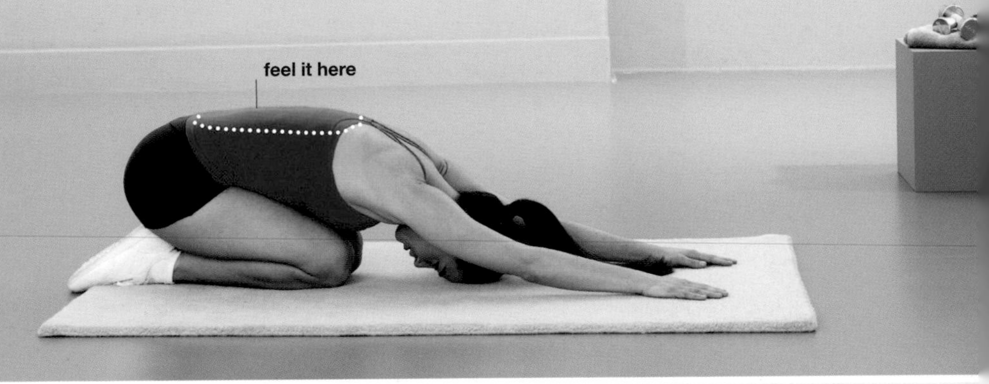

19 **Kneeling Lunge** Come up onto one knee, bending the other one in front of you, foot on the mat. Raise your arms overhead, palms in, head centered between your elbows. Press your hips forward until you feel a stretch in the front of your hip, the hip flexor. Breathe into the stretch and hold. Then sit back into Child's Pose (see above). Repeat the lunge on the other side.

keep hips square to front

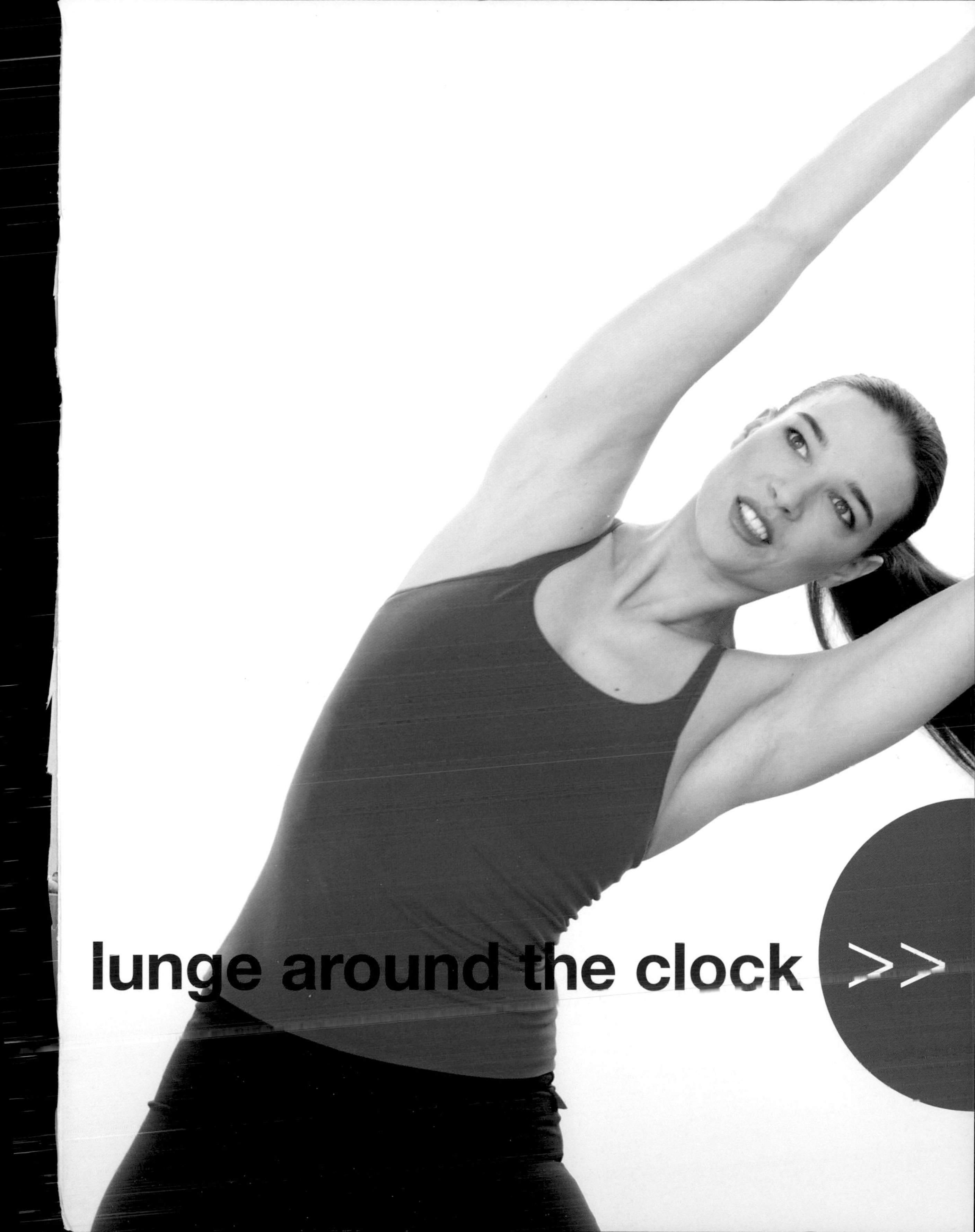

lunge around the clock >>

lunge around the clock at a glan

1

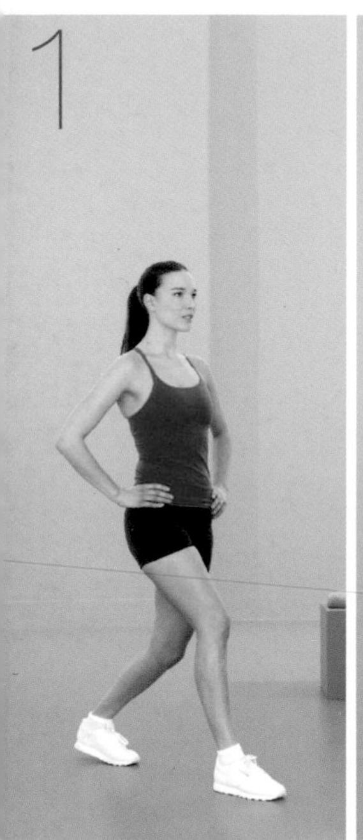

▲ **Warm up,** Front Lunge, page 92

2

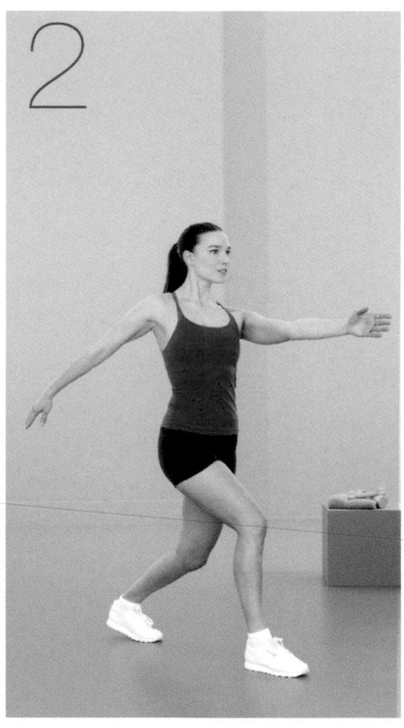

▲ **Warm up,** Opposite Arm Raise, page 92

3

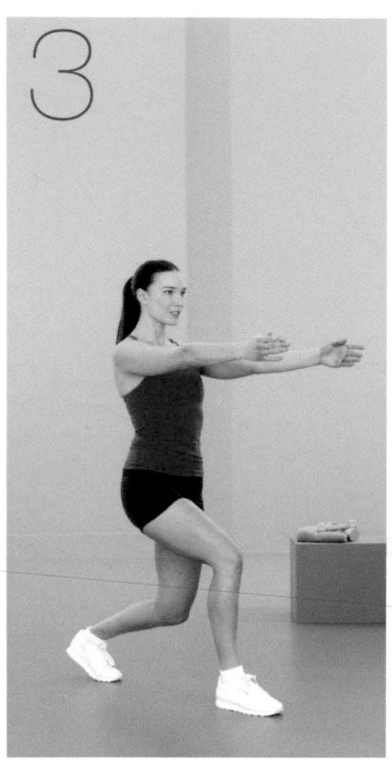

▲ **Warm up,** Arm Reach, page 93

4

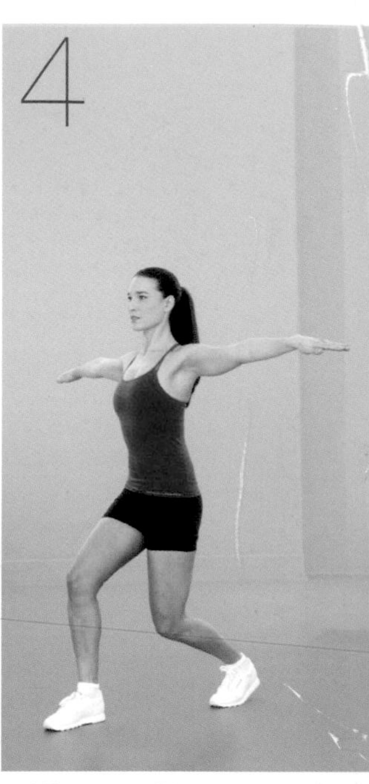

▲ **Warm up,** Diagonal Lunge, page 93

13a

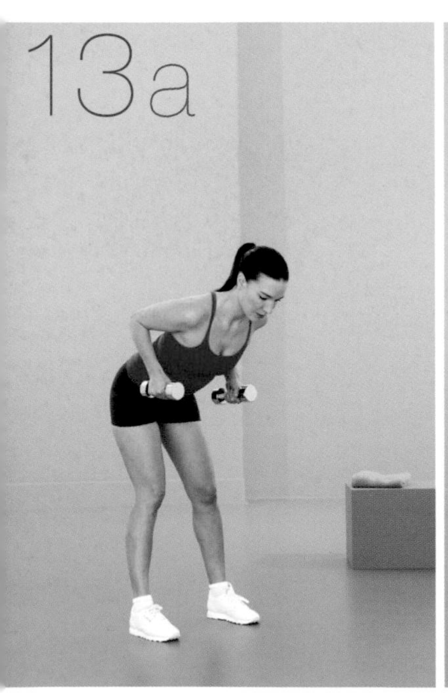

▲ **Resistance,** Bent-Over Row, page 100

13b

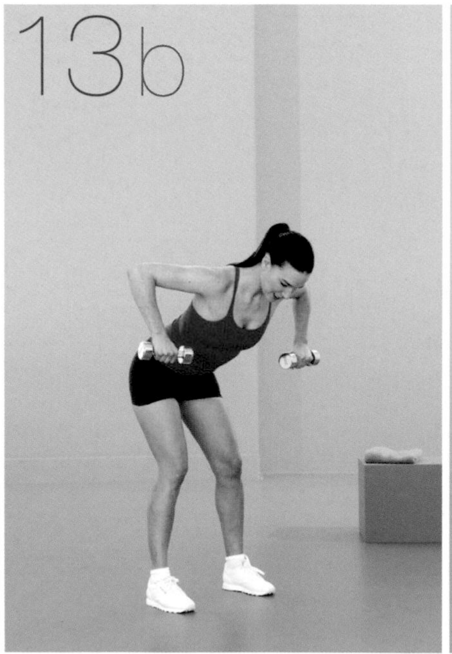

▲ **Resistance,** Bent-Over Row, page 100. Repeat steps 8–10

14a

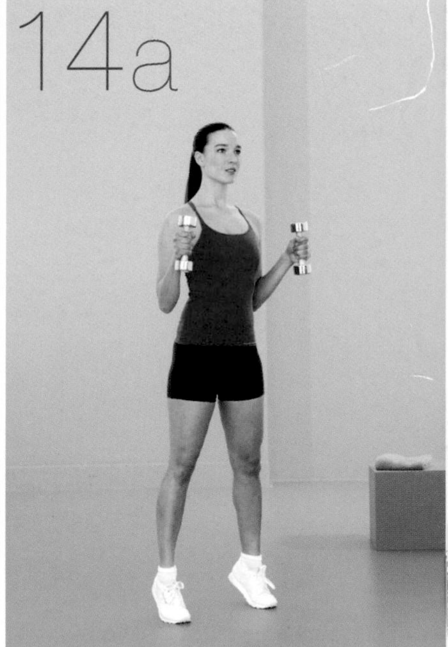

▲ **Resistance,** Lift & Squat, page 101

ce

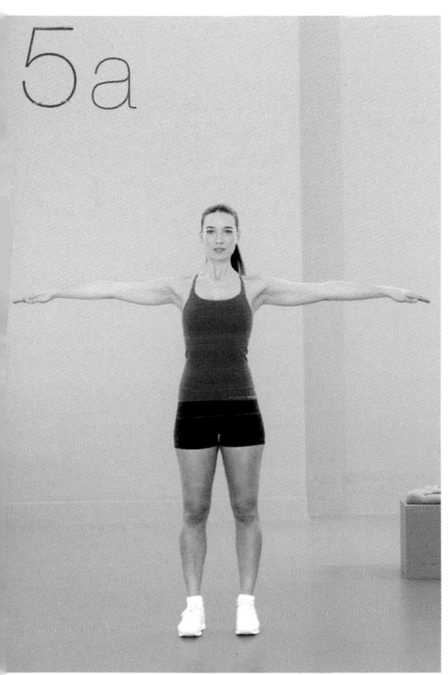

▲ **Warm up,** Side Lunge, page 94

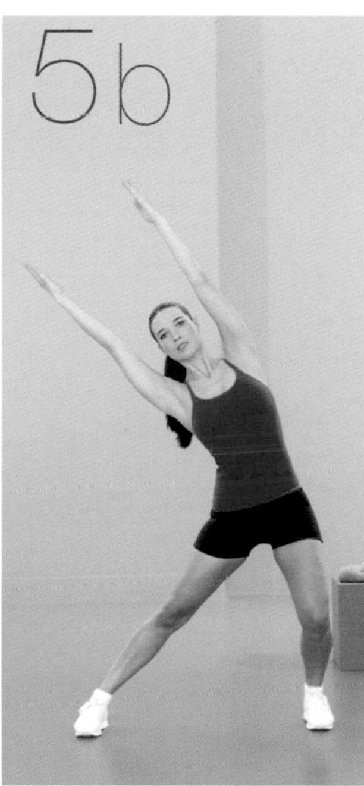

▲ **Warm up,** Side Lunge, page 94

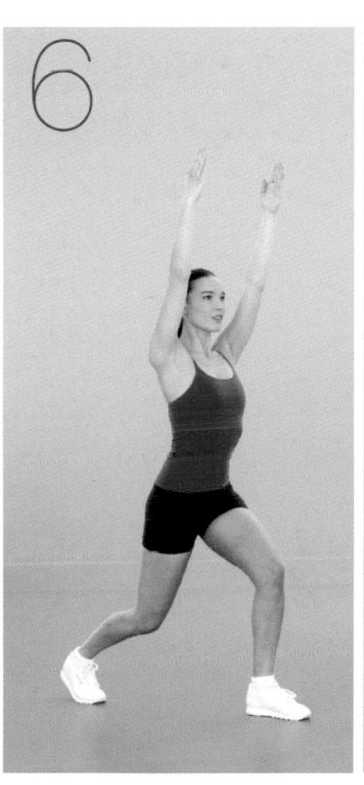

▲ **Warm up,** Reverse Lunge, page 95. Repeat Steps 5–1

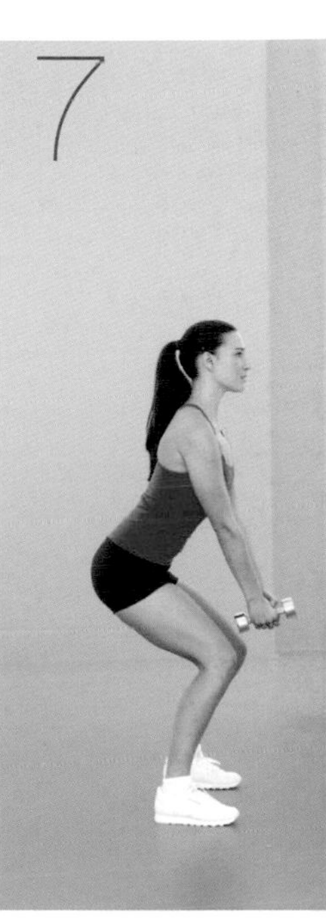

▲ **Resistance,** Wood-Chop Squat, page 95

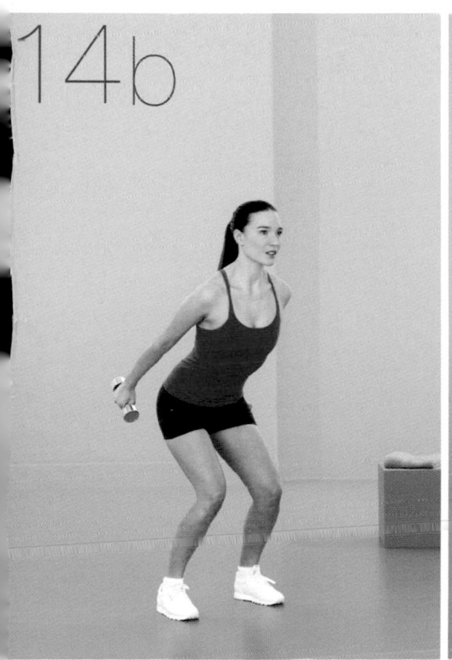

▲ **Resistance,** Lift & Squat, page 101. Repeat Steps 8–10

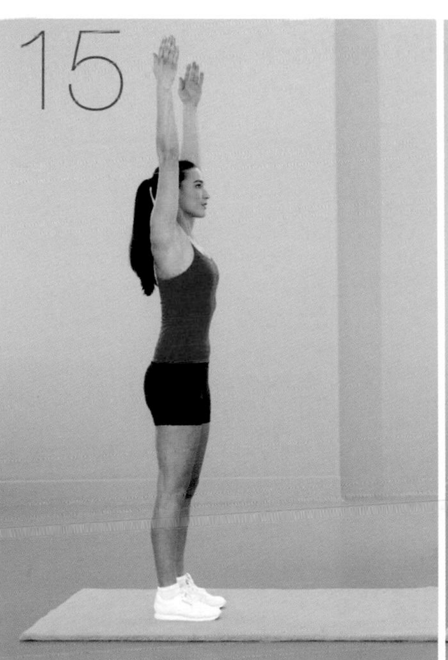

▲ **Cool down,** Upper Body Stretch, page 102

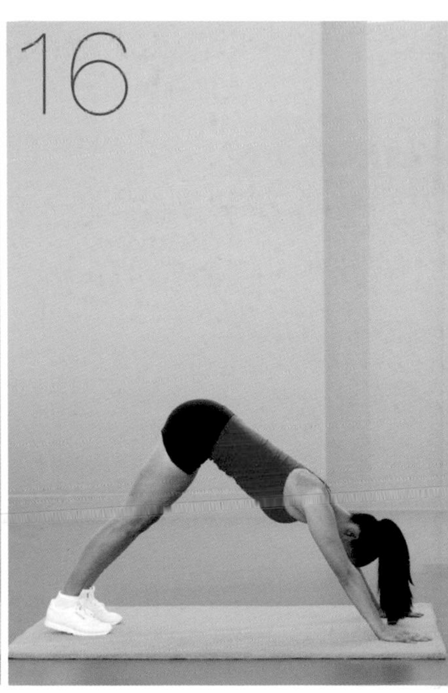

▲ **Cool down,** Down Dog, page 102

20a Cross-Legged Stretch

Sit back on your buttocks and cross your legs comfortably in front. Bend forward from the hips with your back straight, keep the sitbones anchored on the floor, and extend your arms to the front. Breathe deeply and relax into the position.

keep back straight
keep sitbones anchored

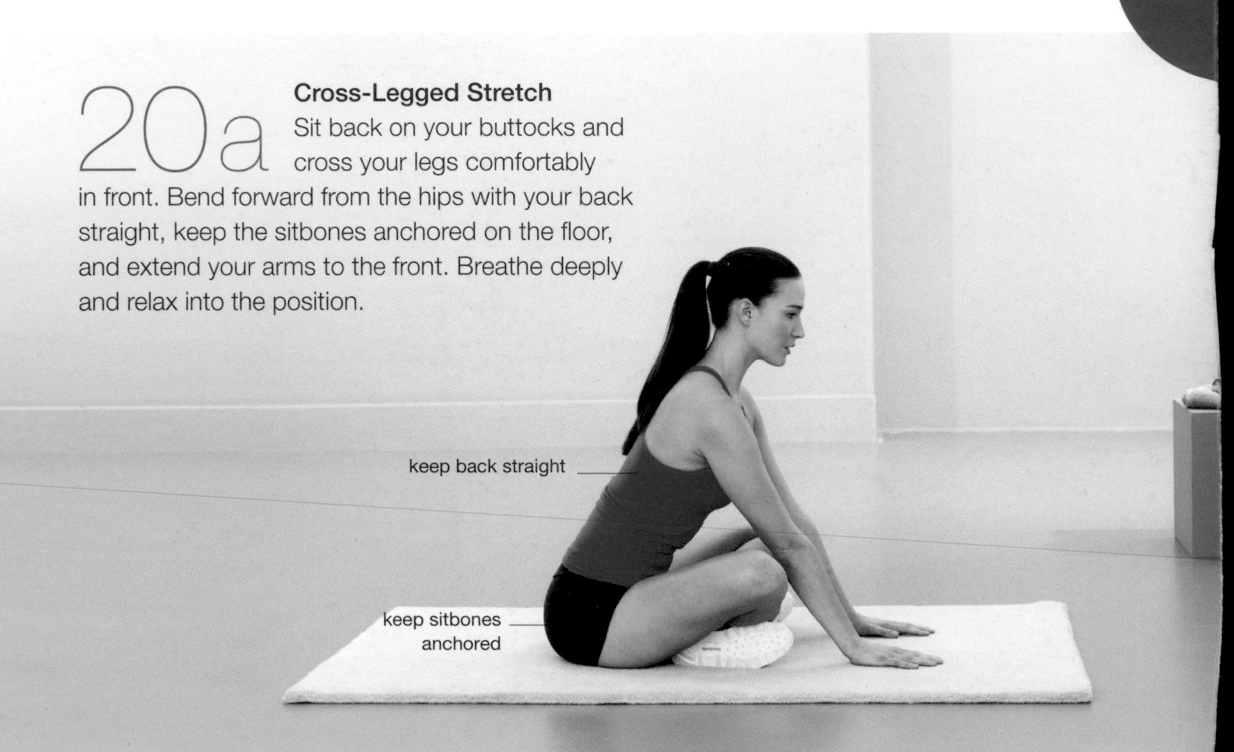

20b

Walk your hands to one side, turning your torso to face that knee. Hold the position briefly and breathe deeply, trying to relax more deeply into the position with each exhalation. Pass through center and repeat on the other side. Remember to keep your sitbones anchored throughout.

position torso to face knee

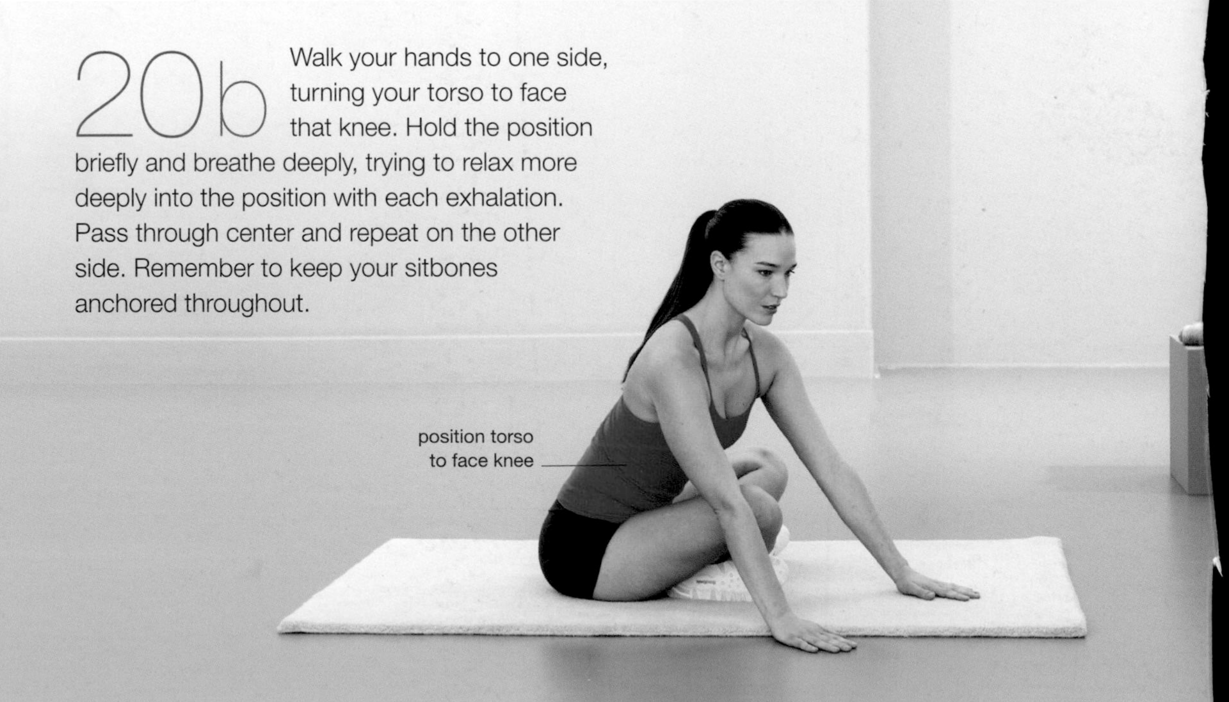

15 minute

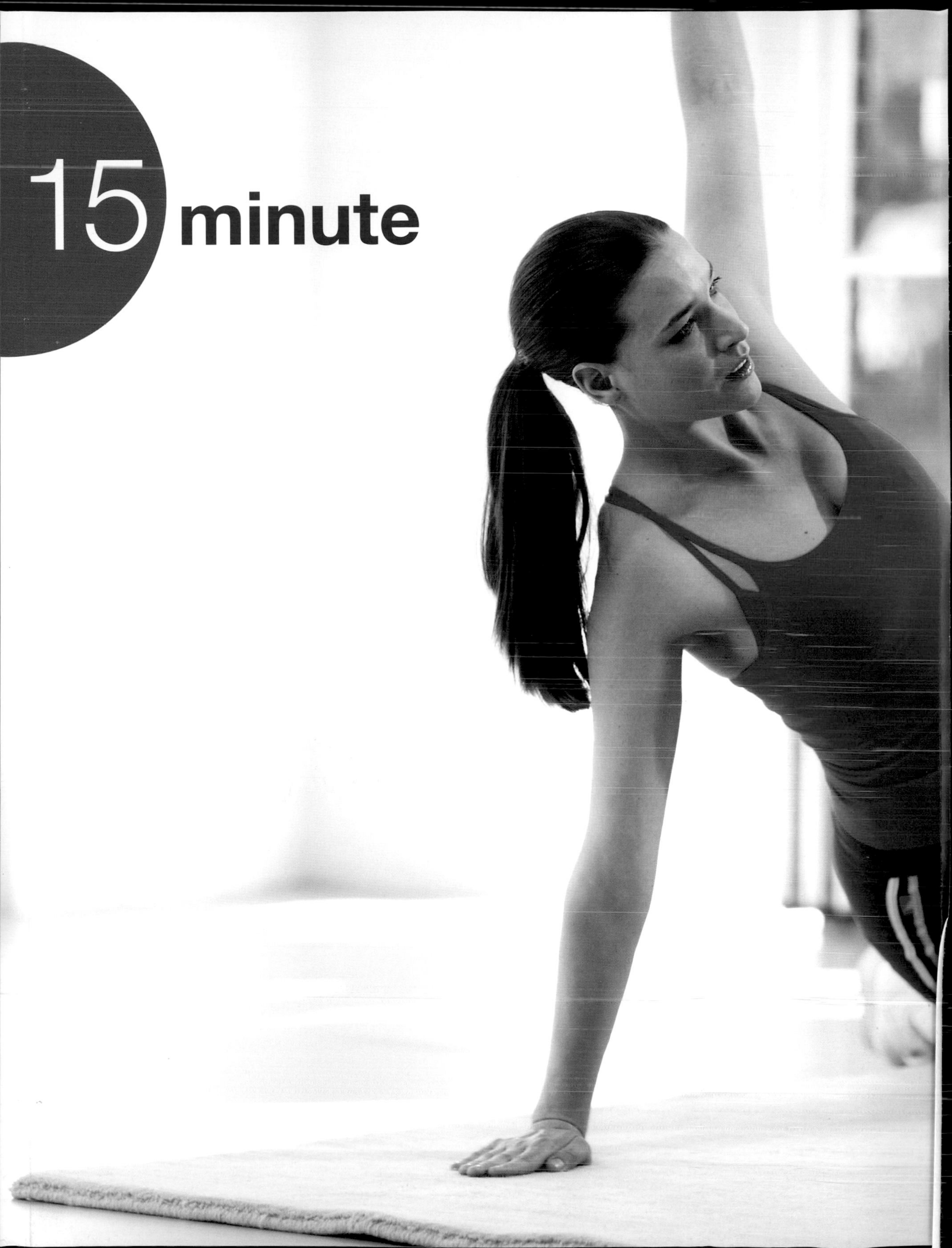

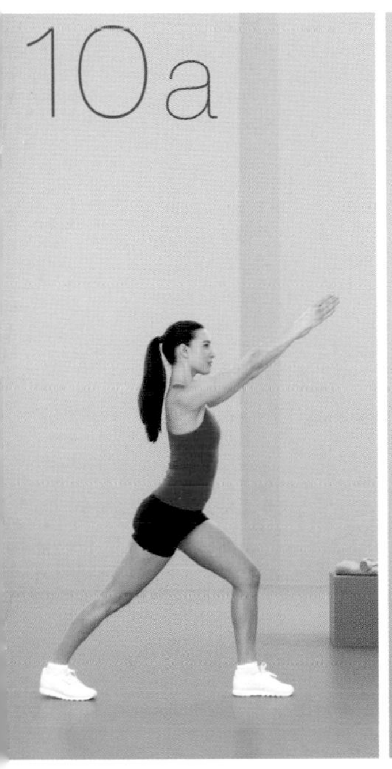

▲ **Cardio,** Push-off Lunge, page 98

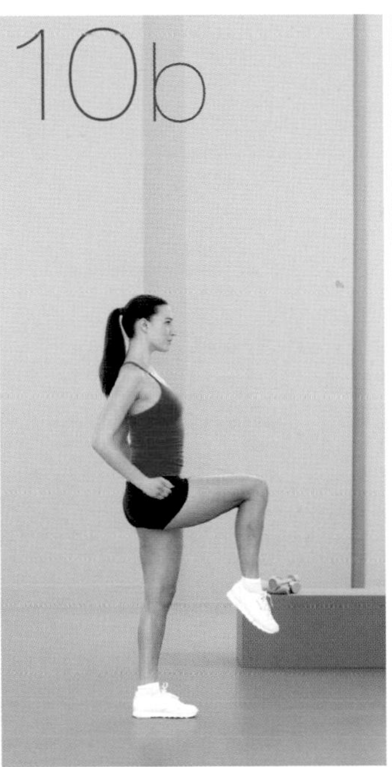

▲ **Cardio,** Push-off Lunge, page 98

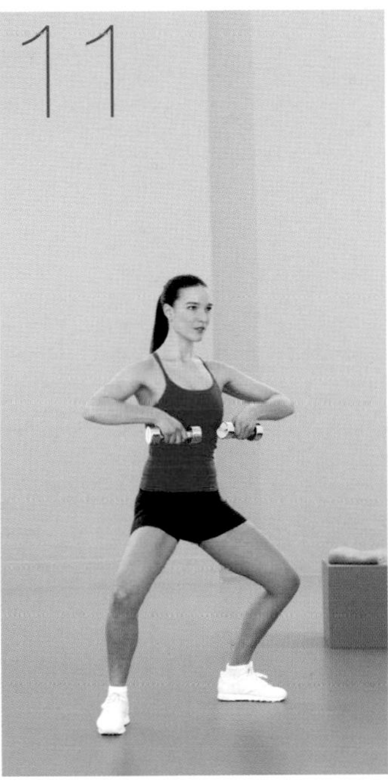

▲ **Resistance,** Plié & Row, page 99. Repeat Steps 8–10

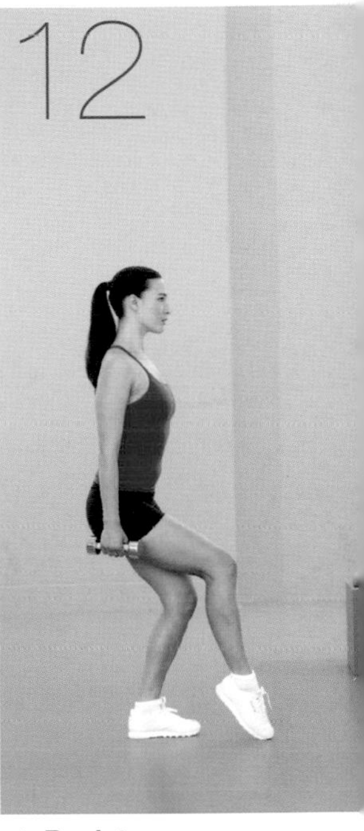

▲ **Resistance,** Balance Squat. Repeat Steps 8–10

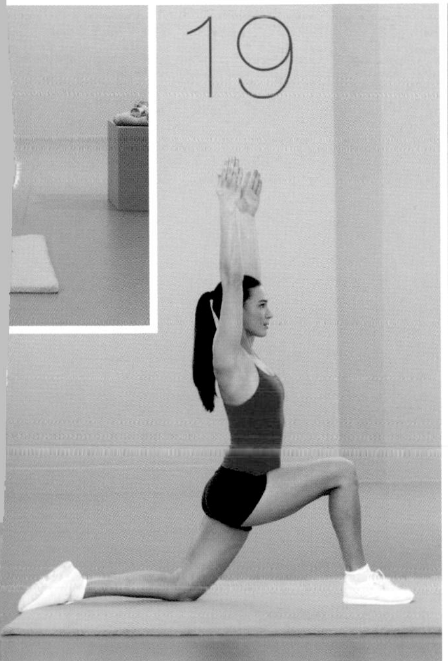

▲ **Cool down,** Kneeling Lunge, page 104

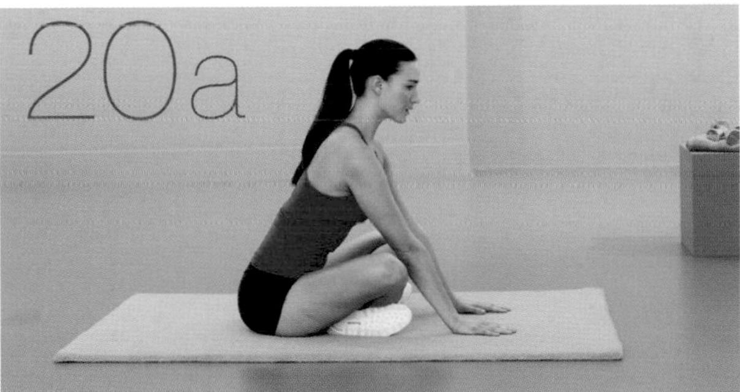

▲ **Cool down,** Cross-Legged Stretch, page 105

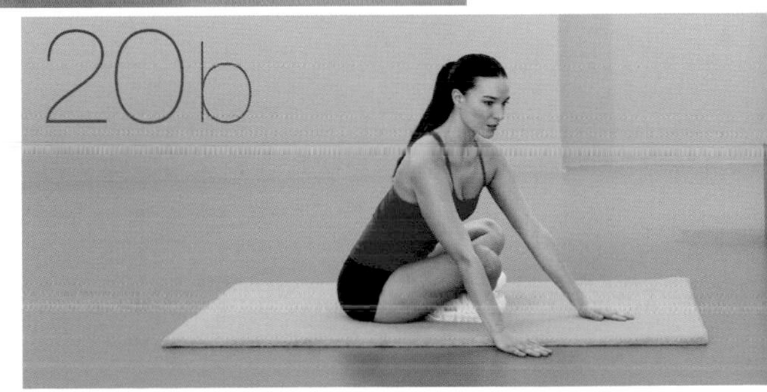

▲ **Cool down,** Cross-Legged Stretch, page 105

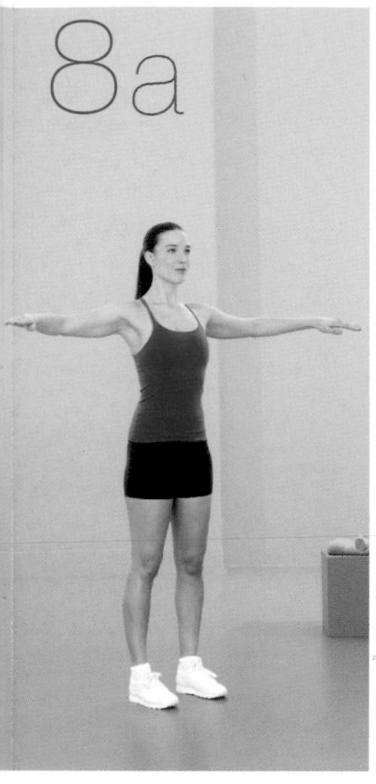

▲ **Cardio,** Curtsy Lunge, page 96

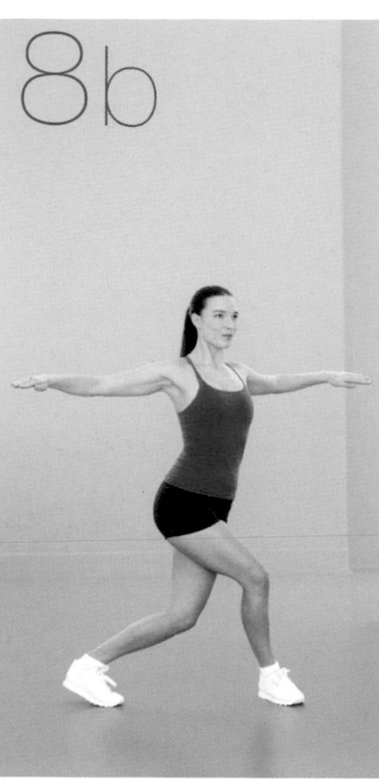

▲ **Cardio,** Curtsy Lunge, page 96

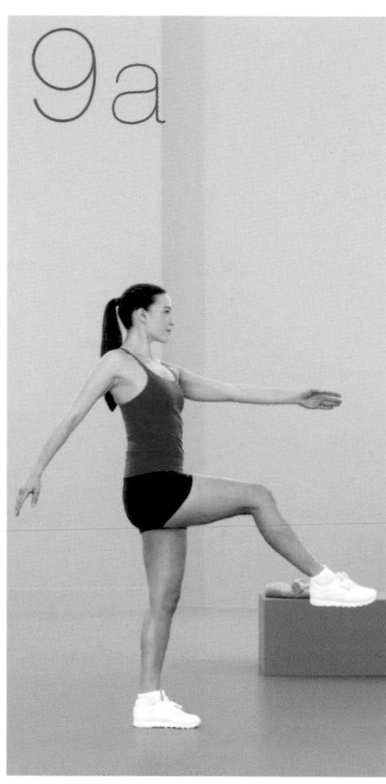

▲ **Cardio,** Charleston Lunge, page 97

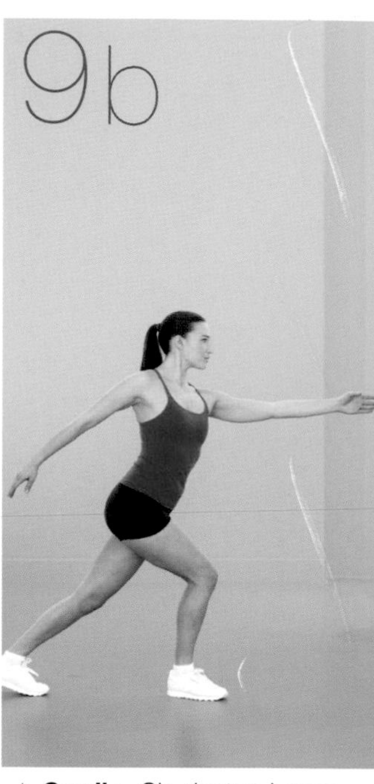

▲ **Cardio,** Charleston Lunge, page 97

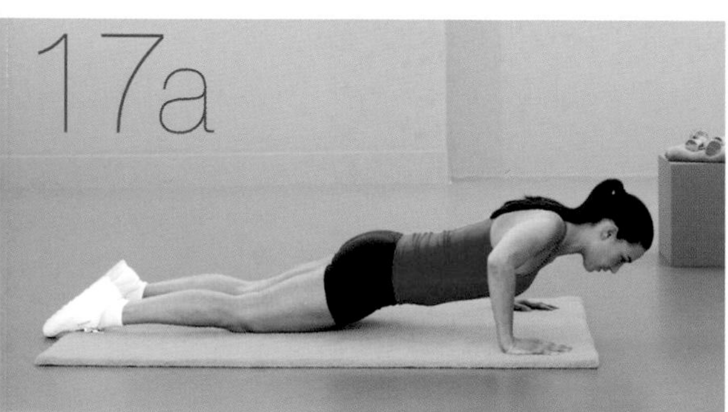

▲ **Cool down,** Half Push-up & Side Plank, page 103

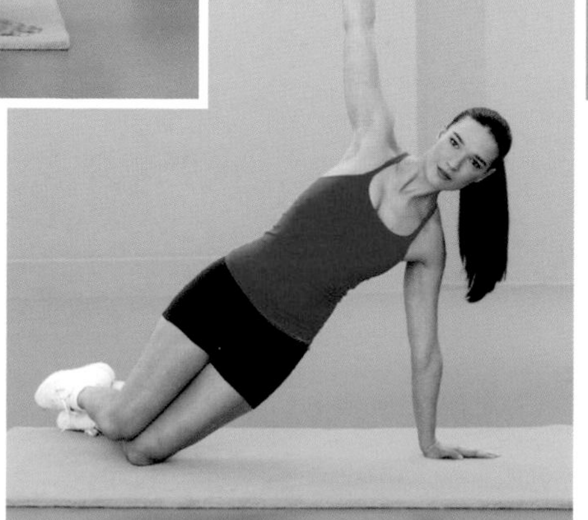

▲ **Cool down,** Half Push-up & Side Plank, page 103

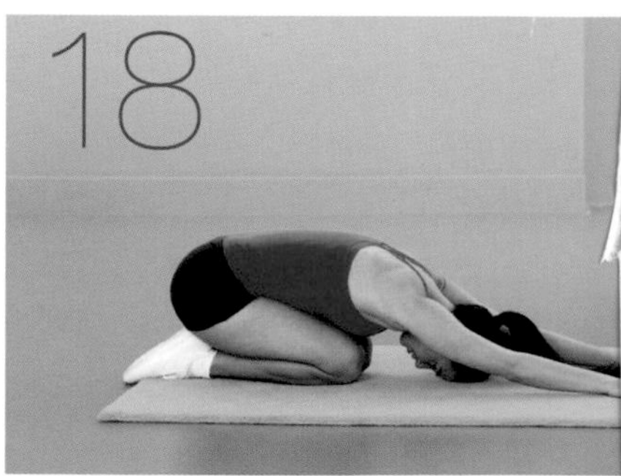

▲ **Cool down,** Child's Pose, page 104

>> **frequently** asked questions

Now you've gathered some exercising experience, but maybe you've stopped seeing obvious results—the same workouts may not have such noticeable effects as they did at the start. Perhaps you need some advice on long-term effects of exercise or keeping bones as healthy as possible. Here are a few questions that may help.

>> I am not seeing great results. Why aren't my muscles developing?

Maybe the weights are not challenging enough. Try lifting heavier weights: the last couple of repetitions should feel somewhat difficult. The *Total Body Workout* formula follows strength-training guidelines, working in the range of 8–12 repetitions. This method develops the muscle by stimulating growth (hypertrophy) of the muscle fibers, which makes it bigger and more powerful.

>> Where will I see the results first?

In four to eight weeks of consistently doing the routines three times a week, your arms and legs will feel firmer and you will see more definition in your muscles. Your shape will improve and your clothing will fit better—you'll have trimmer contours (like a smaller waist) and better posture.

>> What can I expect if I follow the routines for a whole year?

If you do the routines consistently three times a week, and combine them with a modest reduction in your daily caloric intake (250 calories), you can expect to lose about 10 lbs (4.5 kg) of fat and gain about 5 lbs (2.2 kg) of muscle.This will result in a smaller dress size regardless of the amount of actual weight loss. You will have stronger muscles and bones, more stamina, lower blood pressure and cholesterol levels.

>> How can I get the most out of lifting weights?

Proper form, alignment, and mental focus enhance the results. First, take a moment to align your body: Spine straight, shoulder blades down and together, abdominals engaged. Then make sure you are holding the weights properly, with your wrists flat. Focus on the muscle that you are working, and give it an extra "squeeze" as you feel the muscle contract with the movement. It takes time to learn to coordinate the movements gracefully and to develop body awareness of the proper form.

>> Since my new desk job, I've been getting "love handles." Any advice?

Focus on the routines that have more torso twisting and flexing, like Beach Ball (see p42) and Hop, Jig, & Jump (see p66). They will help firm up the obliques: the muscles that run along the sides of your waist. Be sure to include some Bicycle Crunches from the Step-Touch program (see p18) as well. Keep up the cardio to reduce any body fat that is settling there.

>> What exercise is best for keeping bones healthy?

Any weight-bearing exercise will load the bones. The pull of the muscle on the bone causes bone deposition at that specific site, so you must be sure to do exercises for the entire skeleton—upper and lower body. If you have healthy bones, studies have shown that jumping is very effective at increasing bone density at the hip—just remember to work within safe limits. If you have already been diagnosed with osteoporosis, then you must avoid high-impact exercise such as jumping, and protect the spine by not rounding forward or twisting.

>> I'm no longer seeing results. What should I do?

Keep surprising your muscles by stimulating them in different ways. Incorporate change into your routine. When you do the same routine for more than a couple of months, the cardiovascular and muscular systems stop improving because they don't have to. At any level of fitness you can boost your results by changing the variables. Pick a different workout each time; try doing two or three workouts at a time; change the order of the sequence.

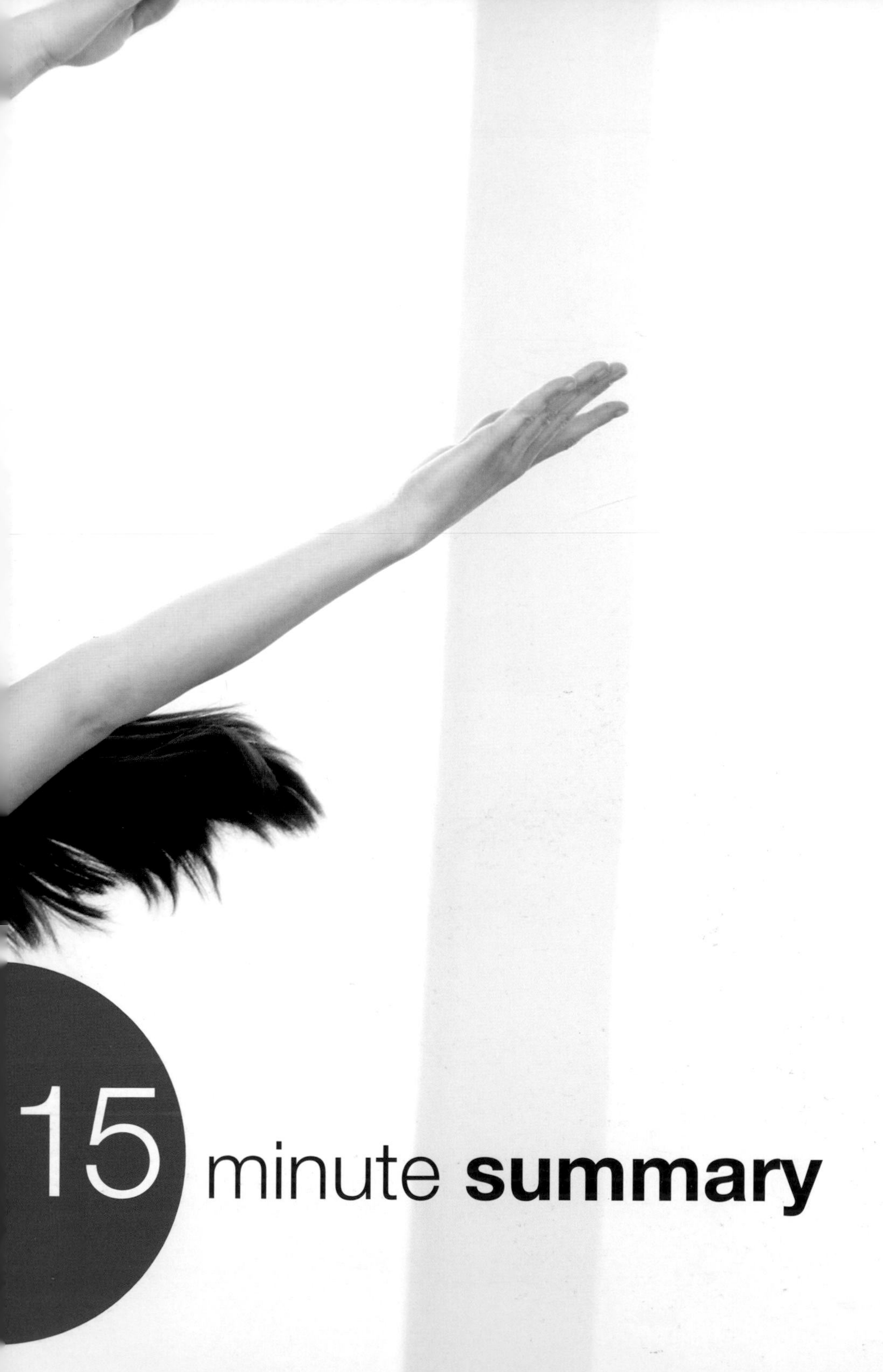

15 minute **summary**

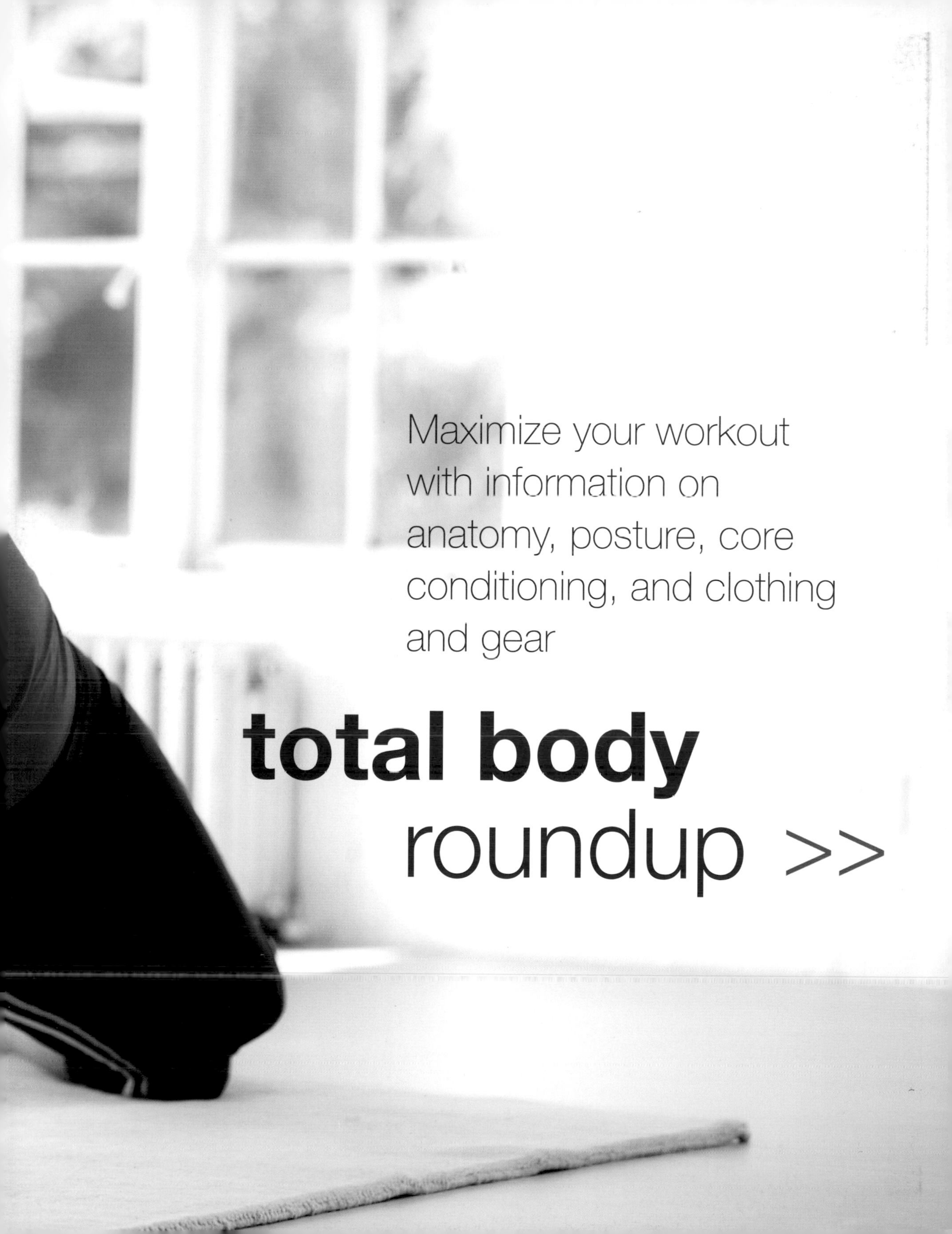

Maximize your workout with information on anatomy, posture, core conditioning, and clothing and gear

total body roundup >>

>> **anatomy** of an exercise

If you know which muscle is working in a particular exercise, you can enhance your effort by mentally focusing on it. This will help you key into the muscular movement and improve your body awareness.

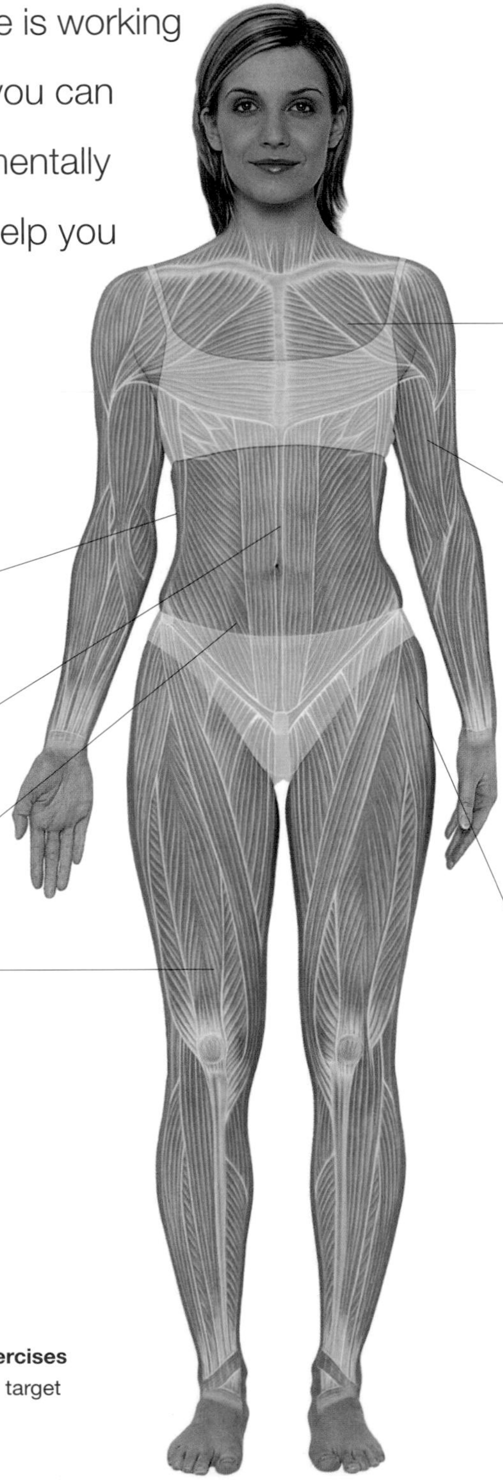

CHEST
Pectorals
Half Push-up & Side Plank, p103

ARMS
Biceps
Lunge & Curl, p27
Squat with Weight Shift, p52
Plié & Curl, p76
Lift & Squat, p101

ABDOMEN
Obliques
Bicycle Crunch,p31
Plank, p30, p57
Lunge & Twist, pp73-74
Half Push-up & Side Plank, p103

Rectus abdominis
Bicycle Crunch, p31
Plank, p30, p57
Half Push-up & Side Plank, p103

Transversus abdominis
Bicycle Crunch, p31

OUTER THIGH
Hip abductor
Lateral Lift, p77

FRONT OF THIGH
Quadriceps
Plié with Lateral Raise, p23
Lunge & Curl, p27
Squat, p28
Plié with Front Raise, p47
Squat with Knee Lift, p50
Lunge & Row, p51
Squat with Weight Shift, p52
Lunge & Twist, pp73-74
Side-Squat Jump, p75
Balance & Press, p76
Plié & Curl, p76

Muscle groups and corresponding exercises
The anatomical illustrations will help you target specific areas that you want to work on.

>> the main muscle groups

- **Hips and thighs** (gluteals, quadriceps, hamstrings, and hip adductors and abductors)
- **Back** (latissimus dorsi, rhomboids, trapezius, and erector spinae)
- **Chest** (pectorals)
- **Shoulders** (deltoids)
- **Arms** (biceps and triceps)
- **Abdomen** (rectus abdominis, transversus abdominis, and obliques)

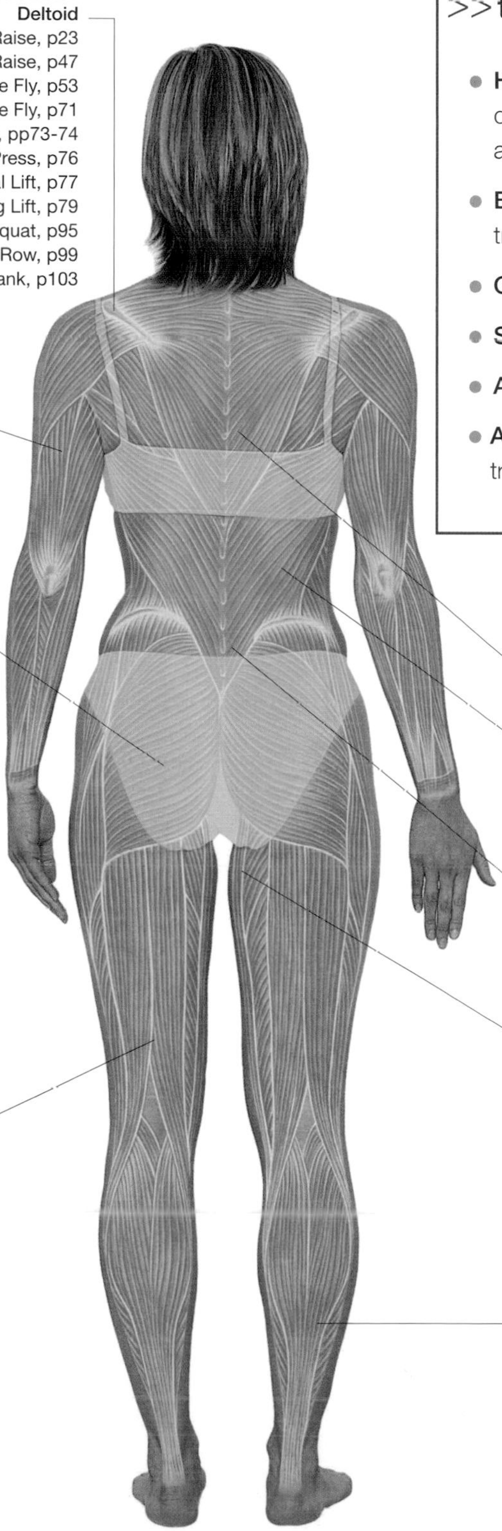

SHOULDER
Deltoid
Plié with Lateral Raise, p23
Plié with Front Raise, p47
Reverse Fly, p53
Hip Hinge & Reverse Fly, p71
Lunge & Twist, pp73-74
Balance & Press, p76
Lateral Lift, p77
Arm & Leg Lift, p79
Wood-Chop Squat, p95
Plié & Row, p99
Half Push-up & Side Plank, p103

ARMS
Triceps
Triceps Kick Back, p28
Triceps Double Kick Back, p53
Lift & Squat, p101
Half Push-up & Side Plank, p103

BUTTOCKS
Gluteals/Glutes
Plié with Lateral Raise, p23
Lunge & Curl, p27
Squat, p28
Plié with Front Raise, p47
Squat with Knee Lift, p50
Lunge & Row, p51
Squat with Weight Shift, p52
Hip Hinge & Reverse Fly, p71
Lunge & Twist, pp73-74
Side-Squat Jump, p75
Plié & Curl, p76
Arm & Leg Lift, p79
Wood-Chop Squat, p95
Plié & Row, p99
Balance Squat, p99
Lift & Squat, p101

BACK OF THIGH
Hamstrings
Plié with Lateral Raise, p23
Lunge & Curl, p27
Squat, p28
Plié with Front Raise, p47
Squat with Knee Lift, p50
Lunge & Row, p51
Squat with Weight Shift, p52
Hip Hinge & Reverse Fly, p71
Lunge & Twist, pp73-74
Side-Squat Jump, p75
Plié & Curl, p76
Wood-Chop Squat, p95
Plié & Row, p99
Balance Squat, p99
Lift & Squat, p101

BACK
Rhomboids & Trapezius
Bent-Over Row, p100

Latissimus dorsi
One-Arm Row, p27
Lunge & Row, p51
Lunge & Twist, pp73-74
Bent-Over Row, p100

Erector spinae
Arm & Leg Lift, p79

INNER THIGH
Hip adductor
Plié with Lateral Raise, p23
Plié with Front Raise, p47
Plié & Curl, p76
Plié & Row, p99

LOWER LEG, CALF
Squat with Weight Shift, p52
Side-Squat Jump, p75
Lift & Squat, p101

>> **posture** and alignment

Standing properly counteracts the constant force of gravity on the body, reducing stress on the spine and ensuring that the joints work efficiently. Resistance training combined with stretching can help correct muscular imbalances and maintain the alignment of your skeletal frame.

Poor posture can strain your joints and ultimately lead to headaches, neck and shoulder tension, sciatica, and hip and knee pain. In addition, shortened muscles are more at risk of injury caused by even simple movements. Improving your posture can bring relief from all these conditions, and also aid in quieting the mind, as practiced in the art of meditation. Good posture and poor posture are both habits that develop from making repeated movement patterns. Get in the routine of doing a few simple exercises that will ultimately serve you for life.

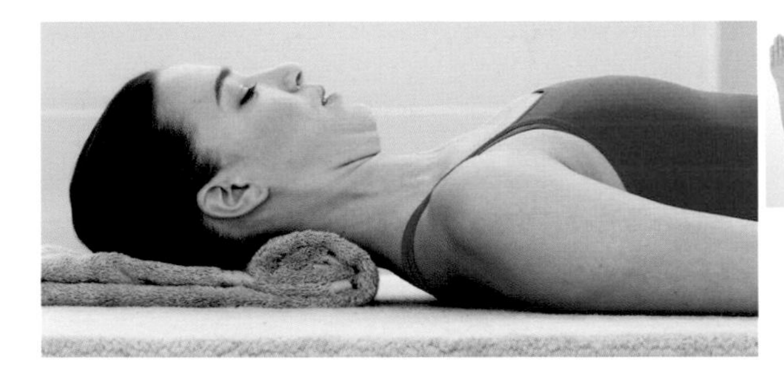

Neck Press To strengthen the neck: lie on your back with your knees bent, feet flat on the floor. Put a small towel roll under your neck. Exhale on a count of 5 as you press the back of your neck into the towel. Do 10 times. Release.

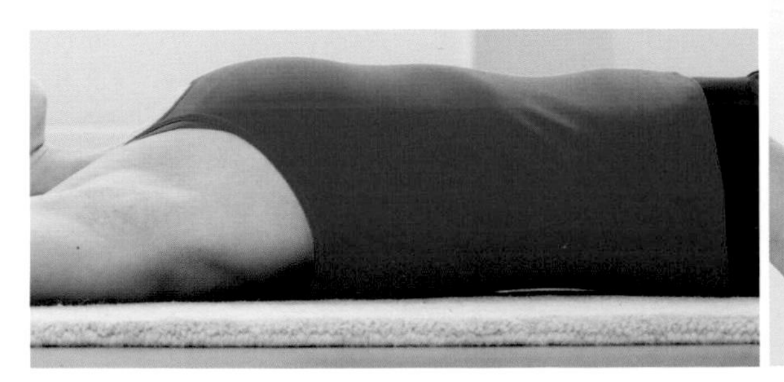

Neutral spine alignment This is midway between a full arch and a flat back. Lie on your back with your knees bent; do a strong pelvic tilt, then release halfway, allowing the natural curve in the lower back.

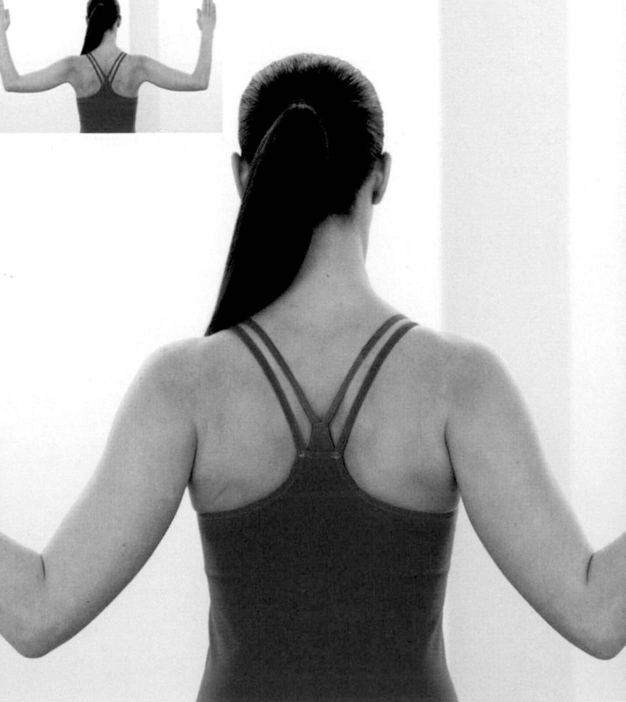

Anchoring the shoulder blades Hold your arms out to your sides, with the elbows bent (top left). To form a "W", inhale, then squeeze the shoulder blades down and together as you let your breath out slowly. Repeat 10 times daily.

Proper alignment

What is good posture? The correct way to stand is with all the body's segments stacked from head to shoulders to hips, knees, and feet. An easy, reliable way to assess posture is to attach a weighted length of string to the ceiling (to a light fixture, for example) so that it forms a straight line. When you stand next to it sideways, the center of your ear, shoulder, hip, knee, and ankle should form a line. Do this with a partner to check each other's posture. The most common problems are forward head (with the chin jutting out), rounded shoulders, protruding abdomen, excessive curve in the lower back, and hyperextended knees.

To check your alignment from the front, stand before a mirror with your feet parallel, hip width apart. Feel your weight on the balls, outer edges, and heels of your feet. Make sure that your knees are not locked or hyperextended. Putting your little fingers on your hipbones and your thumbs on the bottom of your ribcage, align your ribs with the top of your hips, with your pelvis in neutral, i.e. not tilted forward or backward. Lift your chest, sliding your shoulder blades down and together against the back of your rib cage, and center your head right on top of the spinal column.

Improving posture

To restore and maintain the normal curves of the spine, take a deep breath into the belly, and gradually lengthen the spine by lifting the top of your head toward the ceiling. Stretching the space between the ribs and the hips, and decompressing the spine, draw air up into the chest cavity. As you exhale, hold the height and stay tall.

The Neck Press (see far left, top) and the "Ws" (see near left) strengthen the muscles of the midback to keep it straight, and are helpful in reversing a forward slouch. To maintain a slight curve in your lower back, you can practice neutral spine alignment (see far left).

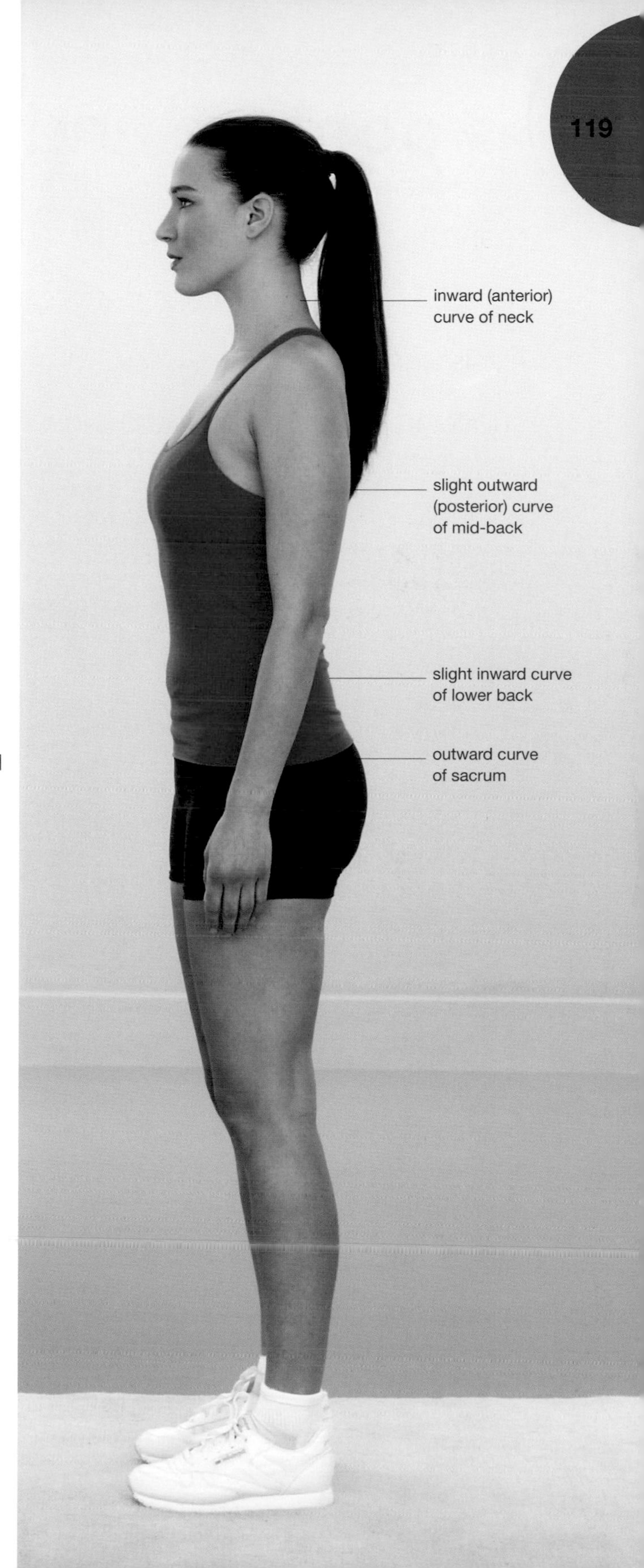

Proper alignment, side view The correct way to stand is with all the body's segments stacked from head to shoulders, to hips, knees, and feet.

>> **core** conditioning

A strong core is the foundation for quality of movement in the whole body. Core conditioning combines strengthening, stretching, balance, and alignment training of the muscles that control your torso. They act to stabilize your hips, shoulders, and trunk.

Core training is an integrated approach to working the core muscles of your torso and pelvis, and training them to function as a unit instead of in isolation. An example of an isolation exercise is the Reverse Fly (p53). When you combine this exercise with the Hip Hinge (p71) it becomes core training, as the muscles of your hips flex and extend your torso; your spinal and abdominal muscles stabilize the trunk; and your mid-back and shoulder muscles perform the upper body movement.

Improving balance

An important aspect of core conditioning is balance training. With proper alignment, your weight-bearing joints are "stacked" for balance. Your balance centers—eyes, ears, and feet—work together to sense imbalance and correct posture. Your ability to balance peaks around age 20 and normally remains excellent though early- to mid-40s. In the mid-40s, it begins a subtle process of deterioration, happening so slowly that it is almost imperceptible. Everyone has the ability to improve their balance, which reduces the risk of falling. Quicker reaction time, along with your ability to recover from a stumble or to change direction, can prevent an injury. If you are just beginning to work on balance, start with an exercise like this one (see right), which is done in a static position. Stand with your feet in a straight line. Focus your eyes on something directly in front of you, and come up on your toes, using your arms to help find your balance. If this is too easy, try shutting your eyes!

Balance To maintain your balance, think of pulling up through the abdomen and lengthening through the spine. This will activate your core muscles.

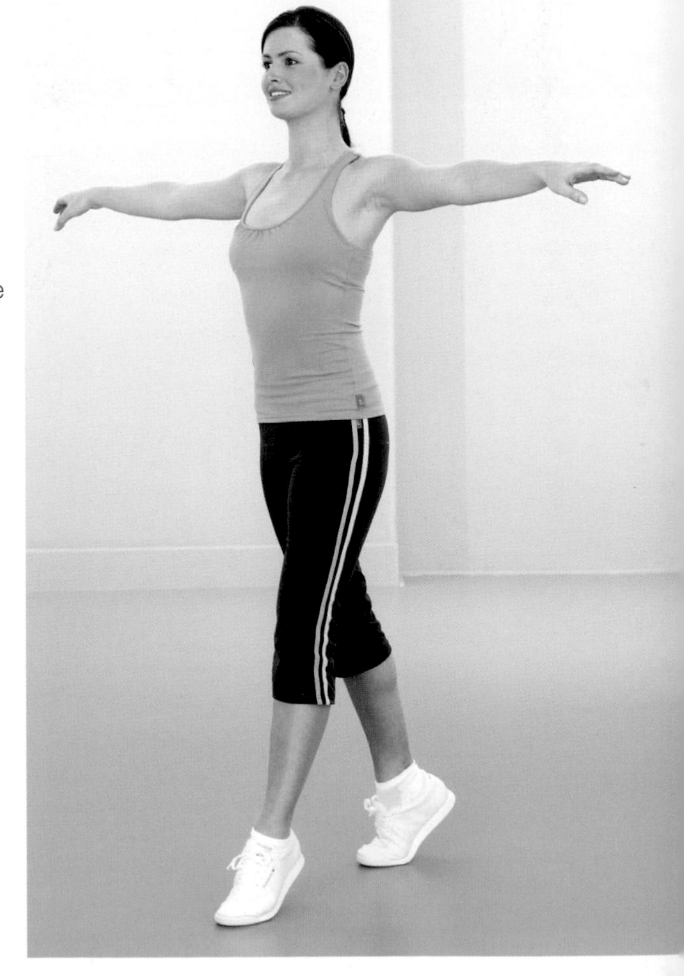

The next challenge is to add movement for dynamic balance, such as in the Lunge Walk (see below). Now you must maintain your balance as you are moving. The muscles of your hips, shoulders, and trunk engage to perform the movement and at the same time keep your upper body vertical, ribs stacked over hips for balance. This is a good example of training a movement rather than a body part, which is the essential concept behind core training. One major core group, the abdominals, will be working throughout the exercises of *Total Body Workout*, although it may not be obvious at first. As opposed to doing endless crunches on the floor, these exercises will activate your abdominals to stabilize your torso while performing multiple actions, help you maintain proper alignment in different positions against gravity, and enable you to twist and flex your trunk in the standing position.

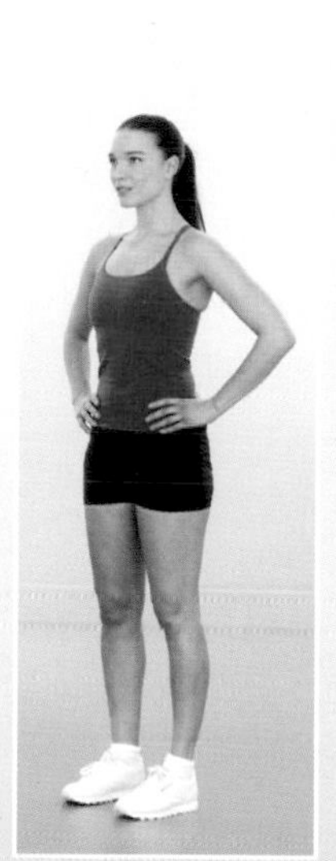

Lunge Walk

1 Stand in the ready position, feet together, with your weight on the right, supporting, leg. Resting your hands lightly on your waist, inhale as you step forward into a lunge with your left foot.

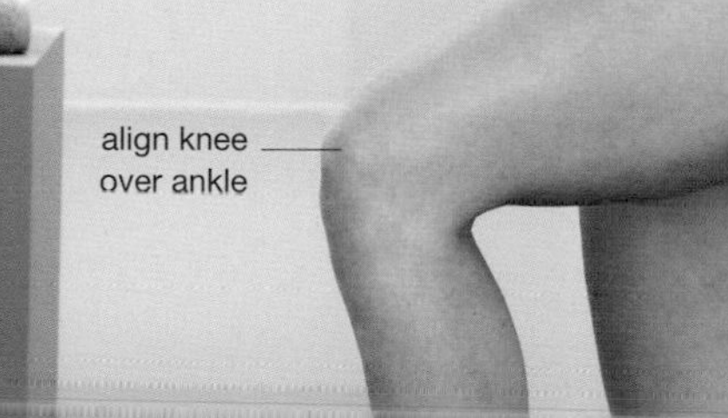

keep upper body vertical

align knee over ankle

keep back heel lifted

2 Exhale as you step forward with your back leg, bringing your feet together. Change the lead leg for the next lunge, traveling forward with each front lunge.

>> **equipment** & clothing

I recommend a ball and two pairs of free weights (also called hand weights, or dumbbells), either 3 lb (1 kg) and 5 lb (2 kg), or 5 lb (2 kg) and 8 lb (4 kg), depending on your starting level. An exercise mat is also useful to provide cushioning as well as traction for some of the exercises.

My preferences and recommendations in your choices of equipment are based on quality, economy, and safety of use.

What to wear

Wear comfortable clothing that you can move in; some people prefer formfitting clothing because it makes it easier to monitor body alignment, while others prefer less-revealing loose clothing. Shoes, for example cross-trainers, should be supportive and allow movement in all directions. Running shoes are not a good choice as they are designed primarily for moving forward and backward only.

Free weights

These make resistance training interesting by challenging your balance, coordination, and core stabilization. Since you lift them with individual limbs, it is easy to spot imbalances in the body and to use them to improve symmetry. You can effectively isolate one muscle at a time, or combine movements to challenge whole muscle groups. Free weights are usually solid metal covered in gray

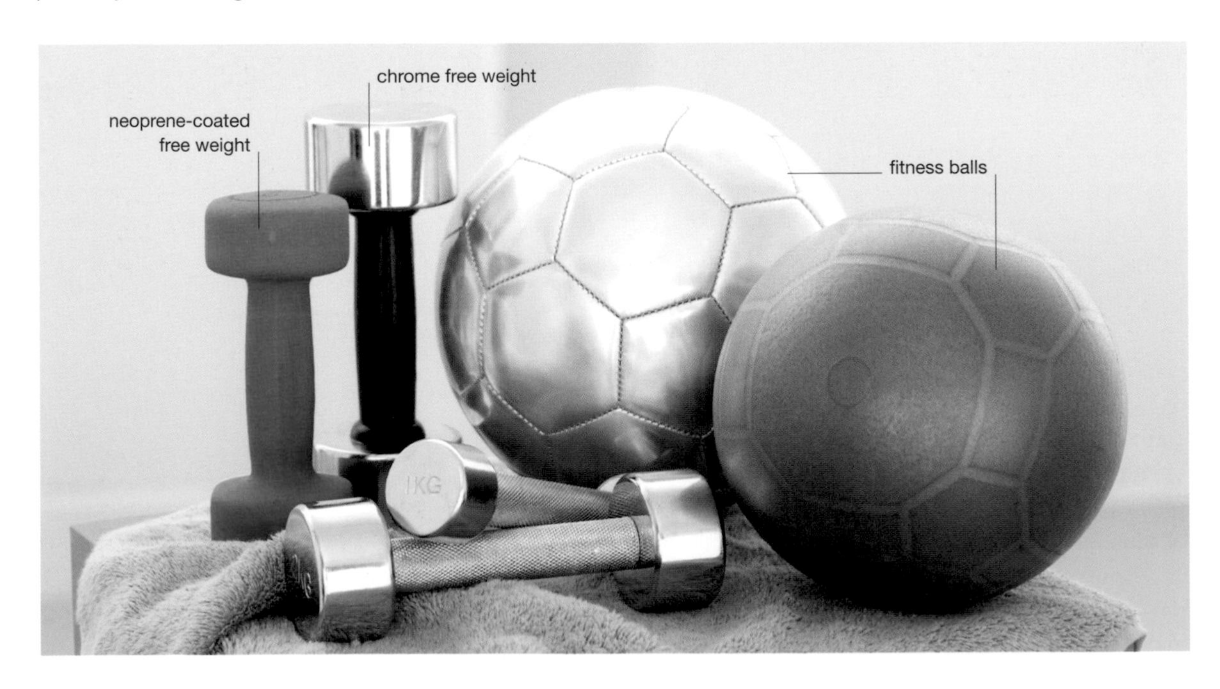

Free weights and balls come in a variety of sizes and finishes. Both weights and balls should be comfortable to hold and easy to use.

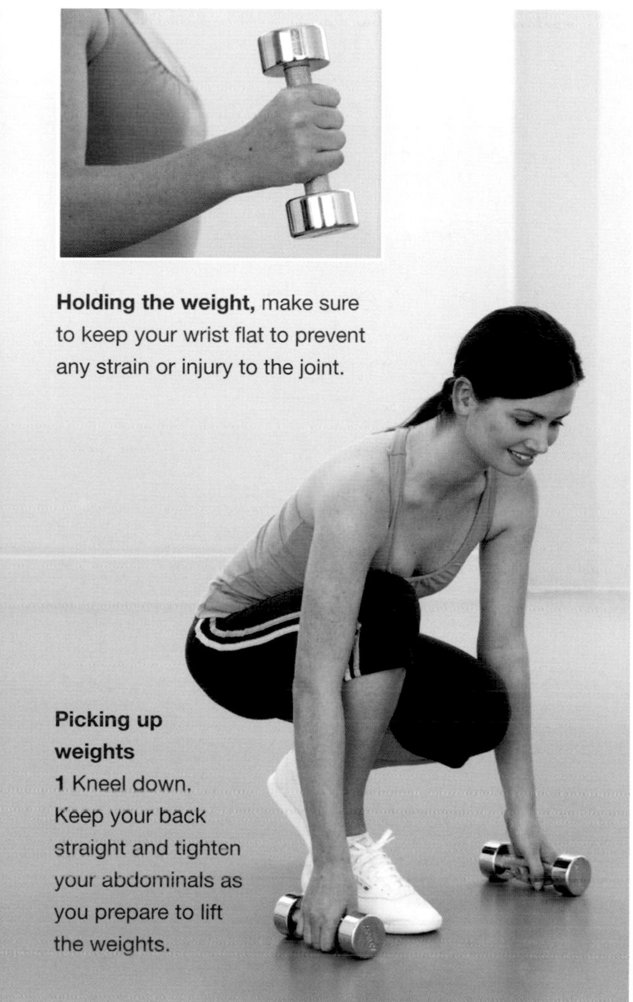

Holding the weight, make sure to keep your wrist flat to prevent any strain or injury to the joint.

Picking up weights
1 Kneel down. Keep your back straight and tighten your abdominals as you prepare to lift the weights.

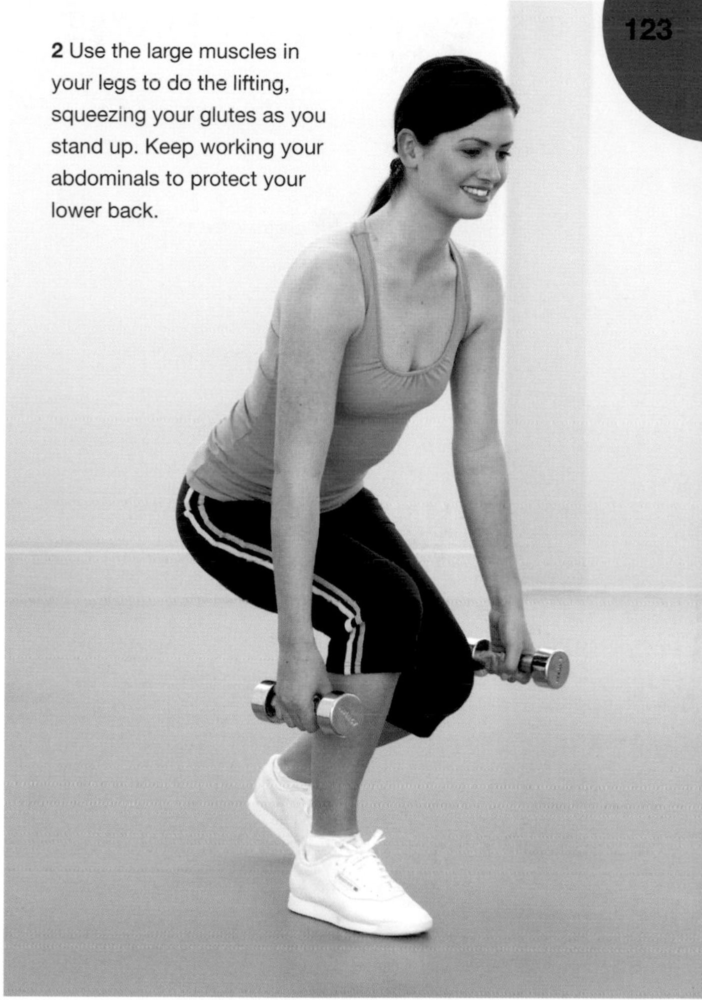

2 Use the large muscles in your legs to do the lifting, squeezing your glutes as you stand up. Keep working your abdominals to protect your lower back.

enamel, chrome, vinyl, neoprene (which contains latex), or rubber. Enamel and chrome coatings chip and flake over time, presenting a small risk. Some people prefer neoprene-coated weights as they are nicer to hold, and do not become slippery with sweat. Free weights are widely available in various weight increments.

Balls

A simple, unweighted beach ball will do just fine, but a weighted "medicine" ball provides resistance for muscle toning. My personal favorites are filled with gel and feel good to the touch. I recommend a weight of 3 lb (1 kg) or 4 lb (1.5 kg) because anything heavier may cause strain in the neck and shoulders from repetitive motions. A convenient size to fit in your hands is 7–10 in (18–25 cm) in diameter, although smaller balls will work too. Anything larger than this might be too unwieldy.

Exercise mats

Exercise mats are readily available in a variety of different densities of foam that either fold or roll up. Of the foldable mats, I prefer the dense foam, which is stiff to touch but surprisingly resilient to use. Of the roll-up mats, I prefer a soft durable foam because it offers comfortable cushioning with a sticky surface to prevent sliding. A yoga "sticky mat" is great for this too, but doesn't offer the same degree of cushioning.

useful resources

The resources below provide some useful contact details which will help to give you a good start in finding high quality exercise equipment. You will also find some organizations and websites with general information on health and fitness if you decide you would like to learn more.

US & Canada

The American College of Sports Medicine
www.acsm.org
ACSM promotes and integrates scientific research, education, and practical applications of sports medicine and exercise science to maintain and enhance physical performance, fitness, health, and quality of life.

The American Council on Exercise
www.acefitness.org
ACE is a nonprofit organization committed to enriching quality of life through safe and effective physical activity. ACE protects all segments of society against ineffective fitness products, programs, and trends through its ongoing public education, outreach, and research. ACE further protects the public by setting certification and continuing education standards for fitness professionals.

The Canadian Society for Exercise Physiology
www.csep.ca/forms.asp
The scientific authority on exercise physiology, health, and fitness in Canada.

Fitness Wholesale
Tel (US): 1-888-FW-ORDER
Tel: 001-330-929-7227
email: fw@fwonline.com
www.fitnesswholesale.com
For weights, exercise mats, and "slomo balls" (unweighted, inflatable balls).

Perform Better
Tel (US): 1-800-556-7464
e-mail: performbetter@ mfathletic.com
www.performbetter.com
This web-based retailer offers a very wide range of all types of fitness equipment.

Power Systems
Tel (US) 1-800-321-6975
email: customerservice@power-systems.com
www.power-systems.com
Offers a range of gear, with a good selection of exercise balls.

Topaz Medical
Tel (US) 1-800-264-5623
email: info@topazusa.com
www.topazusa.com
Specializes in rehabilitation exercise equipment, selling high quality gel-filled medicine balls.

UK

Newitt & Co Ltd
Tel: 01904-468551
email: sales@newitts.com
www.newitts.com
For medicine balls and weights.

Sissel UK Limited
Tel: 01422-885433
email: info@sisseluk.com
www.sisseluk.com
For thick exercise mats and stability balls.

sweatyBetty
Tel: 0800-169-3889
email: internet@sweatyBetty.com
www.sweatyBetty.com
Founded in 1998 by Tamara Hill-Norton, sweatyBetty sells gorgeous clothing for active and

not so active women in boutiques nationwide and online.

Totally Fitness
Tel: 020-7467-5939
email: sales@totally fitness.com
www.totallyfitness.co.uk
For weights and stability balls.

Australia

Elite Fitness Equipment
Tel: (AU) 1800-622-644
email: info@elitefitness.com.au
www.elitefitness.com.au
Provides an extensive selection of fitness gear.

Fernwood Women's Health Club
National Office
Tel: (03) 5443-4555
www.fernwoodfitness.com.au
Fernwood is the largest organization of women-only health clubs in Australia.

Fitness First
www.fitnessfirst.com.au
Tel: 1300-557-799
A global gym operator with 70 locations in Australia.

Health Insite
www.healthinsite.gov.au
Contains a wide range of information on important health topics including sport, exercise, fitness, and injury prevention.

Osteoporosis Australia
Level 1, 52 Parramatta Road
Forest Lodge
NSW 2037
Tel: (02) 9518-8140
www.osteoporosis.org.au

YMCA Australia
www.ymca.org.au
The YMCA delivers health, fitness, recreation, and other services to individuals, families, and communities across the whole of Australia.

Other books by Joan Pagano

Strength Training for Women
(Dorling Kindersley, 2005)
This step-by-step strength-training manual features exercises to help you shape and tone your body. Joan shows you how to get the best out of your workout, improving both your strength and stamina for long-lasting results.

8 Weeks to a Younger Body
(Dorling Kindersley, 2007)
Whatever your actual age, you can beat your body-clock and drop a decade with these specially designed exercises. Find out how to stay young as you increase your personal fitness levels and overall health.

To contact Joan Pagano

Joan Pagano Fitness Group
401 East 89th Street (no. 2M)
New York, NY 10128, USA
email: info@joanpaganofitness.com
www.joanpaganofitness.com

index

acknowledgements

Author's acknowledgements

My deepest gratitude to Linda Rose Iennaco whose expertise in dance, music, and choreography was indispensable to this work, and whose dedication, determination and stamina carried it through to the end. You are amazing!

With heartfelt thanks to my family and friends for their patience and support throughout this project. Thank you, James, for sharing the love; Mom, for sharing the experience; and my sister Lucy for sharing her gift with words.

Thank you, DK, for putting together a winning team. To Mary-Clare Jerram for the opportunity to expand my horizons and Jenny Latham for guiding me along the way. To my editor, Helen Murray, for her delightful encouragement and to Anne Fisher for her keen aesthetics. Special thanks to Ruth Jenkinson for creating magic with her camera and lighting. And to Kerry and Samantha, our lovely models, for grace and style.

Publisher's acknowledgments

Dorling Kindersley would like to thank photographer Ruth Jenkinson and her assistants, James McNaught and Vic Churchill: sweatyBetty for the loan of the exercise clothing; Viv Riley at Touch Studios; the models Kerry Jay and Samantha Johannesson; Roisin Donaghy and Victoria Barnes for the hair and makeup; YogaMatters for lending us the mat and ball. A special thanks to Andrea Bagg and Tara Woolnough for editorial assistance.

about Joan Pagano

Joan Pagano, a Phi Beta Kappa, cum laude graduate of Connecticut College, is certified in health and fitness instruction by the American College of Sports Medicine (ACSM), whose credentials provide the very best measure of competence as a professional. She has worked as a personal fitness trainer on Manhatten's Upper East Side since 1988, providing professional guidance and support to people at all levels of fitness. Through her work, she has created hundreds of training programmes specially tailored for individuals, groups, fitness facilities, schools, hospitals, and corporations.

Today, Joan manages her own staff of fitness specialists, who work together as Joan Pagano Fitness Group. For many years, she served as Director of the Personal Trainer Certification Program at Marymount Manhatten College, where she remains on the faculty as the instructor in fitness evaluation techniques. She is now a nationally recognized provider of education courses for fitness trainers through IDEA (an organization supporting fitness professionals worldwide). Joan is also recognized in the industry as an authority on the benefit of exercise for women's health issues such as the menopause, breast cancer, and osteoporosis.